MARRIOTT'S
Practical
Electrocardiography

**TWELFTH
EDITION**

Galen S. Wagner, MD

Associate Professor
Department of Internal Medicine
Duke University Medical Center
Durham, North Carolina

David G. Strauss, MD, PhD

Medical Officer
U.S. Food and Drug Administration
Silver Spring, Maryland
Affiliated Researcher
Karolinska Institutet
Stockholm, Sweden

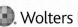 Wolters Kluwer | Lippincott Williams & Wilkins
Health

Philadelphia • Baltimore • New York • London
Buenos Aires • Hong Kong • Sydney • Tokyo

Acquisitions Editor: Julie Goolsby
Product Development Editor: Leanne Vandetty
Production Project Manager: Marian Bellus
Senior Manufacturing Coordinator: Beth Welsh
Marketing Manager: Stephanie Manzo
Design Coordinator: Stephen Druding
Production Service: Absolute Service, Inc.

©2014 by **LIPPINCOTT WILLIAMS & WILKINS, a WOLTERS KLUWER business**
Two Commerce Square
2001 Market Street
Philadelphia, PA 19103 USA
LWW.com

11th Edition© 2008 by LIPPINCOTT WILLIAMS & WILKINS
10th Edition© 2001 by LIPPINCOTT WILLIAMS & WILKINS

This work was completed outside of Dr. Strauss' duties at the U.S. Food and Drug Administration (FDA). This book reflects the views of the authors and should not be construed to represent FDA's views or policies.

Printed in China

Library of Congress Cataloging-in-Publication Data

Wagner, Galen S., author.
  Marriott's practical electrocardiography. — Twelfth edition / Galen S. Wagner, David G. Strauss.
     p. ; cm.
  Practical electrocardiography
  Includes bibliographical references and index.
   ISBN 978-1-4511-4625-7 (alk. paper)
  I. Strauss, David G., author. II. Title. III. Title: Practical electrocardiography.
  [DNLM: 1. Electrocardiography. 2. Heart Diseases—diagnosis. WG 140]
  RC683.5.E5
  616.1′207547—dc23
                            2013036495

Care has been taken to confirm the accuracy of the information presented and to describe generally accepted practices. However, the authors, editors, and publisher are not responsible for errors or omissions or for any consequences from application of the information in this book and make no warranty, expressed or implied, with respect to the currency, completeness, or accuracy of the contents of the publication. Application of the information in a particular situation remains the professional responsibility of the practitioner.

   The authors, editors, and publisher have exerted every effort to ensure that drug selection and dosage set forth in this text are in accordance with current recommendations and practice at the time of publication. However, in view of ongoing research, changes in government regulations, and the constant flow of information relating to drug therapy and drug reactions, the reader is urged to check the package insert for each drug for any change in indications and dosage and for added warnings and precautions. This is particularly important when the recommended agent is a new or infrequently employed drug.

   Some drugs and medical devices presented in the publication have Food and Drug Administration (FDA) clearance for limited use in restricted research settings. It is the responsibility of the health care provider to ascertain the FDA status of each drug or device planned for use in their clinical practice.

To purchase additional copies of this book, call our customer service department at (800) 638-3030 or fax orders to (301) 223-2320. International customers should call (301) 223-2300.

Visit Lippincott Williams & Wilkins on the Internet: at LWW.com. Lippincott Williams & Wilkins customer service representatives are available from 8:30 am to 6 pm, EST.

10 9 8 7 6 5 4 3 2 1

CCS1113

Dedicated to Marilyn Wagner, Mya Sjogren, and
Molly and Michael Strauss

Contents

SECTION I: BASIC CONCEPTS

SECTION II: ABNORMAL WAVE MORPHOLOGY

SECTION III: ABNORMAL RHYTHMS

Digital Contents

 Use a QR reader app on your smartphone or tablet to scan QR codes throughout this edition and access bonus animations and videos, or visit http://solution.lww.com (see details on inside front cover).

Chapter 14

Chapter 17

Chapter 18

Chapter 19

 This symbol, where it appears throughout this edition, indicates that bonus self-help learning digital content is available on the companion website.

A Self Help Learning Tool in ECG Education

Tobin H. Lim, MD and Galen S. Wagner, MD

Intraventricular Conduction Abnormalities
    Normal Conduction
  Left Fascicular Blocks
    Left Anterior Fascicular Block
    Left Posterior Fascicular Block
  Bundle-Branch Blocks
    Left-Bundle-Branch Block
    Right-Bundle-Branch Block
  Bifascicular Block
    Right-Bundle-Branch Block and Left Anterior Fascicular Block
  Trifascicular Block
    Right-Bundle-Branch Block and Left-Bundle-Branch Block
Myocardial Ischemia and Infarction
  Anteroseptal
  Extensive Anterior
  Midanterior
  Lateral
  Inferolateral
  Inferior
  Extensive Inferior

Contributors

Ljuba Bacharova, MD, PhD

International Laser Centre
Bratislava, Slovak Republic

Raymond R. Bond, PhD

School of Computing and Mathematics
University of Ulster
Northern Ireland, United Kingdom

Esben A. Carlsen, BSc

Medicine
Faculty of Health and Medical Sciences
University of Copenhagen
Copenhagen, Denmark

E. Harvey Estes, Jr., MD

Professor Emeritus
Department of Community and Family Medicine
Duke University Medical Center
Durham, North Carolina

Dewar D. Finlay, PhD

School of Engineering
University of Ulster
Northern Ireland, United Kingdom

Marcel Gilbert, MD

Professor of Medicine
Laval University
Quebec City, Quebec, Canada

Wesley K. Haisty, Jr., MD
Emeritus Associate
Professor of Medicine/Cardiology
Wake Forest University Health Sciences
Winston-Salem, North Carolina

Vivian Paola Kamphuis, BSc
Leiden University Medical Center
Leiden, The Netherlands

Tobin H. Lim, MD
Department of Medicine
University of Utah Health Care
Salt Lake City, Utah

Henry J. L. Marriott, MD*
Clinical Professor
Emory University
Atlanta, Georgia
University of Florida
Gainesville, Florida
University of South Florida College of Medicine
Tampa, Florida
Director, Marriott Heart Foundation
Riverview, Florida

Charles W. Olson, MSEE
Huntington Station, New York

Jacob Simlund
Department of Clinical Physiology
Karolinska Institutet and Karolinska University Hospital
Stockholm, Sweden

David G. Strauss, MD, PhD
Medical Officer
U.S. Food and Drug Administration
Silver Spring, Maryland
Affiliated Researcher
Karolinska Institutet
Stockholm, Sweden

*deceased

Albert Y. Sun, MD

Assistant Professor of Medicine
Codirector, Inherited Arrhythmias Program
Clinical Cardiac Electrophysiology
Duke University Medical Center
Durham, North Carolina

Peter M. van Dam, PhD

Cognitive Neuroscience
Radboud University Nijmegen
Nijmegen, The Netherlands

Galen S. Wagner, MD

Associate Professor
Department of Internal Medicine
Duke University Medical Center
Durham, North Carolina

Foreword

Barney Marriott was one of those bigger-than-life icons who populated the 20th century. To those who knew him at all, he was simply Barney. Born on the eve of St. Barnabas' day in 1917 in Hamilton, Bermuda, he was never referred to as Henry J.L. Marriott. Those who did were likely destined to remain strangers . . . but not for long. He was never a stranger to me. I have had the wonderful and rare privilege of spanning the charmed lives and careers of both authors of this book. Galen Wagner, my mentor, friend, and colleague for the past nearly 40 years, has asked me to pen a reminiscence of Barney because, for the last 25 years of Barney's life, he and I were buddies. Therein lies a tale.

Following his early formative years in Bermuda, this "onion," as Bermudans call themselves, went to Oxford as a Rhodes scholar. He enrolled at Brasenose College. The principal of Brasenose was a German named Sonnenschein (later changed to Stallybrass), about whom Barney painted me a picture of respect, awe, and perhaps a little disdain. Traveling to London during the war (not The War), he matriculated at St. Mary's as a medical student, then as a registrar. During our many luncheon outings together, Barney would regale me to stories of St. Mary's. Not uncommonly, the Germans would launch their V-1 missiles called "buzz bombs" (because of their ramjet engines) to rain terror on the English populous, especially London. Barney would laugh in his usually reserved guffaw as he told me that the medical students had been fascinated by these weapons. The V-1 missiles emitted a characteristic high-pitched "clack-clack-clack" as they approached the city, then silence as the missiles entered their final path to their target. Barney said that the clacking drew the students to the wide open windows of the anatomy lab on the top floor of St. Mary's, except for Barney, who, not quite ready to meet his maker, had dived under the cadaver dissection table seeking some sort of premortem protection provided by his postmortem colleague. Happily for all concerned, there were no acute casualties in the St. Mary's Medical School anatomy lab during those wartime adventures.

In another tale of St. Mary's, Sir Alexander Fleming had performed his initial studies into the isolation and first clinical use of penicillin in that institution. By the time of Barney's registrar years, the original "penicillin lab" had become a registrar's on-call room. Barney was the registrar on the Penicillin Service, where he and his attending made fateful decisions about who was to receive the new life-saving antibiotic and who was not. Dr. Marriott's attending of that era was George Pickering, later knighted and a much later successor to Osler as Regius Professor of Medicine at the Radcliffe Infirmary at Oxford.

Following the war, Barney came to the United States. After a fellowship year in allergy at Johns Hopkins Children's Center, Barney moved across town to the University of Maryland. As a young faculty member there and director of the Arthritis Clinic, Dr. Marriott was drafted into the role of teaching and supervising ECGs, a job he embraced with a fervor that was infectious and illuminating. By the late 1950s, Barney had grown tired of Baltimore and its cold, wet winters. He accepted a position at Tampa General Hospital in 1961 as director of Medical Education, where he remained for several years.

In 1965, Dr. Marriott was approached by Frank LaCamera of the Rogers Heart Foundation to relocate across the bay to St. Petersburg, where he began his series of seminars on ECG interpretation. Many greats of cardiology nationally and internationally were invited to speak at these seminars. Regardless, it was Barney who set the curriculum and the informality that characterized his personal approach to teaching. Those landmark courses put Barney and his talents in front of literally tens of thousands of doctors and nurses around the world for the next 40 years. All the while, he published over 17 books, mostly on electrocardiography. His scholarly writing was not limited to books. His list of published scientific papers is prodigious. *The New England Journal of Medicine* alone published papers spanning over 50 years of his vibrant productivity. Barney's love of language is apparent in one of his least well-recognized contributions. For many years, Dr. Marriott was the author of the Medical Etymology section of *Stedman's Medical Dictionary*. He reveled in and revered English and its many quirky words and grammatical rules.

In addition to his visiting professorships at Emory and the University of Florida, the University of South Florida (USF) in Tampa was fortunate to have Barney on its volunteer clinical faculty beginning in the 1980s. Monthly or quarterly, Barney would bring a mountain of carousel slide trays to our evening conferences. It was the glorious, now bygone era of big pharma. The fellows and faculty alike would be repeatedly skewered by Barney's rapier-like witticisms as he led and pushed us to be better ECG readers. His acumen and sharpness for his task and his boundless enthusiasm were hallmarks of the conferences. Aphorisms such as "Every good arrhythmia has at least three possible interpretations" poured forth like the sangria that fueled raucous audience participation. Barney's old friends from around the United States and the world would drop by to be toasted and roasted by the master. David Friedberg, an immigrant to the United States from South Africa, was one of the first I encountered. Later, Bill Nelson joined our faculty at USF and became a suitable stage partner and foil for Barney. One particularly memorable evening, Leo Schamroth himself, from South Africa, joined Barney, David, and me for an evening at Bill Nelson's home, where we argued about concealed conduction and AV block late into the night.

As the decades in the Tampa Bay region wore on, Barney and his companion, Jonni Cooper, RN, spent more time at their place in Riverview, Florida, where he had a large library and workspace for his many books and teaching projects. Chief among those books was his personal favorite, *Practical Electrocardiography*, a bestseller up to today. It remained a single-author volume through the eight editions he wrote. He graciously facilitated Galen Wagner's evolution of print and electronic formats through the subsequent editions. In those first eight editions, beginning in 1954, Barney loved to write with his uniquely conversational style, unlike just about any textbook that you might find in a medical bookstore. *Practical Electrocardiography* was and remains, however, a very special, now multiformat text suitable for students of all ages and skills at ECG interpretation.

Barney and I continued our monthly lunches as he and Bill Nelson and I put together his last book, *Concepts and Cautions in Electrocardiography*. Barney's health held on until his terminal bout with lung cancer; we increased the frequency of those meetings as his health declined. To the very end, he remained gracious, charming, curious, and firmly attached to his ECGs. Every week, tracings continued to come to him from former students around the globe. On my Thursdays with Barney, my task was to bring the Guinness so that we could chat, look at ECGs together, lift a few pints, and reminisce a bit. He reminded me, as his life ebbed away, that being bitter and holding grudges was "a useless waste of time." It was a lesson for all of us. His legacy remains much more than the eponymic moniker for this volume. Pour me another Guinness. Cheers, Barney.

Douglas D. Schocken, MD
Durham, North Carolina
July 2013

Preface

Barney Marriott created *Practical Electrocardiography* in 1954 and nurtured it through eight editions. After assisting him with the 8th edition, Galen Wagner enthusiastically accepted the challenge of writing the subsequent editions. The 9th edition had extensive revisions to the text, the 10th edition had almost completely new illustrations, and the 11th edition had further text and figure updates and also an accompanying DVD with interactive animations. For this 12th edition, David Strauss joined Galen as coauthor. Galen and David have been working together on electrocardiographic teaching and research challenges for the past 9 years.

One of the strengths of *Marriott's Practical Electrocardiography* through its more than 50-year history has been its lucid foundation for understanding the basis for ECG interpretation. Again, in this revision, we have attempted to retain the best of the Marriott tradition—emphasis on the concepts required for everyday ECG interpretation and the simplicities, rather than complexities, of the ECG recordings. Tobin Lim coauthored many of the 11th edition chapters and served as the primary developer of the digital content associated with that edition.

Tobin Lim's input continues into this 12th edition, and David Strauss has led even further into the electronic-based interactive learning experiences. More than 30 of the figures that evolved through previous editions have now been converted through the creative expertise of Mark Flanders into animated movies accessed via QR codes embedded in the book. David has also collaborated with electrocardiographic educators who are especially skilled in e-based education to add interactive video content to many of the 12th edition chapters. These include Raymond Bond and Dewar Finlay in Chapter 2, Charles (Bill) Olson in the new Chapter 4, and Peter van Dam in Chapter 9.

The chapters are in the same order as in the 11th edition; however, two new chapters have been added. In Chapter 4, Bill Olson, Harvey Estes, Vivian Kamphuis, and Esben Carlsen contribute to the introduction of "The Three-Dimensional Electrocardiogram"; and in Chapter 8, Albert Sun presents "Inherited Arrhythmia Disorders." Each of the now 24 chapters is divided (as indicated in the table of contents) into discrete, compact "learning units." Each learning unit begins on a new page to provide blank space for the reader's notes. The purpose of the learning units is to make this book easier to use by allowing the reader to be selective regarding the material to be considered at a particular time. Because the modern student of electrocardiography is primarily oriented to a visual perspective, we have typically begun each page with an illustration.

The four chapters in Section I (Basic Concepts) provide an introductory orientation to electrocardiography. In Chapter 1 ("Cardiac Electrical Activity"), we include a basic perspective for those with no previous experience in reading ECGs. The reader is asked to consider, "What can this book do for me?" and "What can I expect from myself after I have completed this book?" Also in Chapter 1, the magnetic resonance images of the normal heart in the thorax provide orientation to the relationship between the cardiac structures and the body surface ECG recording sites. Animated video has been added to many of the illustrations to enhance understanding of the basic electrophysiologic principles of electrocardiography. Jacob Simlund provided a new perspective on QT interval correction in Chapter 3.

In the nine chapters of Section II (Abnormal Wave Morphology), the standard 12-lead ECG recordings have been modified from their typical format. Single cardiac cycles are included for each of the standard leads to show how the morphology of the ECG waveforms characteristically appears in each of these 12 different views of the cardiac electrical activity. Ljuba Bacharova added her enthusiasm of studying left-ventricular hypertrophy to Chapter 5 ("Chamber Enlargement"). There have been extensive revisions of the four chapters on myocardial ischemia and infarction (Chapters 9 to 12) because of the many recent advances in understanding their electrocardiographic manifestations. A broad spectrum of health care providers are being challenged to learn the ECG interpretive skills required for rapid prehospital diagnosis and management of patients with acute coronary syndrome.

The Marriott legacy is particularly strong in Section III (Abnormal Rhythms). Barney Marriott and Galen Wagner worked extensively in the preparation for the 9th edition to retain his methodical and innovative approach while including the more recent concepts. In the 10th edition, Galen organized perspectives from clinical electrophysiologists into a practical classification of the various tachyarrhythmias. In the 11th and 12th editions, in-depth electrophysiologic principles were added to enhance understanding of the basic pathophysiology. Ten-second rhythm strips from three simultaneously recorded ECG leads are typically used for the illustrations. Chapter 23 ("Artificial Cardiac Pacemakers") has been extensively revised by Wesley (Ken) Haisty because of the current availability of a wide variety of sophisticated devices.

Marcel Gilbert, an electrophysiologist at Laval University in Quebec, provided the ECG illustrations for all of the chapters on tachyarrhythmias and contributed to rewriting Chapter 18 ("Reentrant Junctional Tachyarrhythmias") and Chapter 19 ("Reentrant Ventricular Tachyarrhythmias").

Ken Haisty, an electrophysiologist at Wake Forest University in Winston-Salem, and Tobin Lim share authorship with Galen Wagner of Chapter 23 ("Artificial Cardiac Pacemakers"). It had become clear that advances in pacing had made the chapter in the 11th edition obsolete.

We coordinated our communication with LWW personnel, which included editorial support from Julie Goolsby (Acquisitions Editor) and Leanne Vandetty (Product Development Editor), digital media support from Freddie Patane (Art Director, Media) and Mark Flanders (Creative Media Director, BioMedia Communications), production support from Marian Bellus (Production Project Manager) and Russ Hall (Executive Director, Absolute Service, Inc.), and marketing support from Stephanie Manzo (Marketing Manager).

Our goal for the 12th edition is to continue to preserve the "spirit of Barney Marriott" through the many changes in words and images. He had been a tough but most helpful critic as Galen justified the maintenance of the title *Marriott's Practical Electrocardiography*. Barney passed away during the time of production of the 11th edition, so this is the first edition without his own unique input. However, his long-time Tampa colleague Douglas Schocken provides his warm personal tribute to Barney in the foreword to this 12th edition, and "Dr. Marriott's Systematic Approach to the Diagnosis of Arrhythmias" remains the final chapter.

Galen S. Wagner and David G. Strauss
Durham, North Carolina, and Washington, District of Columbia

SECTION I

Basic Concepts

1

Cardiac Electrical Activity

GALEN S. WAGNER, TOBIN H. LIM, AND
DAVID G. STRAUSS

THE BOOK: MARRIOTT'S PRACTICAL ELECTROCARDIOGRAPHY, 12TH EDITION

What Can This Book Do for Me?

This 12th edition of *Marriott's Practical Electrocardiography* has been specifically designed to provide you with a practical approach to reading *electrocardiograms* (*ECGs*). No previous text or experience is required. You should consider how you learn best before deciding how to approach this book. If you are most comfortable acquiring a basic understanding of a subject even before you encounter a need to use the subject information, you probably want to read the first section (Basic Concepts) carefully. However, if you have found that such understanding is not really helpful to you until you encounter a specific problem, you probably want to quickly scan this first section.

All medical terms are defined in a glossary at the end of each chapter. Each individual "practical concept" is presented in a "Learning Unit." Each Learning Unit begins on a new page with a heading that is underscored with a green line. The Learning Units are listed in the Table of Contents for easy reference. This book will be more useful if you make your own annotations; blank space is provided for this purpose.

The illustrations are fully integrated into the text, eliminating the need for extensive figure legends. A pink background is used for the ECG examples to provide contrast with the recordings, which appear in black. Because ECG reading is a visual experience, most of the book's illustrations are typical examples of the various clinical situations for which ECGs are recorded. Reference to these examples should provide you with support for accurately reading the ECGs you encounter in your own clinical experience.

To better understand the basic concepts the ECG provides, we have added a digital content to the 12th edition to provide the learner with visuospatial orientation of common cardiac abnormalities. The digital content is not a stand-alone educational tool but should be used to visually conceptualize.

What Can I Expect From Myself When I Have "Completed" This Book?

This book is not intended for you to "complete." Rather, it is intended as a reference for the ECG problems you encounter. There will be evidence that this is your book, with dog-eared pages and your own notes in the sections you have already used. Through your experience with this book, you should develop confidence in identifying a "normal" ECG and be able to accurately diagnose the many common ECG abnormalities. You should also have an understanding of the practical aspects of the pathophysiologic basis for each of these common ECG abnormalities.

THE ELECTROCARDIOGRAM

What Is an Electrocardiogram?

An ECG is the recording (*gram*) of the electrical activity (*electro*) generated by the cells of the heart (*cardio*) that reaches the body surface. This electrical activity initiates the heart's muscular contraction that pumps the blood to the body. Each ECG recording *electrode* provides one of the poles of a lead, which gives the view of this electrical activity that it "sees" from its particular position on the body surface. Observation of the 12 views provided by the routine clinical ECG allows you to "move around" this electrical activity just as though you were seeing the heart from various viewpoints. Indeed, reversal of the poles of each lead provides a reciprocal or mirrorlike view. You should probably have your own ECG recorded and then ask an experienced ECG reader to explain it to you. This experience removes the mystery surrounding the ECG and prepares you for the "Basic Concepts" section of this book.

What Does an Electrocardiogram Actually Measure?

The ECG recording plots voltage on its vertical axis against time on its horizontal axis. Measurements along the horizontal axis indicate the overall heart rate, regularity, and the time intervals during electrical activation that move from one part of the heart to another. Measurements along the vertical axis indicate the voltage measured on the body surface. This voltage represents the "summation" of the electrical activation of all of the cardiac cells. Some abnormalities can be detected by measurements on a single ECG recording, but others become apparent only by observing serial recordings over time.

What Medical Problems Can Be Diagnosed With an Electrocardiogram?

Many cardiac abnormalities can be detected by ECG interpretation, including enlargement of heart muscle, electrical conduction blocks, insufficient blood flow, and death of heart muscle due to a coronary thrombosis. The ECG can even identify which of the heart's coronary arteries contains this occlusion when it is still only threatening to destroy a region of heart muscle. The ECG is also the primary method for identifying problems with heart rate and regularity. In addition to its value for understanding cardiac problems, the ECG can be used to aid in diagnosing medical conditions throughout the body. For example, the ECG can reveal abnormal levels of ions in the blood, such as potassium and calcium, and abnormal function of glands such as the thyroid. It can also detect potentially dangerous levels of certain drugs.

Would It Be Helpful to Have My Own Electrocardiogram Recorded?

In the process of learning electrocardiography, it may be useful to have your own ECG recorded. Here is a list of possible reasons why:

- You will be able to understand the importance of ECG lead placement and orientation because you have experienced the electrodes being placed on your body.
- You can carry your ECG with you as reference if an abnormality is ever suspected.
- You can compare it to someone else's ECG to see normal variations.
- You can compare it at different times of your life to see how it changes.
- You can take deep breaths to see how the resulting slight movement of your heart affects your ECG.
- You can move the electrodes to incorrect positions to see how this distorts the recording.

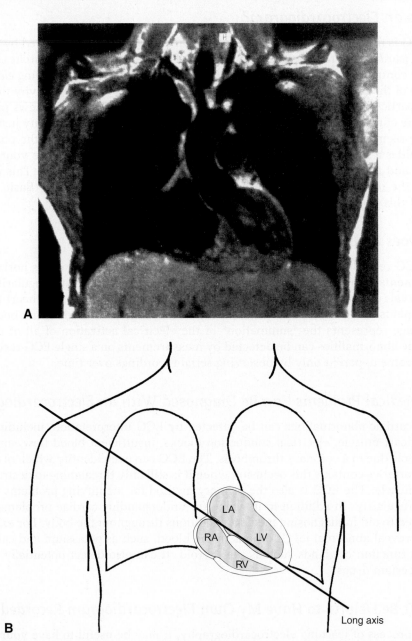

FIGURE 1.1. **A.** Frontal plane magnetic resonance image. **B.** Chambers of the heart. LA, left atrium; LV, left ventricle; RA, right atrium; RV, right ventricle.

The position of the heart within the body determines the "view" of the cardiac electrical activity that can be observed from any site on the body surface. A frontal plane magnetic resonance image of the heart within the thorax is seen in Figure 1.1A. The atria are located in the top or *base* of the heart, and the *ventricles* taper toward the bottom or *apex*. The long axis of the heart, which extends from base to apex, is tilted to the left at its apical end in the schematic drawing of this frontal plane view (see Fig. 1.1B).

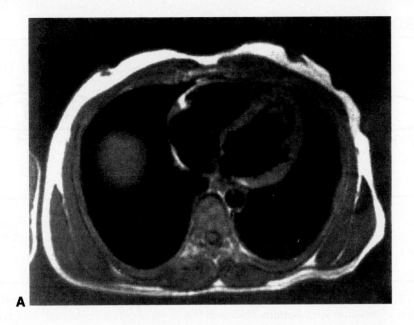

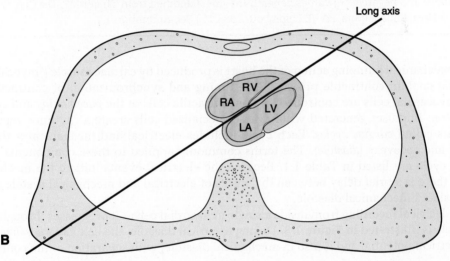

FIGURE 1.2. **A.** Transverse plane magnetic resonance image, as viewed from below. **B.** Chambers of the heart. LA, left atrium; LV, left ventricle; RA, right atrium; RV, right ventricle.

However, the right *atrium*/right ventricle and left *atrium*/left ventricle are not directly aligned with the right and left sides of the body as viewed in the transverse plane magnetic resonance image of the heart within the thorax (Fig. 1.2A). The schematic drawing shows how the right-sided chambers of the heart are located *anterior* to the left-sided chambers, with the result that the interatrial and interventricular septa form a diagonal in this transverse plane view (see Fig. 1.2B).[1,2]

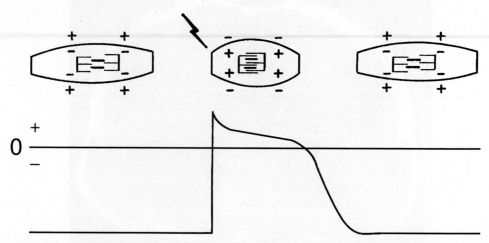

FIGURE 1.3. Cardiac cycle in a single myocardial cell. **Top.** *Lightning bolt:* Electrical impulse; +, positive ions; −, negative ions. **Bottom.** *Horizontal line:* Level of zero (0) potential, with positive (+) values above and negative (−) values beneath the line. (Modified from Thaler MS. *The Only EKG Book You'll Ever Need.* Philadelphia, PA: JB Lippincott; 1988:11.) See Animation 1.1.

The mechanical pumping action of the heart is produced by cardiac muscle ("myocardial") cells that contain contractile proteins. The timing and synchronization of contraction of these myocardial cells are controlled by noncontractile cells of the *pacemaking* and *conduction system*. Impulses generated within these specialized cells create a rhythmic repetition of events called *cardiac cycles*. Each cycle includes electrical and mechanical activation (*systole*) and recovery (*diastole*). The terms commonly applied to these components of the cardiac cycle are listed in Table 1.1. Because the electrical events initiate the mechanical events, there is a brief delay between the onsets of electrical and mechanical systole and of electrical and mechanical diastole.

The electrical recording from inside a single myocardial cell as it progresses through a cardiac cycle is illustrated in Figure 1.3. During electrical diastole, the cell has a *baseline* negative electrical potential and is also in mechanical diastole, with separation of the contractile

Animation 1.1

Table 1.1.	
Terms Describing Cardiac Cycle	
Systole	Diastole
Electrical	
Activation	Recovery
Excitation	Recovery
Depolarization	Repolarization
Mechanical	
Shortening	Lengthening
Contraction	Relaxation
Emptying	Filling

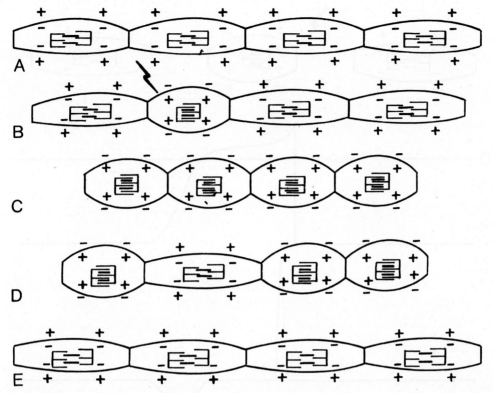

FIGURE 1.4. Cardiac cycle in a series of myocardial cells. The symbols are the same as in Figure 1.3. (Modified from Thaler MS. *The Only EKG Book You'll Ever Need*. Philadelphia, PA: JB Lippincott; 1988:9.) See Animation 1.2.

proteins. At top, a single cardiac cell is shown at three points in time, during which it is relaxed, contracted, and relaxed again. An electrical impulse arriving at the cell allows positively charged ions to cross the cell membrane, causing its *depolarization*. This movement of ions initiates "electrical systole," which is characterized by an *action potential*. This electrical event then initiates mechanical systole, in which the contractile proteins within the myocardial cell slide over each other, thereby shortening the cell. Electrical systole continues until the positively charged ions are pumped out of the cell, causing its *repolarization*. Below the cell is a representation of an internal electrical recording that returns to its negative resting level. The repolarization process begins with an initial brief component that is followed by a "plateau" that varies among myocardial cells. Repolarization is completed by a rapid component. This return of "electrical diastole" causes the contractile proteins within the cell to separate. The cell is then capable of being reactivated when another electrical impulse arrives at its membrane.

The electrical and mechanical changes in a series of myocardial cells (aligned end to end) as they progress through a cardiac cycle are illustrated in Figure 1.4. In Figure 1.4A, the four representative cells are in their resting or repolarized state. Electrically, the cells have negative charges; mechanically, their contractile proteins are separated. An electrical stimulus arrives at the second myocardial cell in Figure 1.4B, causing electrical and then mechanical systole.

The wave of depolarization in Figure 1.4C spreads throughout all the myocardial cells. In Figure 1.4D, the recovery or repolarization process begins in the second cell, which was first to depolarize. Finally, in Figure 1.4E, the wave of repolarization spreads throughout all of the myocardial cells, and they await the coming of another electrical stimulus.[3-6]

Animation 1.2

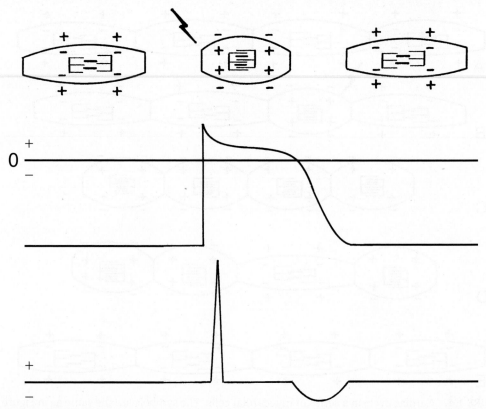

FIGURE 1.5. Single-cell recording combined with an ECG. The symbols are the same as in Figure 1.3. (Modified from Thaler MS. *The Only EKG Book You'll Ever Need*. Philadelphia, PA: JB Lippincott; 1988:11.) See Animation 1.3.

In Figure 1.5, the relationship between the intracellular electrical recording from a single myocardial cell presented in Figure 1.3 is combined with an ECG recording on a "lead" that has its positive and negative electrodes on the body surface. The ECG recording is the summation of electrical signals from all of the myocardial cells. There is a flat baseline in two very different situations: (a) when the cells are in their resting state electrically and (b) when the summation of cardiac electrical activity is directed perpendicular to a line between the positive and negative electrodes. The depolarization of the cells produces a high-frequency ECG *waveform*. Then, between the initial transient and final complete phases of repolarization, the ECG returns to the baseline. Completion of repolarization of the myocardial cells is represented on the ECG by a lower frequency waveform in the opposite direction from that representing depolarization.

Animation 1.3

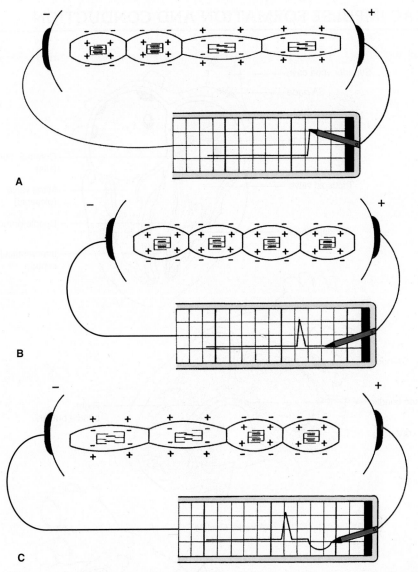

FIGURE 1.6. Single-channel ECG recording. The symbols are the same as in Figure 1.3. *Black semiovals*, electrodes. (Modified from Thaler MS. *The Only EKG Book You'll Ever Need*. Philadelphia, PA: JB Lippincott; 1988:29,31.) See Animation 1.3.

In Figure 1.6, a lead with its positive and negative electrodes has been placed on the body surface and connected to a single-channel ECG recorder. The process of production of the ECG recording by waves of depolarization and repolarization spreading from the negative toward the positive electrode is illustrated. In Figure 1.6A, the first of the four cells shown is electrically activated, and the activation then spreads into the second cell. This spread of depolarization toward the positive electrode produces a positive (upward) *deflection* on the ECG. In Figure 1.6B, all of the cells are in their depolarized state, and the ECG recording returns to its baseline level. In Figure 1.6C, repolarization begins in the same cell in which depolarization was initiated, and the wave of repolarization spreads into the adjoining cell. This produces the oppositely directed negative (downward) waveform on the ECG recording.

Animation 1.3

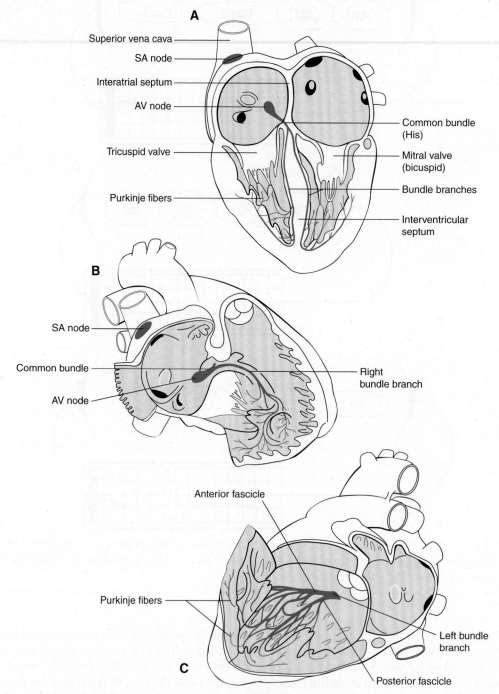

FIGURE 1.7. Special cells of the cardiac pacemaking and conduction system. In **A,** the anterior aspect of all chambers has been removed to reveal the entire AV and ventricular conduction system. In **B,** the lateral aspect of the right atrium and ventricle has been removed. In **C,** the lateral aspect of the left atrium and ventricle has been removed to reveal the right and left bundle branches, respectively. AV, atrioventricular; SA, sinoatrial. (Modified from Netter FH. In: Yonkman FF, ed. *The Ciba Collection of Medical Illustrations. Vol 5: Heart.* Summit, NJ: Ciba–Geigy; 1978:13,49.)

The electrical activation of a single cardiac cell or even of a small group of cells does not produce enough voltage to be recorded on the body surface. Clinical electrocardiography is made possible by the activation of large groups of atrial and ventricular myocardial cells, whose numbers are of sufficient magnitude for their electrical activity to be recorded on the body surface.

Myocardial cells normally lack the ability for either spontaneous formation or rapid conduction of an electrical impulse. They depend on special cells of the *cardiac pacemaking* and *conduction system* that are located strategically through the heart for these functions (Fig. 1.7). These cells are arranged in *nodes, bundles, bundle branches,* and branching networks of *fascicles.* The cells that form these structures lack contractile capability, but they can generate spontaneous electrical impulses (act as pacemakers) and alter the speed of electrical conduction throughout the heart. The intrinsic pacemaking rate is most rapid in the specialized cells in the atria and slowest in those in the ventricles. This intrinsic pacemaking rate is altered by the balance between the sympathetic and parasympathetic components of the autonomic nervous system.[7-10]

Figure 1.7 illustrates three different anatomic relationships between the cardiac pumping chambers and the specialized pacemaking and conduction system: Anterior precordium with less tilt (see Fig. 1.7A), right anterior precordium looking onto the interatrial and interventricular septa through the right atrium and ventricle (see Fig. 1.7B), and left posterior thorax looking onto the septa through the left atrium and ventricle (see Fig. 1.7C). The *sinoatrial* (SA) or *sinus node* is located high in the right atrium, near its junction with the *superior vena cava.* The SA node is the predominant cardiac pacemaker, and its highly developed capacity for autonomic regulation controls the heart's pumping rate to meet the changing needs of the body. The *atrioventricular* (AV) *node* is located low in the right atrium, adjacent to the interatrial *septum.* Its primary function is to slow electrical conduction sufficiently to asynchronize the atrial contribution to ventricular pumping. Normally, the AV node is the only structure capable of conducting impulses from the atria to the ventricles because these chambers are otherwise completely separated by nonconducting fibrous and fatty tissue.[11-13]

In the atria, the electrical impulse generated by the SA node spreads through the myocardium without needing to be carried by any specialized conduction bundles. Electrical impulses reach the AV node where the impulse is delayed before continuing to the intraventricular conduction pathways.

The intraventricular conduction pathways include a *common bundle* (bundle of His) that leads from the AV node to the summit of the interventricular septum as well as the right and left bundle branches of the bundle of His, which proceed along the septal surfaces of their respective ventricles. The left bundle branch fans out into fascicles that proceed along the left septal endocardial surface and toward the two papillary muscles of the mitral valve. The right bundle branch remains compact until it reaches the right *distal* septal surface, where it branches into the interventricular septum and toward the free wall of the right ventricle. These intraventricular conduction pathways are composed of fibers of *Purkinje cells,* which have specialized capabilities for both pacemaking and rapid conduction of electrical impulses. Fascicles composed of Purkinje fibers form networks that extend just beneath the surface of the right and left ventricular *endocardium.* After reaching the ends of these Purkinje fascicles, the impulses then proceed more slowly from endocardium to *epicardium* throughout the right and left ventricles.[14-16] This synchronization process allows activation of the myocardium at the base to be delayed until the apical region has been activated. This sequence of electrical activation is necessary to achieve the most efficient cardiac pumping because the pulmonary and aortic outflow valves are located at the ventricular bases.

RECORDING LONG-AXIS (BASE–APEX) CARDIAC ELECTRICAL ACTIVITY

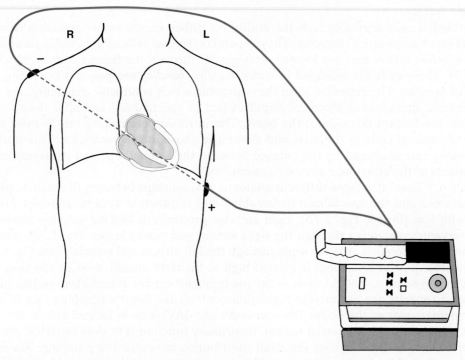

FIGURE 1.8. Optimal sites for recording long-axis cardiac electrical activity. *Black semi-ovals* represent the electrodes. L, left; R, right. See Animation 1.4.

The schematic frontal plane view of the heart in the thorax is shown in Figure 1.1B, with the negative and positive electrodes located where the long axis of the heart intersects with the body surface. The optimal body surface sites for recording long-axis (base–apex) cardiac electrical activity are located where the extensions of the long axis of the heart intersect with the body surface (Fig. 1.8). The negative electrode on the right shoulder and the positive electrode on the left lower chest are aligned from the cardiac base to apex parallel to the interatrial and interventricular septa. This long-axis "ECG lead" is oriented similarly to a lead termed "aVR" on the standard 12-lead ECG (see Chapter 2). However, the lead in Figure 1.8 would actually be lead –aVR because, for lead aVR, the positive electrode is placed on the right arm. Both the positive and negative electrodes are attached to a single-channel ECG recorder that produces predominantly upright *waveforms* on the ECG, as explained later in this unit (see also Chapter 2).

Animation 1.4

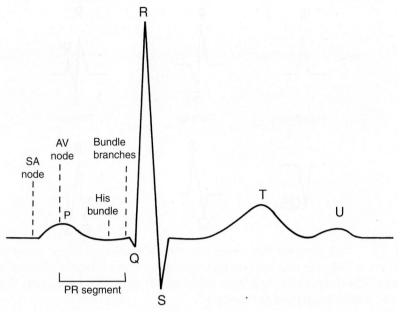

FIGURE 1.9. Wave forms. P, atrial activation; Q, R, and S, ventricular activation; T and U, ventricular recovery. AV, atrioventricular; SA, sinoatrial. See Animation 1.5.

The long-axis recording in Figure 1.8 has been magnified to illustrate the sequence of activation in structures of the pacemaking and conduction system (Fig. 1.9). The initial wave of a cardiac cycle represents activation of the atria and is called the *P wave*. Because the SA node is located in the right atrium, the first part of the P wave represents the activation of this chamber. The middle section of the P wave represents completion of right-atrial activation and initiation of left-atrial activation. The final section of the P wave represents completion of left-atrial activation. Activation of the AV node begins by the middle of the P wave and proceeds slowly during the final portion of the P wave. The wave representing electrical recovery of the atria is usually too small to be seen on the ECG, but it may appear as a distortion of the PR segment. The bundle of His and bundle branches are activated during the PR segment but do not produce waveforms on the body surface ECG.

The next group of waves recorded is termed the *QRS complex*, representing the simultaneous activation of the right and left ventricles. On this long-axis recording, the P wave is entirely positive and the QRS complex is predominantly positive.

Animation 1.5

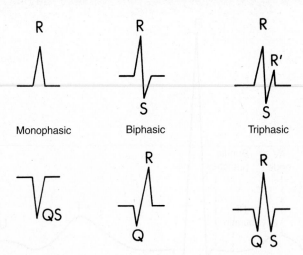

FIGURE 1.10. QRS complex waveforms and their alphabetical terms. (From Selvester RH, Wagner GS, Hindman NB. The development and application of the Selvester QRS scoring system for estimating myocardial infarct size. *Arch Intern Med.* 1985;145:1879, with permission. Copyright 1985, American Medical Association.) See Animation 1.5.

The QRS complex may normally appear as one (*monophasic*), two (*diphasic*), or three (*triphasic*) individual waveforms (Fig. 1.10). By convention, a negative wave at the onset of the QRS complex is called a *Q wave*. The predominant portion of the QRS complex recorded from this long-axis viewpoint is normally positive and is called the *R wave*, regardless of whether or not it is preceded by a Q wave. A negative deflection following an R wave is called an *S wave*. When a second positive deflection occurs, it is termed *R'* (R prime). A monophasic negative QRS complex should be termed a *QS wave* (see Fig. 1.10, left). Biphasic complexes are either RS or QR (see Fig. 1.10, center), and triphasic complexes are RSR' or QRS (see Fig. 1.10, right). Occasionally, more complex patterns of QRS waveforms occur (see Chapter 3).

Animation 1.5

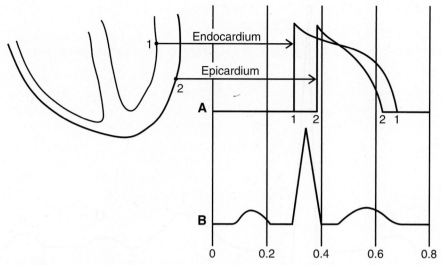

FIGURE 1.11. **A.** Action potential of left-ventricular myocardial cells. **B.** Long-axis body surface ECG waveforms. See Animation 1.6.

The wave in the cardiac cycle that represents recovery of the ventricles is called the *T wave*. The frontal plane view of the right and left ventricles (as in Fig. 1.7A) is presented along with schematic recordings from left-ventricular myocardial cells on the endocardial and epicardial surfaces (Fig. 1.11). The numbers below the recordings refer to the time (in seconds) required for these sequential electrical events. As stated in the previous Learning Unit, the Purkinje fibers provide electrical activation of the endocardium, initiating a "wave front" of depolarization that spreads through the myocardial wall to the cells on the epicardial surface. Because recovery of the ventricular cells (repolarization) causes an ion flow opposite to that of depolarization, one might expect the T wave to be inverted in relation to the QRS complex, as shown in Figures 1.5 and 1.6. However, epicardial cells repolarize earlier than endocardial cells, thereby causing the wave of repolarization to spread in the direction opposite that of the wave of depolarization (epicardium to endocardium; see Fig. 1.11A). This results in the long-axis body surface ECG waveform (as in Fig. 1.9) with the T wave deflected in a similar direction as the QRS complex (see Fig. 1.11B). The T wave is sometimes followed by another small upright wave (the source of which is uncertain), called the *U wave*, as seen in Figure 1.9.

Animation 1.6

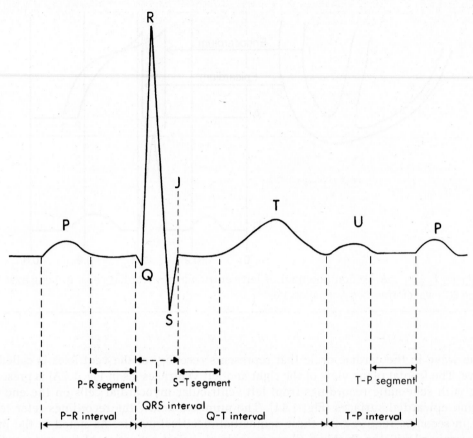

FIGURE 1.12. Magnified cardiac long-axis viewpoint of ECG segments and time intervals. See Animation 1.7.

The magnified recording from Figure 1.9 is again presented with the principal ECG segments (P-R and S-T) and time intervals (P-R, QRS, Q-T, and T-P) as displayed in Figure 1.12. The time from the onset of the P wave to the onset of the QRS complex is called the *PR interval*, regardless of whether the first wave in this QRS complex is a Q wave or an R wave. This interval measures the time between the onset of activation of the atrial and ventricular myocardium. The designation *PR segment* refers to the time from the end of the P wave to the onset of the QRS complex. The *QRS interval* measures the time from the beginning to the end of ventricular activation. Because activation of the thick left-ventricular free wall and interventricular septum requires more time than does activation of the right-ventricular free wall, the terminal portion of the QRS complex represents the balance of forces between the basal portions of these thicker regions.

The *ST segment* is the interval between the end of ventricular activation and the beginning of ventricular recovery. The term *ST segment* is used regardless of whether the final wave of the QRS complex is an R or an S wave. The junction of the QRS complex and the ST segment is called the *J point*.[17] The interval from the onset of ventricular activation to the end of ventricular recovery is called the *QT interval*. This term is used regardless of whether the QRS complex begins with a Q or an R wave.

At low heart rates in a healthy person, the PR, ST, and TP segments are at approximately the same level (*isoelectric*). The TP segment between the end of the T or U wave and beginning of the P wave is typically used as the *baseline* for measuring the amplitudes of the various waveforms.[18–20]

Animation 1.7

RECORDING SHORT-AXIS (LEFT VERSUS RIGHT) CARDIAC ELECTRICAL ACTIVITY

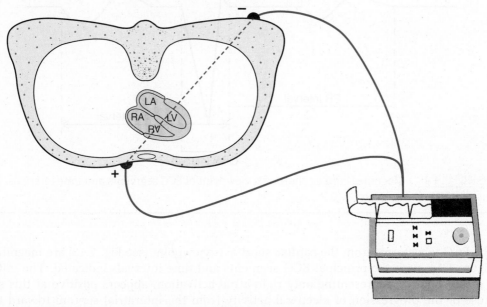

FIGURE 1.13. Optimal recording sites for left- versus right-sided cardiac electrical activity, as viewed from above. *Black semi-ovals* represent the electrodes LA, left atrium; LV, left ventricle; RA, right atrium; RV, right ventricle. See Animation 1.8.

It is often important to determine whether an abnormality originates from the left or right side of the heart. The optimal sites for recording left- versus right-sided cardiac electrical activity are located where the extensions of the short axis of the heart intersect with the body surface as illustrated in the schematic transverse plane view (Fig. 1.13). The negative electrode on the left posterior thorax (back) and the positive electrode on the right anterior thorax (right of sternum) are aligned perpendicular to the interatrial and interventricular septa, and they are attached to a single-channel ECG recorder. This short-axis "ECG lead" is oriented similarly to a lead termed "V1" on the standard 12-lead ECG (see Chapter 2). The positive electrode for lead V1 is placed on the anterior thorax in the fourth intercostal space at the right edge of the sternum. The typically diphasic P and T waves and the predominantly negative QRS complex recorded by electrodes at these positions are indicated on the ECG recording.

Animation 1.8

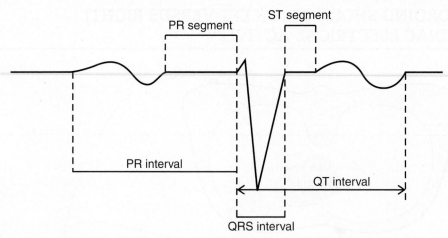

FIGURE 1.14. Magnified cardiac short-axis viewpoint of ECG segments and time intervals. See Animation 1.9 and Animation 1.10.

The ECG waveforms from the cardiac short-axis viewpoint (see Fig. 1.13) are magnified in Figure 1.14, with the principal ECG segments and time intervals indicated. The initial part of the P wave, representing only right-atrial activation, appears positive at this site because of the progression of electrical activity from the interatrial septum toward the right-atrial free wall and the positive electrode. The final part of the P wave, representing only left-atrial activation, appears negative because of progression of electrical activity from the interatrial septum toward the left-atrial free wall and the negative electrode. This activation sequence produces a diphasic P wave.

The initial part of the QRS complex represents the progression of activation in the interventricular septum. This movement is predominantly from the left toward the right side of the septum, producing a positive (R wave) deflection at this left- versus right-sided recording site. The midportion of the QRS complex represents progression of electrical activation through the left- and right-ventricular myocardium. Because the posteriorly positioned left-ventricular free wall is much thicker than the anteriorly placed right-ventricular free wall, its activation predominates over that of the latter, resulting in a deeply negative deflection (S wave). The final portion of the QRS complex represents the completion of activation of the left-ventricular free wall and interventricular septum. This posteriorly directed excitation is represented by the completion of the S wave. The T wave is typically biphasic in this short-axis view, and there is no U wave.

Animation 1.9   Animation 1.10

Action potential: the electrical potential recorded from within a cell as it is activated by an electrical current or impulse.

Anterior: located toward the front of the body.

Apex: the region of the heart where the narrowest parts of the ventricles are located.

Atrioventricular (AV) node: a small mass of tissue situated in the inferior aspect of the right atrium, adjacent to the septum between the right and left atria. Its function is to slow impulses traveling from the atria to the ventricles, thereby synchronizing atrial and ventricular pumping.

Atrium: a chamber of the heart that receives blood from the veins and passes it along to its corresponding ventricle.

Base: the broad top of the heart where the atria are located.

Baseline: see **Isoelectric line**.

Bundle branches: groups of Purkinje fibers that emerge from the common bundle (of His); the right bundle branch rapidly conducts electrical impulses to the right ventricle, while the left bundle branch conducts impulses to the left ventricle.

Cardiac cycle: a single episode of electrical and mechanical activation and recovery of a myocardial cell or of the entire heart.

Cardiac pacemaking and conduction system: groups of modified myocardial cells strategically located throughout the heart and capable of forming an electrical impulse and/or of conducting impulses particularly slowly or rapidly.

Common bundle (of His): a compact group of Purkinje fibers that originates at the AV node and rapidly conducts electrical impulses to the right and left bundle branches.

Deflection: a waveform on the ECG; its direction may be either upward (positive) or downward (negative).

Depolarization: the transition in which there becomes minimal difference between the electrical charge and potential on the inside versus the outside of the cell. In the resting state, the cell is polarized, with the inside of the cell markedly negative in comparison to the outside. Depolarization is then initiated by a current that alters the permeability of the cell membrane, allowing positively charged ions to cross into the cell.

Diastole: the period in which the electrical and mechanical aspects of the heart are in their baseline or resting state: electrical diastole is characterized by repolarization and mechanical diastole by relaxation. During mechanical diastole, the cardiac chambers are filling with blood.

Diphasic: consisting of two components.

Distal: situated away from the point of attachment or origin; the opposite of proximal.

Electrocardiogram (ECG): the recording made by the electrocardiograph, depicting the electrical activity of the heart.

Electrode: an electrical contact that is placed on the skin and is connected to an ECG recorder.

Endocardium: the inner aspect of a myocardial wall, adjacent to the blood-filled cavity of the adjacent chamber.

Epicardium: the outer aspect of a myocardial wall, adjacent to the pericardial lining that closely envelops the heart.

Fascicle: a small bundle of Purkinje fibers that emerges from a bundle or a bundle branch to rapidly conduct impulses to the endocardial surfaces of the ventricles.

Isoelectric line: a horizontal line on an ECG recording that forms a baseline; representing neither a positive nor a negative electrical potential.

J point: junction of the QRS complex and the ST segment.

Lateral: situated toward either the right or left side of the heart or of the body as a whole.

Monophasic: consisting of a single component, being either positive or negative.

P wave: the first wave depicted on the ECG during a cardiac cycle; it represents atrial activation.

PR interval: the time from onset of the P wave to onset of the QRS complex. This interval represents the time between the onsets of activation of the atrial and the ventricular myocardium.

PR segment: the time from the end of the P wave to the onset of the QRS complex.

Purkinje cells or fibers: modified myocardial cells that are found in the distal aspects of the pacemaking and conduction system, consisting of the common bundle, the bundle branches, the fascicles, and individual strands.

Q wave: a negative wave at the onset of the QRS complex.

QRS complex: the second wave or group of waves depicted on the ECG during a cardiac cycle; it represents ventricular activation.

QRS interval: the time from the beginning to the end of the QRS complex, representing the duration required for activation of the ventricular myocardial cells.

QS: a monophasic negative QRS complex.

QT interval: the time from the onset of the QRS complex to the end of the T wave. This interval represents the time from the beginning of ventricular activation to the completion of ventricular recovery.

R wave: the first positive wave appearing in a QRS complex; it may appear at the onset of the QRS complex or following a Q wave.

R' wave: the second positive wave appearing in a QRS complex.

Repolarization: the transition in which the inside of the cell becomes markedly positive in relation to the outside. This condition is maintained by a pump in the cell membrane, and it is disturbed by the arrival of an electrical current.

Septum: a dividing wall between the atria or between the ventricles.

Sinoatrial (SA) node: a small mass of tissue situated in the superior aspect of the right atrium, adjacent to the entrance of the superior vena cava. It functions as the dominant pacemaker, which forms the electrical impulses that are then conducted throughout the heart.

ST segment: the interval between the end of the QRS complex and the beginning of the T wave.

Superior: situated above and closer to the head than another body part.

Superior vena cava: one of the large veins that empties into the right atrium.

Systole: the period in which the electrical and mechanical aspects of the heart are in their active state: electrical systole is characterized by depolarization and mechanical systole by contraction. During mechanical systole, blood is being pumped out of the heart.

T wave: the final major wave depicted on the ECG during a cardiac cycle; it represents ventricular recovery.

Triphasic: consisting of three components.

U wave: a wave on the ECG that follows the T wave in some individuals; it is typically small and its source is uncertain.

Ventricle: a chamber of the heart that receives blood from its corresponding atrium and pumps the blood it receives out into the arteries.

Waveform: electrocardiographic representation of either the activation or recovery phase of electrical activity of the heart.

■ REFERENCES

1. De Vries PA, Saunders JB. Development of the ventricles and spiral outflow tract of the human heart. *Contrib Embryol.* 1962;37:87.
2. Mall FP. On the development of the human heart. *Am J Anat.* 1912;13:249.
3. Hoffman BF, Cranefield PF. *Electrophysiology of the Heart.* New York, NY: McGraw-Hill; 1960.
4. Page E. The electrical potential difference across the cell membrane of heart muscle. *Circulation.* 1962;26:582–595.
5. Fozzard HA, ed. *The Heart and Cardiovascular System: Scientific Foundations.* New York, NY: Raven; 1986.
6. Guyton AC. Heart muscle: the heart as a pump. In: Guyton AC, ed. *Textbook of Medical Physiology.* Philadelphia, PA: WB Saunders; 1991.
7. Rushmer RF. Functional anatomy and the control of the heart, part I. In: Rushmer RF, ed. *Cardiovascular Dynamics.* Philadelphia, PA: WB Saunders; 1976:76–104.
8. Langer GA. Heart: excitation—contraction coupling. *Ann Rev Physiol.* 1973;35:55–85.
9. Weidmann S. Resting and action potentials of cardiac muscle. *Ann NY Acad Sci.* 1957;65:663.
10. Rushmer RF, Guntheroth WG. Electrical activity of the heart, part I. In: Rushmer RF, ed. *Cardiovascular Dynamics.* Philadelphia, PA: WB Saunders; 1976.
11. Truex RC. The sinoatrial node and its connections with the atrial tissue. In: Wellens HJJ, Lie KI, Janse MJ, eds. *The Conduction System of the Heart.* The Hague, The Netherlands: Martinus Nijhoff; 1978.

12. Hecht HH, Kossmann CE. Atrioventricular and intraventricular conduction. *Am J Cardiol*. 1973;31:232–244.

13. Becker AE, Anderson RH. Morphology of the human atrioventricular junctional area. In: Wellens HJJ, Lie KI, Janse MJ, eds. *The Conduction System of the Heart*. The Hague, The Netherlands: Martinus Nijhoff; 1978.

14. Meyerburg RJ, Gelband H, Castellanos A, et al. Electrophysiology of endocardial intraventricular conduction: the role and function of the specialized conducting system. In: Wellens HJJ, Lie KI, Janse MJ, eds. *The Conduction System of the Heart*. The Hague, The Netherlands: Martinus Nijhoff; 1978.

15. Guyton AC. Rhythmic excitation of the heart. In: Guyton AC, ed. *Textbook of Medical Physiology*. Philadelphia, PA: WB Saunders; 1991.

16. Scher AM. The sequence of ventricular excitation. *Am J Cardiol*. 1964;14:287.

17. Aldrich HR, Wagner NB, Boswick J, et al. Use of initial ST segment for prediction of final electrocardiographic size of acute myocardial infarcts. *Am J Cardiol*. 1988;61:749–763.

18. Graybiel A, White PD, Wheeler L, et al., eds. The typical normal electrocardiogram and its variations. In: *Electrocardiography in Practice*. Philadelphia, PA: WB Saunders; 1952.

19. Netter FH. Section II, the electrocardiogram. In: *The CIBA Collection of Medical Illustrations*. Vol 5. New York, NY: CIBA; 1978.

20. Barr RC. Genesis of the electrocardiogram. In: Macfarlane PW, Lawrie TDV, eds. *Comprehensive Electrocardiology*. Vol I. New York, NY: Pergamon Press; 1989:139–147.

2

Recording the Electrocardiogram

GALEN S. WAGNER, RAYMOND R. BOND,
DEWAR D. FINLAY, TOBIN H. LIM,
AND DAVID G. STRAUSS

THE STANDARD 12-LEAD ELECTROCARDIOGRAM

Frontal Plane

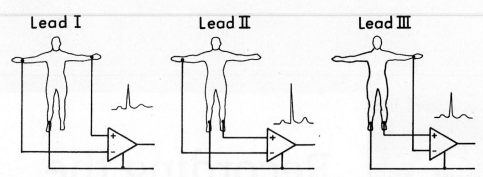

FIGURE 2.1. Einthoven's three original limb leads: (+) positive and (−) negative electrode pairs on distal limb sites. (Modified from Netter FH. *The CIBA Collection of Medical Illustrations. Vol 5. Heart.* Summit, NJ: Ciba-Geigy; 1978:51, with permission.) See Animation 2.1.

The standard electrocardiogram (ECG) utilizes the two viewpoints presented in Chapter 1 (see Figs. 1.8 and 1.13): base–apex (long axis) and left–right (short axis) plus 10 other viewpoints for recording cardiac electrical activity. Each view is provided by recording the electrical potential difference between a positive and a negative pole, referred to as a *lead*. Six of these leads provide views in the *frontal plane* of the body and six provide views in the *transverse (horizontal) plane* of the body. A single recording electrode on the body surface serves as the positive pole of each lead; the negative pole of each lead is provided either by a single recording electrode or by a *central terminal* that averages the input from multiple recording electrodes. The device used for recording the ECG, called the *electrocardiograph*, contains the circuitry that creates the "central terminal," which serves as the negative electrode for the nine standard leads that are termed "V leads."

More than 100 years ago, Einthoven[1] placed recording electrodes on the right and left arms and the left leg and called the recording an *Elektrokardiogramme* (EKG), which is replaced by the anglicized ECG throughout this book. Einthoven's work produced three leads (I, II, and III), each produced by a pair of the limb electrodes, with one electrode of the pair serving as the positive and the other as the negative pole of the lead (Fig. 2.1). The positive poles of these leads were positioned on the body surface to the left and inferiorly so that the cardiac electrical waveforms would appear primarily upright on the ECG. This waveform direction results because the summations of both the atrial and ventricular electrical forces are generally directed toward the apex of the heart. For lead I, the left arm electrode provides the positive pole and the right arm electrode provides the negative pole. Lead II, with its positive electrode on the left leg and its negative electrode on the right arm, provides a long-axis view of the cardiac electrical activity only slightly different from that presented in Chapter 1 (see Figs. 1.8, 1.9, and 1.12). Lead III has its positive electrode on the left leg and its negative electrode on the left arm. An electrode placed on the right leg is used to ground the system.

Animation 2.1

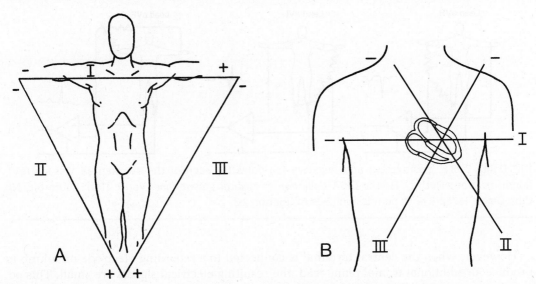

FIGURE 2.2. Leads I, II, and III with positive and negative electrode poles. **A.** Einthoven triangle. **B.** Einthoven triangle in relation to the schematic heart. See Animation 2.2.

The three ECG leads (I, II, and III) form an equiangular (60-degree) triangle known as the *Einthoven triangle* (Fig. 2.2A). Consideration of these three leads so that they intersect in the center of the cardiac electrical activity but retain their original spatial orientation provides a triaxial reference system for viewing the cardiac electrical activity (see Fig. 2.2B). These are the only leads in the standard 12-lead ECG that are recorded using only two body surface electrodes. They are typically called "bipolar leads," but indeed, the other nine leads are also bipolar. Their negative poles are provided by the central terminal.

The 60-degree angles between leads I, II, and III create wide gaps among the three views of the cardiac electrical activity. Wilson and coworkers[2] developed a method for filling these gaps without additional body surface electrodes: They created a central terminal, by connecting the three limb electrodes on the right and left arms and the left leg. An ECG lead using this central terminal as its negative pole and a recording electrode on the body surface as its positive pole is termed a *V lead*, as stated above.

Animation 2.2

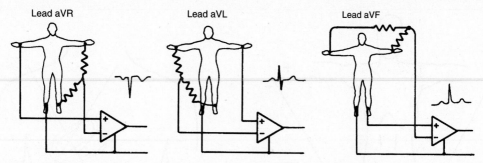

FIGURE 2.3. Positive (+) and negative (−) poles for each of the augmented V leads (aV). (Modified from Netter FH. *The CIBA Collection of Medical Illustrations. Vol 5. Heart.* Summit, NJ: Ciba-Geigy; 1978:51, with permission.) See Animation 2.3.

However, when the central terminal is connected to a recording electrode on a limb to produce an additional frontal plane lead, the resulting electrical signals are small. This occurs because the electrical signal from the recording electrode is partially cancelled when both the positive electrode and one of the three elements of the negative electrode are located on the same extremity. The amplitude of these signals may be increased or "augmented" by disconnecting the central terminal from the electrode on the limb serving as the positive pole. Such an augmented V lead is termed an *aV lead*. The alternating lines in the figure indicate resistors on the connections between two of the recording electrodes that produce the negative poles for each of the aV leads. For example, lead aVR fills the gap between leads I and II by recording the potential difference between the right arm and the average of the potentials on the left arm and left leg (Fig. 2.3). Lead aVR, like lead II, provides a long-axis viewpoint of the cardiac electrical activity but with the opposite orientation from that provided by lead II, as presented in Chapter 1, Figure 1.8. The gap between leads II and III is filled by lead aVF, and the gap between leads III and I is filled by lead aVL. The three aV frontal plane leads were introduced by Goldberger.[3]

Animation 2.3

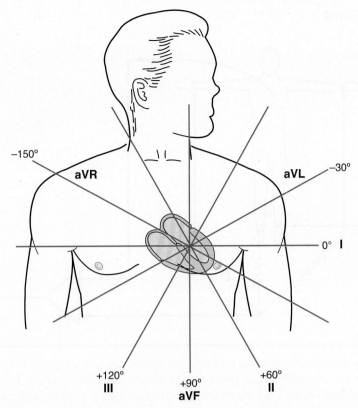

FIGURE 2.4. Frontal plane limb leads that are named according to the locations of their positive electrodes. See Animation 2.4.

Figure 2.2B is reproduced with the addition of the three aV leads to the triaxial reference system, producing a hexaxial system (Fig. 2.4) for viewing the cardiac electrical activity in the frontal plane. Five of the six leads of this system are separated by angles of only 30 degrees. The exception is lead aVR, because its positive electrode on the right arm is oriented to −150 degrees. This provides a 360-degree perspective of the frontal plane similar to the positions of the 2, 3, 5, 6, 7, and 10 on the face of a clock. By convention, the degrees are arranged as shown. With lead I (located at 0 degrees) used as the reference lead, positive designations increase in 30-degree increments in a clockwise direction to +180 degrees, and negative designations increase by the same increments in a counterclockwise direction to −180 degrees. Lead II appears at +60 degrees, lead aVF at +90 degrees, and lead III at +120 degrees. Leads aVL and aVR have designations of −30 and −150 degrees, respectively. The negative poles of each of these leads complete the "clock face."

Modern electrocardiographs, using digital technology, record leads I and II only and then calculate the voltages in the remaining limb leads in real time on the basis of Einthoven law: I + III = II.[1] The algebraic outcome of the formulas for calculating the voltages in aV leads from leads I, II, and III are:

$$aVR = -\tfrac{1}{2}(I + II)$$
$$aVL = I - \tfrac{1}{2}(II)$$
$$aVF = II - \tfrac{1}{2}(I)$$

Thus,

$$aVR + aVL + aVF = 0$$

Animation 2.4

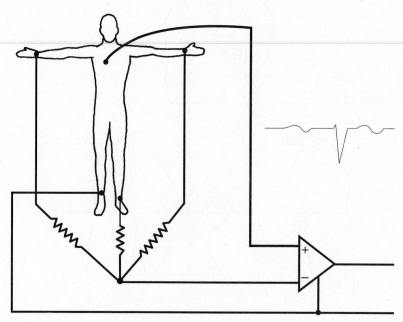

FIGURE 2.5. Heart chambers, as viewed from below. LA, left atrium; LV, left ventricle; RA, right atrium; RV, right ventricle. Black semiovals are electrodes. (Modified from Netter FH. *The CIBA Collection of Medical Illustrations. Vol 5. Heart.* Summit, NJ: Ciba-Geigy; 1978:51, with permission.)

The standard 12-lead ECG includes the six frontal plane leads of the hexaxial system and six additional leads relating to the *transverse plane* of the body. These additional leads, introduced by Wilson, are produced by using the central terminal of the hexaxial system as the negative pole and an electrode placed at various positions on the anterior and left lateral chest wall as the positive pole.[4-8] Because the positions of these latter leads are immediately in front of the heart, they are termed *precordial*. Because the positive poles of these leads are provided from an electrode that is not included in the central terminal, no "augmentation" of the recorded wave forms is required. The six additional leads used to produce the 12-lead ECG are labeled V1 through V6. Figure 2.5 shows lead V1, with its positive pole on the right anterior precordium and its negative pole in the center of the cardiac electrical activity. Therefore, this lead provides a short-axis view of cardiac electrical activity that is useful for distinguishing left versus right location of various abnormal conditions as described (see Fig. 1.13). The wavelike lines in the figure indicate resistors in the connections between the recording electrodes on the three limb leads that produce the negative poles for each of the V leads.

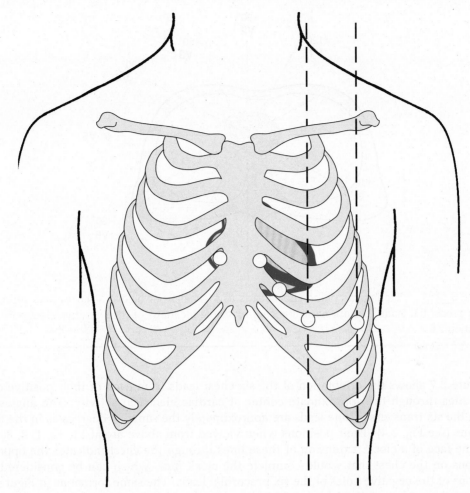

FIGURE 2.6. Bony landmarks for electrode positions. Black circles and *semicircle* are electrodes. *Dashed vertical lines* are the midclavicular (through lead V4) and anterior axillary (through lead V5) lines. (Modified from Thaler MS. *The Only EKG Book You'll Ever Need.* Philadelphia, PA: JB Lippincott; 1988:41.)

The body surface positions of each of these electrodes is determined by bony landmarks on the thorax (Fig. 2.6). The clavicles should be used as a reference for locating the first rib. The space between the first and second ribs is called the first *intercostal space*. The V1 electrode is placed in the fourth intercostal space just to the right of the *sternum*. The V2 electrode is placed in the fourth intercostal space just to the left of the sternum (directly anterior to the center of cardiac electrical activity), and electrode V4 is placed in the fifth intercostal space on the *midclavicular line*. Placement of electrode V3 is then halfway along a straight line between electrodes V2 and V4. Electrodes V5 and V6 are positioned directly lateral to electrode V4, with electrode V5 in the *anterior axillary line* and electrode V6 in the *midaxillary line*. In women, electrodes V4 and V5 should be positioned on the chest wall beneath the breast.

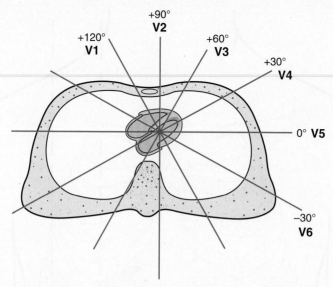

FIGURE 2.7. Transverse plane chest leads as viewed from below. *Solid red lines* represent the six precordial leads that are named according to the locations of their positive electrodes. See Animation 2.5.

Figure 2.7 shows the orientation of the six chest leads from each of their positive electrode sites through the approximate center of cardiac electrical activity. The angles between the six transverse plane leads are approximately the same 30 degrees as in the frontal plane (see Fig. 2.4). Their positions when viewed from above are at 11, 12, 1, 2, 3, and 4 on the face of a clock. Extension of these lines through the chest indicates the opposite positions on the chest that would complete the clock face, which can be considered the locations of the negative poles of the six precordial leads. The same format as in Figure 2.4 indicates the angles on the clock face.

Animation 2.5

CORRECT AND INCORRECT ELECTRODE PLACEMENTS

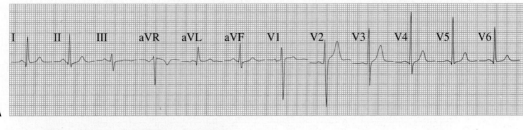

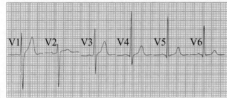

FIGURE 2.8. **A.** Normal ECG. **B.** Precordial lead reversal.

A single cardiac cycle from each of the standard 12 ECG leads of a healthy individual, recorded with all nine recording electrodes positioned correctly, is shown in Figure 2.8A. An accurate electrocardiographic interpretation is possible only if the recording electrodes are placed in their proper positions on the body surface. The three frontal plane electrodes (right arm, left arm, and left leg) used for recording the six limb leads should be placed at distal positions on the designated extremity. It is important to note that when more *proximal* positions are used, particularly on the left arm,[9] marked distortion of the QRS complex may occur. The distal limb positions provide "clean" recordings when the individual maintains the extremities in "resting" positions.

There can be many errors in the placement of the 9 ECG electrodes. This includes reversal of any pair of the six chest electrodes. Reversal of the positions of the V1 and V2 electrodes produces the recording shown in Figure 2.8B.

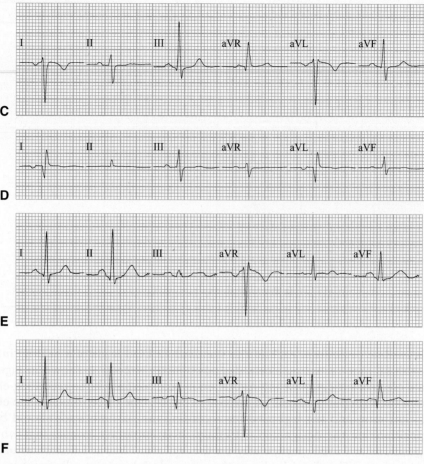

FIGURE 2.8. *(continued)* **C–F.** Limb lead reversals.

Figures 2.8C through 2.8F present examples of ECG recordings produced by incorrect placement of a limb electrode on the same individual, as described. The most common error in frontal plane recording results from reversal of two of the electrodes. One example of this is reversal of the right and left arm electrodes (see Fig. 2.8C). In this instance, lead I is inverted, leads II and III are reversed, leads aVR and aVL are reversed, and lead aVF is correct. Another example that produces a characteristic ECG pattern is reversal of the right leg grounding electrode with one of the arm electrodes. Extremely low amplitudes of all waveforms appear in lead II when the right arm electrode is on the right leg (see Fig. 2.8D) and in lead III when the left arm electrode is on the right leg (see Fig. 2.8E). These amplitudes are so low because the potential difference between the two legs is almost zero. Left arm and leg electrode reversal is the most difficult to detect; lead III is inverted and leads I and II and aVL and aVF are reversed (see Fig. 2.8F).

However, a more common error in transverse plane recording involves failure to place the individual electrodes according to their designated landmarks (see Fig. 2.6). Precise identification of the bony landmarks for proper electrode placement may be difficult in women, obese individuals, and persons with chest wall deformities. Even slight alterations of the position of these electrodes may significantly distort the appearance of the cardiac waveforms. Comparison of serial ECG recordings relies on precise electrode placement.

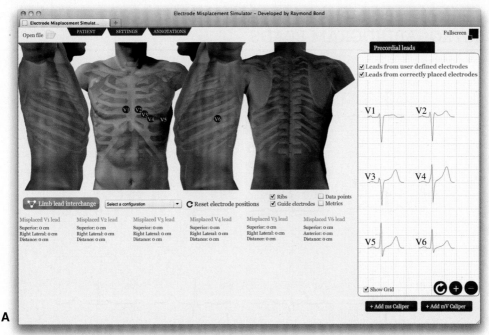

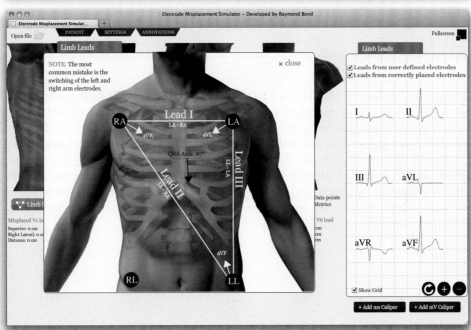

FIGURE 2.9. The electrode misplacement simulation software developed by Raymond Bond. **(A)** shows the six precordial electrodes and their corresponding leads and **(B)** shows the four limb electrodes and the corresponding limb leads. Using this software, electrodes can be moved/misplaced while viewing the effects this has on the 12-lead ECG. See Video 2.1 and the accompanying simulation program can be directly accessed at http://goo.gl/zlZoCe.

Video 2.1

Figure 2.9 shows ECG simulation software that allows the user to interchange and misplace electrodes. The accompanying video illustrates the effects of misplacement of precordial (Fig. 2.9A) and limb (Fig. 2.9B) electrodes.

ALTERNATIVE DISPLAYS OF THE 12 STANDARD ELECTROCARDIOGRAM LEADS

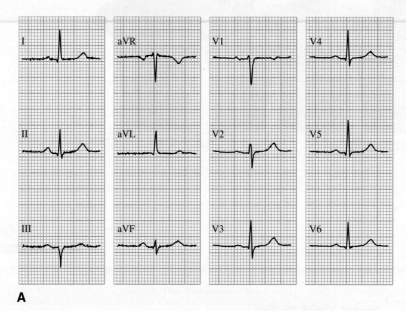

A

FIGURE 2.10. **A.** Classical display.

Alternative displays of the 12-lead ECG may also improve ECG diagnostic capability of the ECG to waveform morphology. Each lead provides its unique view of the cardiac electrical activity, but only the six chest leads are typically displayed in their spatially ordered sequence. The six limb leads are displayed in their two classical sequences (two columns of three leads—I, II, and III and aVR, aVL, and aVF; Fig. 2.10A). This limitation in the standard display becomes most clinically important for the diagnosis of acute myocardial ischemia and infarction; ST-segment elevation in two or more spatially adjacent leads is the cornerstone for an ST-segment elevation myocardial infarction (STEMI) (see Chapters 11 and 12).

Cabrera Sequence

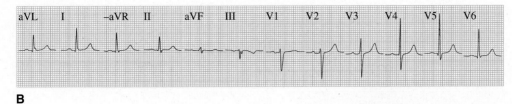

B

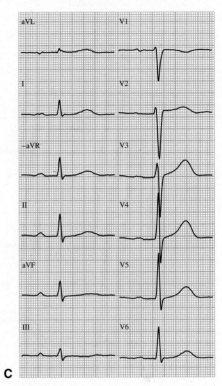

C

FIGURE 2.10. *(continued)* **B.** Single horizontal display. **C.** Parallel vertical displays.

Only in Sweden and scattered other places are the six frontal plane leads integrated into the single orderly sequence from aVL to III, as described by Cabrera.[10] Note that lead aVR in the classical sequence is inverted to –aVR in the orderly sequence to provide another long-axis orientation as lead II. The "10" position on the clock face of lead aVR is replaced by the "4" position of lead –aVR. This lead sequence provides six individual spatially contiguous leads (aVL to III) and five pairs of spatially contiguous leads (aVL and I; I and –aVR; –aVR and II; II and aVF; aVF and III) in the frontal as well as in the transverse plane. This alternative limb lead display was endorsed in the 2000 ESC/ACC consensus guidelines.[11]

The orderly sequence of frontal plane leads followed by the transverse plane leads provides a *panoramic display*[12] of cardiac electrical activity proceeding from left (aVL) to right (III) and then from right (V1) to left (V6; see Fig. 2.10B). The Swedish version of the panoramic display recorded at double paper speed (50 mm per second) is shown in Figure 2.10C.

This display of the 12-lead ECG provides orderly views covering a 150-degree arc in both frontal and transverse planes, which encompasses views of a majority of the left-ventricular myocardium. However, there are some left-ventricular walls in which *ischemia* and infarction can occur that lie outside these arcs, as presented in Chapter 9.

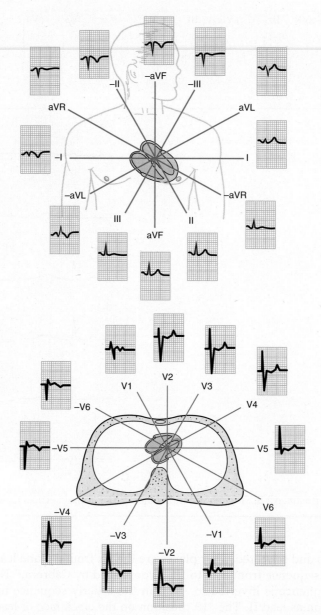

FIGURE 2.11. Clock faces. **Top.** Frontal plane, as seen from the front. **Bottom.** Transverse plane, as seen from below. See Animation 2.6.

Just as lead –aVR in the Cabrera sequence provides an alternative to lead aVR in the classical sequence, the remaining inverted leads provide 11 additional views of the cardiac electrical activity. Thus, the "12-lead ECG" can potentially serve as a "24-lead ECG."

Figures 2.4 and 2.7 are reproduced with all 24 positive and negative leads of an ECG positioned around the frontal and transverse plane clock faces (Fig. 2.11). When a schematic view of the heart in its anatomic position is displayed in the center of the clock, all 24 views provide complete panoramic displays in each of the planes.

Animation 2.6

ALTERNATIVE ELECTRODE PLACEMENT

Clinical Indications

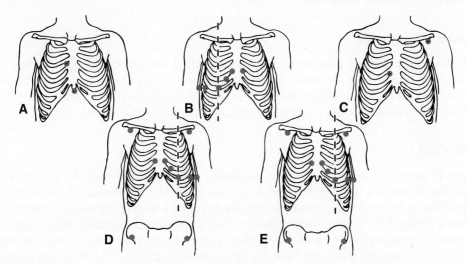

FIGURE 2.12.   Positive and negative poles of a single ECG lead are shown in **A** and **C**. Precordial V electrode locations are shown in **B**, **D**, and **E**. Torso locations of positive electrodes are shown in **D** and **E**. The *vertical dashed line* indicates the midclavicular line in **B**, **D**, and **E**.

Several reasons exist for selecting alternative sites for placement of ECG electrodes: unavailable standard site(s), specific cardiac abnormalities, and continuous monitoring. These sites should be prominently noted on the recording.

Standard Site(s) Unavailable

Standard electrode placement sites may be unavailable because of patient pathology (e.g., amputation or burns) or other impediments (e.g., bandages). In these instances, the electrodes should be positioned as closely as possible to the standard sites and the lead or leads affected by the nonstandard electrode placement clearly designated.

Specific Cardiac Abnormalities

The standard electrode placement sites are not in the optimal position to detect a particular cardiac waveform or abnormality (e.g., P waves obscured within T waves or *situs inversus dextrocardia*). Detection of P waves requires sufficient time between cardiac cycles to provide a baseline between the end of the T wave and the beginning of the QRS complex. In the presence of a rapid cardiac rate (*tachycardia*), alternative electrode placement may produce a lead that reveals recognizable atrial activity (Fig. 2.12A). This may be accomplished by any of the following methods: (a) moving the positive V1 electrode one intercostal space above its standard site, (b) using this site for the positive V1 electrode and the *xiphoid process* of the sternum for the negative V1 electrode, or (c) using a transesophageal site for the positive V1 electrode.

When the congenital position of the heart is rightward (situs inversus dextrocardia), the right and left arm electrodes should be reversed (and the precordial leads should be recorded from rightward-oriented positive electrodes progressing from V1R (V2) to V6R (see Fig. 2.12B). Right-ventricular *hypertrophy* and infarction may best be detected via an electrode in the V3R or V4R position. In infants, in whom the right ventricle is normally more prominent, standard lead V3 is often replaced by lead V4R.

Experimental studies have used body surface maps with multiple rows of electrodes on the anterior and posterior torso to identify specific cardiac abnormalities. This improves the ability to diagnose clinical problems such as left-ventricular hypertrophy or various locations of myocardial infarction.[13]

Continuous Monitoring

The standard electrode placement sites are not ideal for continuous monitoring of cardiac electrical activity (e.g., standard sites produce a recording obscured by skeletal muscle potentials and *artifacts*, especially during ambulatory monitoring). Monitoring may be performed at the bedside, during routine activity, or during exercise stress testing.

Monitoring

There is currently a transition from replacing electrodes for each ECG recording to keeping the electrodes in place for serial recordings. Such "monitoring" has been routine for surveillance in cardiac arrhythmias and during stress testing. However, monitoring is now being adopted for ischemic surveillance. Indeed, the term *diagnostic monitoring* is now used, requiring multiple views of the cardiac electrical activity. Either three orthogonal leads or all 12 standard leads are used for ischemia monitoring. The ECG waveforms are somewhat altered by all monitoring methods. Movement of limb electrodes to torso positions produces altered views for all limb leads and an altered central terminal produced negative pole for all chest leads. In many monitoring methods, the number of chest leads is reduced for efficiency of recording. The missing leads are derived from those recorded, creating further waveform alterations. Therefore, changes observed during monitoring should be viewed in relation to a baseline recording using these leads rather than the standard leads.

Clinical Situation

BEDSIDE. When monitoring for disturbances of cardiac *rhythm*, electrodes should be placed outside the left parasternal area to allow easy access for clinical examination of the heart and possible use of an external defibrillator. A modified lead, modified chest lead V1 (MCL$_1$), with the positive electrode in the same position as lead V1 and the negative electrode near the left shoulder, typically provides good visualization of atrial activity (see Fig. 2.12C) and differentiation of left versus right cardiac activity (see Figs. 1.13 and 1.14).

When monitoring for evidence of ischemia, a complete set of 12 leads may be preferred for recording the ECG. Krucoff and associates[14] described the usefulness of continuous ST-segment monitoring with 12 leads during various unstable coronary syndromes. Some of the major applications of this technique include detection of reoccluded coronary arteries after percutaneous coronary interventions, detection of *reperfusion* and *reocclusion* during acute myocardial infarction,[15,16] and surveillance during *acute coronary syndrome*.

ROUTINE AMBULATORY ACTIVITY. The method of continuous monitoring and recording of cardiac electrical activity is referred to as Holter monitoring[17] after its developer. Originally, only one lead was used. In monitoring for abnormalities of cardiac rhythm, the American Heart Association recommends use of a "V1-type" lead, with the positive electrode in the fourth right intercostal space 2.5 cm from the sternum and the negative electrode below the left clavicle. Currently, three relatively orthogonal leads are used to provide views in all three dimensions (left–right, superior–inferior, and anterior–posterior).

This provides the redundancy for electrocardiographic information should one or more leads fail. The EASI method (described in "Electrode Placement Methods") includes the software for deriving a 12-lead ECG.

EXERCISE STRESS TESTING. ECG monitoring during exercise stress testing is typically performed to diagnose or evaluate cardiac ischemia owing to increased metabolic demand. Typically, all 12 leads are monitored with the limb leads in the torso sites, as originally described by Mason and Likar.[18]

Mason-Likar	SMART	EASI
10 electrodes	6 electrodes	5 electrodes
Less myoelectric noise	Less myoelectric noise	Least myoelectric noise
Less auscultation area	Greater auscultation area	Greater auscultation area

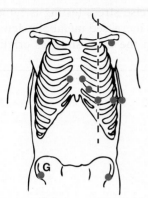 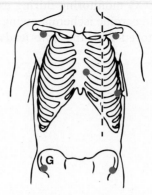 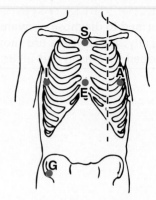

FIGURE 2.13. **A–C.** Electrode placement methods for ECG monitoring. *Circles* represent the electrode positions. *G* indicates position of the ground electrode.

Bony landmarks on the torso provide alternative sites for the right and left arm and leg electrodes that are required for continuous monitoring. Ideally, these sites (a) avoid skeletal muscle artifact, (b) provide stability for the recording electrodes, and (c) record waveforms similar to those from the limb sites. The *Mason–Likar*[18] system (see Fig. 2.12D) and modified Mason–Likar[19] system (see Fig 2.12E) have been used for continuous ST-segment monitoring. The resultant recordings from both, however, have some features that differ from the standard 12-lead recording.[19,20]

Methods other than the original or modified Mason–Likar method for continuous 12-lead ECG monitoring using alternative electrode placement and reduced electrode sites have emerged: (a) reduced electrode sets and (b) EASI. Both are alternative methods of ECG reconstruction based on bipolar orthogonal leads measured through both space and time, called *vectorcardiography*. Transformation of the vectorcardiogram to a 12-lead ECG conversion[21] has shown that the 12-lead ECG can be reconstructed with good approximation using a mathematical transformation matrix.

Reduced electrode sets from the standard 12-lead ECG eliminates excessive electrodes and electrode wires that interfere with precordial examination. This method is based on systematically removing precordial leads that provide redundant information. These fewer, selectively chosen leads contain sufficient diagnostic information for 12-lead reconstruction. Removed precordial leads are reconstructed from existing limb and precordial leads based on general and specific patient coefficients calculated from the patient's existing 12-lead ECG.[22] The Simon Meij Algorithm Reconstruction (SMART) method[22] utilizes Mason–Likar torso sites and the six electrodes required for leads I, II, V2, and V5 for reconstructing precordial leads V1, V3, V4, and V6 (Fig. 2.13).

The EASI system, introduced by Dower et al,[21] uses five electrodes (see Fig. 2.13C). Through mathematical transformations, a reconstructed 12-lead ECG is produced.[21,23] Positions I, E, and A are incorporated from the Frank vectorcardiographic system. E is placed on the inferior-most aspect of the sternal body. I and A are placed on the left and right midaxillary lines, respectively, in the same transverse plane as E. S is placed on the superior-most aspect of the sternal manubrium.

Advantages in using the reconstructive lead placement method (EASI or SMART) over the Mason–Likar are listed in Figure 2.13B and C. Other advantages include continuous monitoring, clear anatomic landmarks for electrode placement (EASI), reproducibility, and time and cost savings (by using fewer electrodes). Thus, it is likely that both reconstructive lead placement methods can be used for diagnostic ECG monitoring of myocardial ischemia and cardiac rhythm abnormalities.

OTHER PRACTICAL POINTS FOR RECORDING THE ELECTROCARDIOGRAM

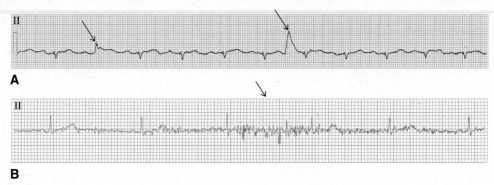

FIGURE 2.14. **A.** Shifting baseline. *Arrows* show movement during the second cycle and between the sixth and seventh cycles. **B.** Noisy baseline. *Arrow* shows the area of maximal baseline deformity.

Care should be taken to ensure that technique is uniform from one ECG recording to another. The following points are important to consider when preparing to record an ECG.

1. Electrodes should be selected for maximum adhesiveness and minimum discomfort, electrical noise, and skin–electrode impedance. The standards for electrodes published by the American Association for Advancement of Medical Instrumentation[24] should be followed.
2. Effective contact between electrode and skin is essential. Sites with skin irritation or skeletal abnormalities should be avoided. The skin should be cleaned with only a dry wipe. Poor electrode contact or slight body movement may produce instability of the baseline recording termed *baseline wander*, when the instability occurs gradually, or *shifting baseline*, when the instability occurs abruptly (Fig. 2.14A shown at half scale for illustrative purposes).
3. Calibration of the ECG signal is typically 1 mV = 10 mm. When large QRS waveform amplitudes require that calibration be reduced to 1 mV = 5 mm, this should be noted to facilitate interpretation.
4. ECG paper speed is typically 25 mm per second, and variations used for particular clinical purposes should be noted. A faster speed may be used to provide a clearer depiction of waveform morphology, and a slower speed may be used to provide visualization of a greater number of cardiac cycles to facilitate rhythm analysis.
5. Electrical artifacts in the ECG may be external or internal. External artifacts introduced by line current (50 or 60 Hz) may be minimized by straightening the lead wires so that they are aligned with the patient's body. Internal artifacts may result from muscle tremors, shivering, hiccups, or other factors, producing a "noisy baseline" (see Fig. 2.14B).
6. It is important that the patient remain supine during recording of the ECG. If another position is clinically required, notation of the altered position should be made. Lying on either side or elevation of the torso may change the position of the heart within the chest. A change in body position may affect the accuracy of an ECG recording[25] similar to a change in electrode placement.

GLOSSARY

Acute coronary syndrome: clinical symptoms suggestive of acute myocardial ischemia/infarction of sufficient severity for an individual to seek emergency care.

Angina: angina pectoris, precordial pressure, or pain caused by cardiac ischemia or lack of blood flow to the heart muscle.

Angioplasty: a procedure using a balloon-tipped arterial catheter to break up atherosclerotic plaques.

Anterior axillary line: a vertical line on the thorax at the level of the anterior aspect of the axilla, which is the area where the arm joins the body.

Artifact: an electrocardiographic waveform that arises from sources other than the myocardium.

aV lead: an augmented V lead (see below) that uses a modified central terminal with inputs from the electrode on the designated limb (R for right arm, L for left arm, and F for left foot) as its positive pole, and the average of the potentials from the leads on the other two limbs as its negative pole.

Baseline wander: a back-and-forth movement of the isoelectric line or baseline, interfering with precise measurement of the various ECG waveforms; sometimes termed *baseline shift* when it is abrupt.

Central terminal: a terminal created by Wilson and colleagues[2] that connects all three limb electrodes through a 5,000-Ω resistor so that it can serve as the negative pole for an exploring positive electrode to form a V lead.

Einthoven triangle: an equilateral triangle composed of limb leads I, II, and III that provides an orientation for electrical information from the frontal plane.

Electrocardiograph: a device used to record the electrocardiogram (ECG).

Frontal plane: a vertical plane of the body (also called the *coronal plane*) that is perpendicular to both the horizontal and sagittal planes.

Hypertrophy: an increase in muscle mass; it most commonly occurs in the ventricles when they are compensating for a pressure (systolic) overload.

Infarct: an area of necrosis in an organ resulting from an obstruction in its blood supply.

Intercostal: situated between the ribs.

Ischemia: an insufficiency of blood flow to an organ that is so severe that it disrupts the function of the organ; in the heart, ischemia is often accompanied by precordial pain and diminished contraction.

Lead: a recording of the electrical potential difference between a positive and a negative body surface electrode. The negative electrode can originate from a combination of two or three electrodes (see V lead and aV lead).

Mason–Likar: a system for alternative lead placement used for recording from the limb leads while the patient is moving about or exercising; in this system, the electrodes are moved from the limbs to the torso.

MCL_1: a modified lead V1 used to enhance visualization of atrial activity.

Midaxillary line: a vertical line on the thorax at the level of the midpoint of the axilla, which is the area where the arm joins the body.

Midclavicular line: a vertical line on the thorax at the level of the midpoint of the clavicle or collarbone.

Panoramic display: the typical ECG display of the precordial leads in their orderly sequence from right to left, with an innovative display of the frontal plane leads from left to right (aVL, I, –aVR, II, aVF, and III). Limb lead aVR is inverted to obtain the same positive leftward orientation as the other five limb leads.

Precordial: situated on the thorax, directly overlying the heart.

Proximal: situated near the point of attachment or origin of a limb; the opposite of distal.

Reocclusion: a recurrence of a complete obstruction to blood flow.

Reperfusion: the restoration of blood circulation to an organ or tissue upon reopening of a complete obstruction to blood flow.

Rhythm: the pattern of recurrence of the cardiac cycle.

Situs inversus dextrocardia: an abnormal condition in which the heart is situated on the right side of the body and the great blood vessels of the right and left sides are reversed.

Sternum: the narrow, flat bone in the middle of the anterior thorax; breastbone.

Tachycardia: a rapid heart rate with a frequency above 100 beats per minute.

Transverse plane: the horizontal plane of the body; it is perpendicular to both the frontal and sagittal planes.

V lead: an ECG lead that uses a central terminal with inputs from leads I, II, and III as its negative pole and an exploring electrode as its positive pole.

Xiphoid process: the lower end of the sternum; it has a triangular shape.

REFERENCES

1. Einthoven W, Fahr G, de Waart A. Uber die richtung und die manifeste grosse der potentialschwankungen im menschlichen herzen und uber den einfluss der herzlage auf die form des elektrokardiogramms. *Pfluegers Arch.*1913;150:275–315. (Translation: Hoff HE, Sekelj P. *Am Heart J.* 1950;40:163–194.)

2. Wilson FN, Macloed AG, Barker PS. The interpretation of the initial deflections of the ventricular complex of the electrocardiogram. *Am Heart J.* 1931;6:637–664.

3. Goldberger E.A simple, indifferent, electrocardiographic electrode of zero potential and a technique of obtaining augmented, unipolar, extremity leads. *Am Heart J.* 1942;23:483–492.

4. Wilson FN, Johnston FD, Macloed AG, et al. Electrocardiograms that represent the potential variations of a single electrode. *Am Heart J.* 1934;9:447–471.

5. Kossmann CE, Johnston FD. The precordial electrocardiogram. I. The potential variations of the precordium and of the extremities in normal subjects. *Am Heart J.* 1935;10:925–941.

6. Joint recommendations of the American Heart Association and the Cardiac Society of Great Britain and Ireland: standardization of precordial leads. *Am Heart J.* 1938;15:107–108.

7. Committee of the American Heart Association for the Standardization of Precordial Leads. Supplementary report. *Am Heart J.* 1938;15:235–239.

8. Committee of the American Heart Association for the Standardization of Precordial Leads. Second supplementary report. *JAMA.* 1943;121:1349–1351.

9. Pahlm O, Haisty WK, Edenbrandt L, et al. Evaluation of changes in standard electrocardiographic QRS waveforms recorded from activity-compatible proximal limb lead positions. *Am J Cardiol.* 1992;69:253–257.

10. Cabrera E. *Bases Electrophysiologiques de l'Electrocardiographie, ses Applications Clinique.* Paris, France: Masson; 1948.

11. The Joint European Society of Cardiology/American College of Cardiology Committee. Myocardial infarction redefined—a consensus document of the joint ESC/ACC committee for the redefinition of myocardial infarction. *J Am Coll Cardiol.* 2000;36:959–969 and *Eur Heart J.* 2000;21:1502–1513.

12. Anderson ST, Pahlm O, Selvester RH, et al. A panoramic display of the orderly sequenced twelve lead electrocardiogram. *J Electrocardiol .* 1994;27:347–352.

13. Kornreich F, Rautaharju PM, Warren J, et al. Identification of best electrocardiographic leads for diagnosing myocardial infarction by statistical analysis of body surface potential maps. *Am J Cardiol.* 1985;56:852–856.

14. Krucoff MW, Parente AR, Bottner RK, et al. Stability of multilead ST segment "fingerprints" over time after percutaneous transluminal coronary angioplasty and its usefulness in detecting reocclusion. *Am J Cardiol.* 1988;61:1232–1237.

15. Krucoff MW, Wagner NB, Pope JE, et al. The portable programmable microprocessor driven realtime 12 lead electrocardiographic monitor: a preliminary report of a new device for the noninvasive detection of successful reperfusion of silent coronary reocclussion. *Am J Cardiol.* 1990;65:143–148.

16. Krucoff MW, Croll MA, Pope JE, et al. Continuously updated 12 lead ST segment recovery analysis for myocardial infarct artery patency assessment and its correlation with multiple simultaneous early angiographic observations. *Am J Cardiol.* 1993;71:145–151.

17. Holter NJ. New method for heart studies. *Science.* 1961;134:1214–1220.

18. Mason RE, Likar I. A new system of multiplelead exercise electrocardiography. *Am Heart J.* 1966;71:196–205.

19. Sevilla DC, Dohrmann ML, Somelofski CA, et al. Invalidation of the resting electrocardiogram obtained via exercise electrode sites as a standard 12-lead recording. *Am J Cardiol.* 1989;63:35–39.

20. Pahlm O, Haisty WK, Edenbrandt L, et al. Evaluation of changes in standard electrocardiographic QRS waveforms recorded from activity-compatible proximal limb lead positions. *Am J Cardiol.* 1992;69:253–257.

21. Dower GE, Yakush A, Nazzal SB, et al. Deriving the 12-lead electrocardiogram from four (EASI) electrodes. *J Electrocardiol.* 1988;21:S182.

22. Nelwan SP, Kors JA, Meij SH, et al. Reconstruction of 12-Lead electrocardiograms from reduced lead sets. *J Electrocardiol*. 2004;37:11–18.

23. Dower GE. *EASI 12-Lead Electrocardiography*. Point Roberts (Walsh): Totemite Inc.; 1996.

24. A Report for Health Professionals by a Task Force of the Council on Clinical Cardiology, AHA. Instrumentation and practice standards for electrocardiographic monitoring in special care units. *Circulation*. 1989;79:464–471.

25. Sutherland DJ, McPherson DD, Spencer CA, et al. Effects of posture and respiration on body surface electrocardiogram. *Am J Cardiol*. 1983;52:595–600.

3

Interpretation of the Normal Electrocardiogram

GALEN S. WAGNER, TOBIN H. LIM,
DAVID G. STRAUSS, AND JACOB SIMLUND

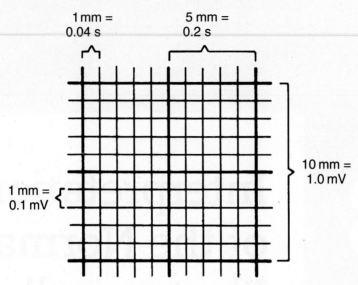

FIGURE 3.1.   Grid lines on standard ECG paper.

Every electrocardiogram (ECG) has nine features that should be examined systematically:

1. Rate and regularity;
2. P-wave morphology;
3. PR interval;
4. QRS complex morphology;
5. ST-segment morphology;
6. T-wave morphology;
7. U-wave morphology;
8. QTc interval; and
9. Rhythm.

Rate, regularity, and *rhythm* are commonly grouped together. However, to accurately assess rhythm, it is necessary to consider not only rate and regularity but also the various waveforms and intervals.

Determination of the ECG features requires understanding of the grid markings provided on the ECG paper (Fig. 3.1). The paper shows thin lines every 1 mm and thick lines every 5 mm. The thin lines, therefore, form small (1 mm) squares and the thick lines form large (5 mm) squares. The horizontal lines facilitate measurements of the various intervals and determination of cardiac rate. At the standard paper speed of 25 mm per second, the thin lines occur at 0.04-second (40-millisecond) intervals and thick lines occur at 0.20-second (200-millisecond) intervals. The vertical lines facilitate measurements of waveform amplitudes. At the standard calibration of 10 mm per mV, the thin lines are at 0.1-mV increments and the thick lines are at 0.5-mV increments. Therefore, each small square is 0.04 second × 0.1 mV, and each large square is 0.20 second × 0.5 mV.

Much of the information provided by the ECG is contained in the morphologies of three principal waveforms: (a) the P wave, (b) the QRS complex, and (c) the T wave. It is helpful to develop a systematic approach to the analysis of these waveforms by considering their:

1. General *contours*,
2. *Durations*,
3. Positive and negative *amplitudes*, and
4. *Axes* in the frontal and transverse planes.

The guidelines for measuring and estimating these four parameters for each of the three principal ECG waveforms are presented in this chapter. The definitions of the various waveforms and intervals were presented in Chapter 1 in the context of describing ECG recordings of base-to-apex and left- versus right-sided cardiac activity.

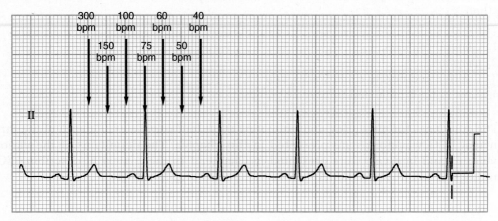

<u>FIGURE 3.2.</u>   Lead II. bpm, beats per minute.

The cardiac rhythm is rarely precisely regular. Even when electrical activity is initiated normally in the sinus node, the rate is affected by the autonomic nervous system. When an individual is at rest, minor variations in autonomic balance are produced by the phases of the respiratory cycle. A glance at the sequence of cardiac cycles is sufficient to determine whether the cardiac rate is essentially regular or irregular. Normally, there are equal numbers of P waves and QRS complexes. Either of these may be used to determine cardiac rate and regularity. When in the presence of certain abnormal cardiac rhythms, the numbers of P waves and QRS complexes are not the same. Atrial and ventricular rates and regularities must be determined separately.

If there is essential regularity in the cardiac rhythm, cardiac rate can easily be determined by counting the number of large squares between cycles. Because each square indicates one fifth of a second and there are 300 fifths of a second in a minute (5 × 60), it is necessary only to determine the number of large squares between consecutive cycles and divide this number by 300. It is most convenient to select the peak of a prominent ECG waveform that occurs on a thick line and then count the number of large squares until the same waveform recurs in the following cycle. When this interval is only one fifth of a second (0.2 second), the cardiac rate is 300 beats per minute; if the interval is two fifths of a second (0.4 second), the cardiac rate is 150 beats per minute; if the interval is three fifths of a second (0.6 second), the cardiac rate is 100 beats per minute, and so forth. Lead II is displayed in Figure 3.2 with the second QRS complex following the onset of the initial QRS complex after four large squares (heart rate = 75 beats per minute).

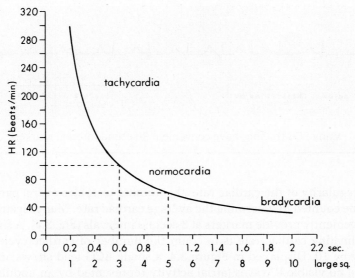

FIGURE 3.3. Intervals between ECG waveforms can be used to estimate cardiac rate.

When the cardiac rate is <100 beats per minute, it is sufficient to consider only the large squares on the ECG paper. When the rate is >100 beats per minute (tachycardia), however, small differences in the observed rate may alter the assessment of the underlying cardiac rhythm, and the number of small squares must also be considered (Fig. 3.3). This illustrates the importance of considering the small squares (0.04 second or 40 milliseconds) rather than the large squares (0.2 second or 200 milliseconds) for estimating rates in the tachycardic range, where small differences in the number of intervals between cardiac cycles result in large differences in the estimated rate. Because there are five small squares in each large square, the number of small squares between successive waveforms of the same type must be divided into 1,500 (6 squares = 250 beats per minute, 7 squares = 214 beats per minute, etc.). Rate determination is facilitated by the use of cardiac "rate rulers," which are easily obtained from pharmaceutical company representatives.

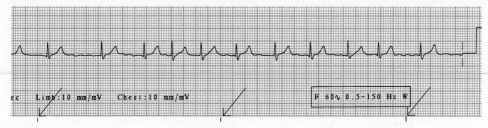

FIGURE 3.4. Many ECG tracings have convenient 3-second interval markers *(arrows)*.

If there is irregularity of the cardiac rate, the number of cycles over a particular interval of time should be counted to determine the average cardiac rate. Many electrocardiographic recordings conveniently provide markers at 3-second intervals (Fig. 3.4). A simple and quick method for estimating cardiac rate is to count the number of cardiac cycles in 6 seconds and to multiply by 10. Displayed in Figure 3.4, a single ECG lead shows an irregular ventricular rate and no visible P waves (atrial activity represented by an undulating baseline). The heart rate is estimated at 100 beats per minute because there are 10 ECG waveforms in 6 seconds.

P-WAVE MORPHOLOGY

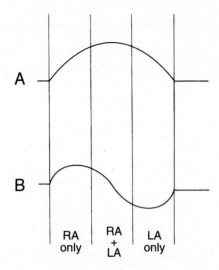

RA only | RA + LA | LA only

FIGURE 3.5. Typical normal P wave. **A.** Long-axis lead. **B.** Short-axis lead. LA, left atrium; RA, right atrium.

At either slow or normal heart rates, the small, rounded P wave is clearly visible just before the taller, more peaked QRS complex. At more rapid rates, however, the P wave may merge with the preceding T wave and become difficult to identify. Four steps should be taken to define the morphology of the P wave, as follows.

General Contour

The P-wave contour is normally smooth and is either entirely positive or entirely negative (see Fig. 1.9; monophasic) in all leads except V1 and possibly V2. In the short-axis view provided by lead V1, which best distinguishes left- versus right-sided cardiac activity, the divergence of right- and left-atrial activation typically produces a biphasic P wave (see Fig. 1.14). The contributions of right- and left-atrial activation to the beginning, middle, and end of the P wave are indicated in Figure 3.5. Typical appearances of a normal P wave in a long-axis lead such as II (see Fig. 3.5A) and a short-axis lead such as V1 (see Fig. 3.5B) are illustrated.

P-Wave Duration

The P-wave duration is normally <0.12 second. Displayed in Figure 3.5, the P-wave duration is divided into thirds (vertical lines) to indicate the relative times of activation in the right and left atria.

Positive and Negative Amplitudes

The maximal P-wave amplitude is normally no more than 0.2 mV in the frontal plane leads and no more than 0.1 mV in the transverse plane leads.

Axis in the Frontal and Transverse Planes

The P wave normally appears entirely upright in leftward- and inferiorly oriented leads such as I, II, aVF, and V4 to V6. It is negative in aVR because of the rightward orientation of that lead and is variable in other standard leads. The direction of the P wave, or its axis in the frontal plane, should be determined according to the method for determining the axis of an ECG waveform presented later in the section "Morphology of the QRS Complex." The normal limits of the P-wave axis are between 0 degrees and +75 degrees.[1]

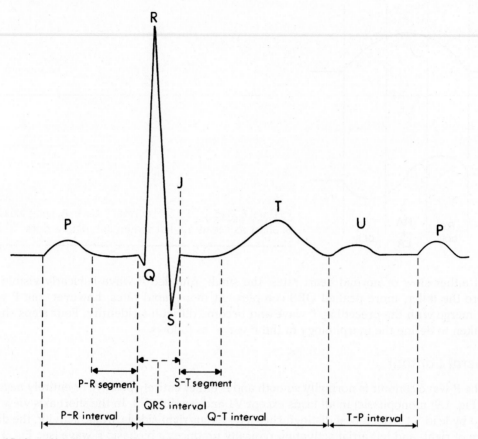

Magnified cardiac long-axis viewpoint of ECG segments and time intervals.

The PR interval measures the time required for an electrical impulse to travel from the atrial myocardium adjacent to the sinoatrial (SA) node to the ventricular myocardium adjacent to the fibers of the Purkinje network (see Fig. 1.12, repeated here). This duration is normally from 0.10 to 0.21 second. A major portion of the PR interval reflects the slow conduction of an impulse through the atrioventricular (AV) node, which is controlled by the balance between the sympathetic and parasympathetic divisions of the autonomic nervous system. Therefore, the PR interval varies with the heart rate, being shorter at faster rates when the sympathetic component predominates, and vice versa. The PR interval tends to increase with age[2]:

In childhood: 0.10 to 0.12 second
In adolescence: 0.12 to 0.16 second
In adulthood: 0.14 to 0.21 second

MORPHOLOGY OF THE QRS COMPLEX

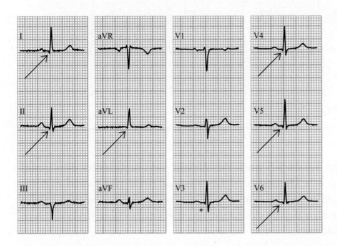

FIGURE 3.6. Normal 12-standard ECG presented in the classical format. *Arrows*, small Q waves; *asterisk*, minute Q wave.

In developing a systematic approach to waveform analysis, the following steps should be taken to determine the morphology of the QRS complex.

General Contour

The QRS complex is composed of higher frequency signals than are the P and T waves, thereby causing its contour to be peaked rather than rounded. Positive and negative components of the P and T waves are simply termed *positive* and *negative deflections*, whereas those of the QRS complex are assigned specific labels, such as "Q wave" (see Fig. 1.10).

Q Waves

In some leads (V1, V2, and V3), the presence of any Q wave should be considered abnormal, whereas in all other leads (except rightward-oriented leads III and aVR), a "normal" Q wave is very small. The upper limit of normal for such Q waves in each lead is illustrated in Figure 3.6 and indicated in Table 3.1.[3]

Table 3.1.

Normal Q-Wave Duration Limits

	Limb Leads		Precordial Leads	
Lead	Upper Limit(s)		Lead	Upper Limit(s)
I	<0.03		V1	Any Q[a]
II	<0.03		V2	Any Q[a]
III	None		V3	Any Q[a]
aVR	None		V4	<0.02
aVL	<0.03		V5	<0.03
aVF	<0.03		V6	<0.03

[a]In these leads, any Q wave is abnormal.

Modified from Wagner GS, Freye CJ, Palmeri ST, et al. Evaluation of a QRS scoring system for estimating myocardial infarct size. I. Specificity and observer agreement. *Circulation.* 1982;65:345, with permission.

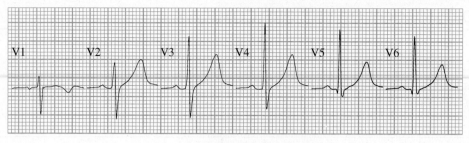

FIGURE 3.7. Panoramic display of the precordial leads.

The absence of small Q waves in leads V5 and V6 should be considered abnormal. A Q wave of any size is normal in leads III and aVR because of their rightward orientations (see Fig. 2.4). Q waves may be enlarged by conditions such as local loss of myocardial tissue (infarction), enlargement (hypertrophy or dilatation) of the ventricular myocardium, or abnormalities of ventricular conduction.

R Waves

Because the precordial leads provide a panoramic view of the cardiac electrical activity progressing from the thinner right ventricle across the thicker left ventricle, the positive R wave normally increases in amplitude and duration from lead V1 to lead V4 or V5 (Fig. 3.7). Reversal of this sequence, with larger R waves in leads V1 and V2, can be produced by right-ventricular hypertrophy, and accentuation of this sequence, with larger R waves in leads V5 and V6, can be produced by left-ventricular hypertrophy. Loss of normal R-wave progression from lead V1 to lead V4 may indicate loss of left-ventricular myocardium, as occurs with myocardial infarction (see Chapter 12).

S Waves

The S wave also has a normal sequence of progression in the precordial leads. It should be large in V1, larger in V2, and then progressively smaller from V3 through V6 (see Fig. 3.7). As with the R wave, this sequence could be altered by hypertrophy of one of the ventricles or myocardial infarction.

QRS Complex Duration

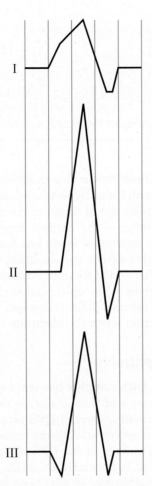

FIGURE 3.8. QRS complexes. *Vertical grid lines,* 0.04-second time intervals.

The duration of the QRS complex is termed the *QRS interval,* and it normally ranges from 0.07 to 0.11 second (see Fig. 1.12). The duration of the complex tends to be slightly longer in males than in females.[4] The QRS interval is measured from the beginning of the first-appearing Q or R wave to the end of the last-appearing R, S, R′, or S′ wave. Figure 3.8 illustrates the use of three simultaneously recorded limb leads (I, II, and III) to identify the true beginning and end of the QRS complex. An isoelectric period of approximately 0.02 second is apparent in lead II at the beginning of the QRS complex, and an isoelectric period of approximately 0.01 second is apparent in lead III at the end of the QRS complex. Note that only lead I reveals the true QRS duration (0.12 second).

Such multilead comparison is necessary; either the beginning or the end of the QRS complex may be isoelectric (neither positive nor negative) in a particular lead, causing an apparently shorter QRS duration. This isoelectric appearance occurs whenever the summation of ventricular electrical forces is perpendicular to the involved lead. The onset of the QRS complex is usually quite apparent in all leads, but its ending at the junction with the ST segment (termed the J point) is often indistinct, particularly in the precordial leads.

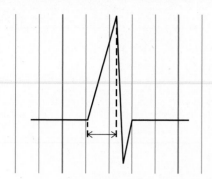

FIGURE 3.9. Magnified QRS complex. *Vertical grid lines,* 0.04-second time intervals. *Double-headed arrow,* length indicates the duration (0.05 second of intrinsicoid deflection).

The QRS interval has no lower limit that indicates abnormality. Prolongation of the QRS interval may be caused by left-ventricular hypertrophy, an abnormality in intraventricular impulse conduction, or a ventricular site of origin of the cardiac impulse.

The duration from the beginning of the earliest appearing Q or R wave to the peak of the R wave in several of the precordial leads has been termed the *intrinsicoid deflection* (Fig. 3.9). Electrical activation of the myocardium begins at the endocardial insertions of the Purkinje network. The end of the intrinsicoid deflection represents the time at which the electrical impulse arrives at the epicardial surface as viewed by that particular lead. The deflection is called an *intrinsic* deflection when the electrode is on the epicardial surface and an *intrinsicoid* deflection when the electrode is on the body surface.[5]

Positive and Negative Amplitudes

The amplitude of the overall QRS complex has wide normal limits. It varies with age, increasing until about age 30 years and then gradually decreasing. The amplitude is generally larger in males than in females. Overall QRS amplitude is measured between the peaks of the tallest positive and negative waveforms in the complex. It is difficult to set an arbitrary upper limit for normal voltage of the QRS complex; peak-to-peak amplitudes as high as 4 mV are occasionally seen in normal individuals. Factors that contribute to higher amplitudes include youth, physical fitness, slender body build, intraventricular conduction abnormalities, and ventricular enlargement.

An abnormally low QRS amplitude occurs when the overall amplitude is no more than 0.5 mV in any of the limb leads and no more than 1.0 mV in any of the precordial leads. The QRS amplitude is decreased by any condition that increases the distance between the myocardium and the recording electrode, such as a thick chest wall or various intrathoracic conditions that decrease the electrical signal that reaches the electrode.

Axis in the Frontal and Transverse Planes

The QRS axis represents the average direction of the total force produced by right- and left-ventricular depolarization. Although the Purkinje network facilitates the spread of the depolarization wavefront from the apex to the base of the ventricles (see Chapter 1), the QRS axis is normally in the positive direction in the frontal plane leads (except aVR) because of the endocardial-to-epicardial spread of depolarization in the thicker walled left ventricle.

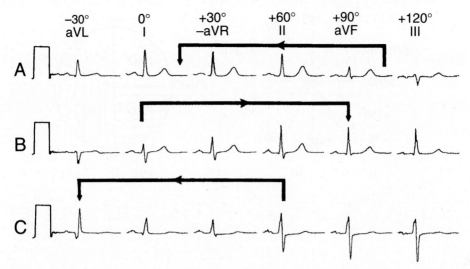

FIGURE 3.10.   Identifying the QRS complex frontal plane axis. **A.** *Vertical line without arrow:* Frontal plane QRS transitional lead location. **A–C.** *Long horizontal line with arrow:* 90 degrees movement away from the transitional lead in the direction of the tallest R wave. *Vertical line with arrow:* axis location, +15 degrees in **A**; +90 degrees in **B**; and −30 degrees in **C**.

In the frontal plane, the full 360-degree circumference of the hexaxial reference system is provided by the positive and negative poles of the six limb leads (see Fig. 2.4); in the transverse plane, it is provided by the positive and negative poles of the six precordial leads (see Fig. 2.7). It should be noted that the leads in both planes are not separated by precisely 30 degrees. In the frontal plane, the scalene Burger triangle has been shown more applicable then the equilateral Einthoven triangle.[6] Of course, body shape and electrode placement determine the spacing between contiguous leads.

Identification of the frontal plane axis of the QRS complex would be easier if the six leads were displayed in their orderly sequence (see Fig. 2.10B and 2.10C) than in their typical classical sequence. A simple method for identifying the QRS complex frontal plane axis with the limb leads in orderly sequence is illustrated in Figure 3.10.[7] Note that there is no truly transitional lead in Figure 3.10A, indicating that the QRS transition is located between leads aVF and III.

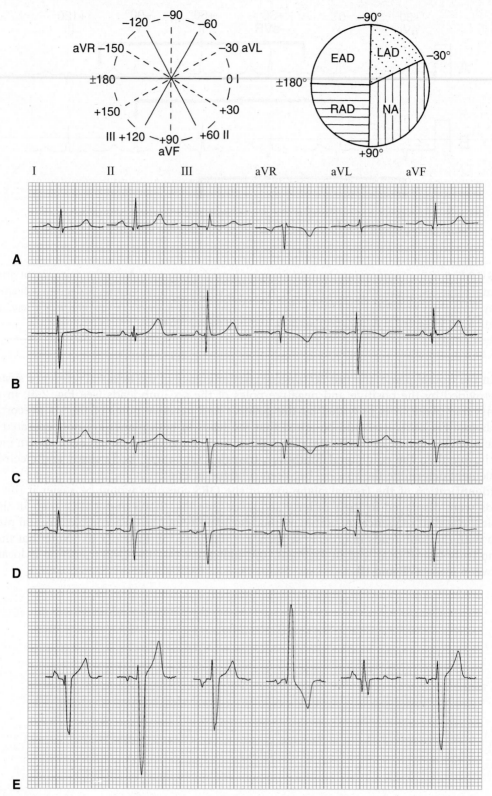

FIGURE 3.11. **A.** +60 degrees. **B.** +150 degrees. **C.** −30 degrees. **D.** −60 degrees. **E.** −120 degrees.

When the classical frontal plane ECG display is used, a three-step method is required for determining the overall axis of the QRS complex:

1. Identify the transitional lead (the lead perpendicular to the waveform axis) by locating the lead in which the QRS complex has the most nearly equal positive and negative components. These positive and negative components may vary from miniscule to quite prominent.
2. Identify the lead that is oriented perpendicular to the transitional lead by using the hexaxial reference system (Fig. 3.11, top left).
3. Consider the predominant direction of the QRS complex in the lead identified in step 2. If the direction is positive, the axis is the same as the positive pole of that lead. If the direction is negative, the axis is the same as the negative pole of the lead. Note that the positive poles of each lead are labeled with the lead name in Figure 3.11.

The frontal plane axis of the QRS complex is normally directed leftward and either slightly superiorly or inferiorly in the region between −30 degrees and +90 degrees (see Fig. 3.11, top right). Therefore, the QRS complex is normally predominantly positive in both leads I and II (see Fig. 3.11A). However, if the QRS complex is negative in lead I but positive in lead II, its axis is deviated rightward, to the region between +90 degrees and ±180 degrees (*right-axis deviation*; see Fig. 3.11B). If the QRS complex is positive in lead I but negative in lead II, its axis is deviated leftward to the region between −30 degrees and −120 degrees (*left-axis deviation*; see Fig. 3.11C, D). Right-ventricular enlargement may produce right-axis deviation and left-ventricular enlargement may produce left-axis deviation of the QRS complex. The axis of the QRS complex is rarely directed completely opposite to its normal direction (−90 to ±180 degrees) with a predominantly negative QRS orientation in both leads I and II (*extreme axis deviation*; see Fig. 3.11E).

Using this method for determining the direction of the axis of the QRS complex in the frontal plane permits no more than a "rounding" of the direction to the nearest multiple of 30 degrees. Although automated ECG analysis provides axis designation to the nearest degree, the manual method described here is sufficient for clinical purposes.

The normal frontal plane axis of the QRS complex is rightward in the neonate, moves to a vertical position during childhood, and then moves to a more leftward position during adulthood.[8] In normal adults, the electrical axis of the QRS complex is almost parallel to the anatomic base-to-apex axis of the heart in the direction of lead II. However, these axes are more vertical in thin individuals and more horizontal in heavy individuals. This same normal growth-dependent rightward-to-leftward movement of the QRS axis that is seen in the frontal plane is also apparent in the transverse plane, but the transverse plane shows the anterior-to-posterior movement of the axis that is not visible in the frontal plane. In the adult, the transitional lead is usually V3 or V4, and the lead oriented perpendicular to this transitional lead is therefore lead V6 or V1, respectively. Because the normal predominant direction of the QRS complex is positive in lead V6 and negative in lead V1, the axis of the QRS complex in the transverse plane in the adult is typically between 0 degrees and −60 degrees.

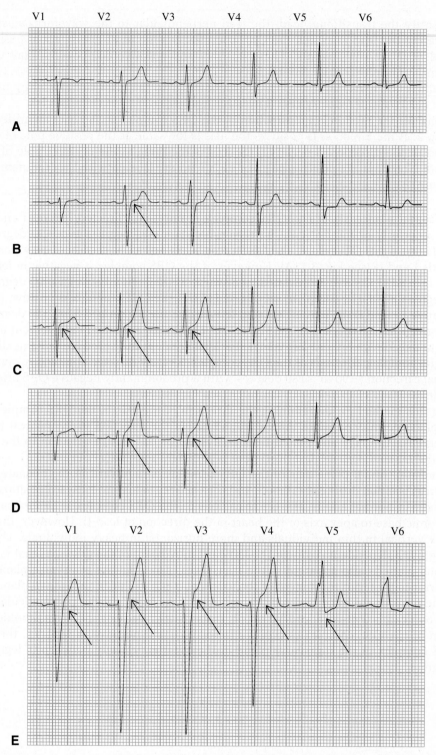

FIGURE 3.12. **A.** Normal ECG. **B–D.** Normal variant ECGs. **E.** Abnormal ECG. *Arrows,* ST-segment deviations in precordial leads.

The ST segment represents the period during which the ventricular myocardium proceeds through the preliminary two phases of repolarization: Phases 1 and 2, following its depolarization in Phase 0 (see Chapter 1, Fig. 1.3). These are the phases considered: early repolarization. At its junction with the QRS complex (J point), the ST segment typically forms a distinct angle with the downslope of the R wave or upstroke of the S wave, and then proceeds nearly horizontally until it curves gently into the T wave. The length of the ST segment is influenced by factors that alter the duration of ventricular activation. Points along the ST segment are designated with reference to the number of milliseconds beyond the J point, such as "J + 20," "J + 40," and "J + 60."

The first section of the ST segment is normally located at the same horizontal level as the baseline formed by the TP segment that fills the space between electrical cardiac cycles (Fig. 3.12A). Slight upsloping, downsloping, or horizontal depression of the ST segment may occur as a normal variant (see Fig. 3.12B). Another normal variant of the ST segment appears when there is altered early repolarization within the ventricles.[9] This causes displacement of the ST segment by as much as 0.1 mV in the direction of the ensuing T wave (see Fig. 3.12C). Occasionally, the ST segment in young males may show even greater elevation in leads V2 and V3 (see Fig. 3.12D).[9] The appearance of the ST segment may also be altered when there is an abnormally prolonged QRS complex (see Fig. 3.12E).

T-WAVE MORPHOLOGY

In continuing the systematic approach to waveform analysis, the steps taken in examining the morphology of the T wave are as follows.

General Contour

Both the shape and axis of the normal T wave resemble those of the P wave (see Figs. 1.9 and 1.14). The waveforms in both cases are smooth and rounded and are positively directed in all leads except aVR, where they are negative, and V1, where they are biphasic (initially positive and terminally negative). Slight "peaking" of the T wave may occur as a normal variant.

T-Wave Duration

The duration of the T wave itself is not usually measured, but it is instead included in the QT interval discussed in the "QTc Interval" learning unit.

Positive and Negative Amplitudes

The amplitude of the T wave, like that of the QRS complex, has wide normal limits. It tends to diminish with age and is larger in males than in females. T-wave amplitude tends to vary with QRS amplitude and should always be greater than that of the U wave if the latter is present. T waves do not normally exceed 0.5 mV in any limb lead or 1.5 mV in any precordial lead. In females, the upper limits of T-wave amplitude are about two thirds of these values. The T-wave amplitude tends to be lower at the extremes of the panoramic views (see Fig. 2.10B) of both the frontal and transverse planes. The amplitude of the wave at these extremes does not normally exceed 0.3 mV in leads aVL and III or 0.5 mV in leads V1 and V6.[8]

Axis in the Frontal and Transverse Planes

The axis of the T wave should be evaluated in relation to that of the QRS complex. The rationale for the similar directions of the waveforms of these two ECG features, despite their representing the opposite myocardial electrical events of activation and recovery, has been presented in Chapter 1. The methods presented earlier for determining the axis of the QRS complex in the two ECG planes should be applied for determining the axis of the T wave. The term *QRS–T angle* is used to indicate the number of degrees between the axes of the QRS complex and the T wave in the frontal and transverse planes.[10]

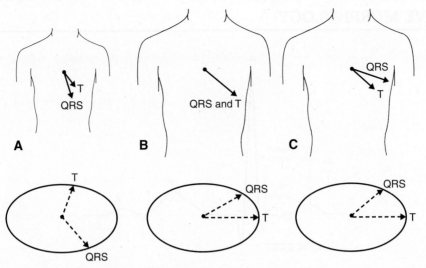

FIGURE 3.13. **A.** Young child. **B.** Young adult. **C.** Elderly adult. *Solid arrows*, directions of QRS axis. *Dashed line arrows*, directions of T axis.

The axis of the T wave in the frontal plane tends to remain constant throughout life, whereas the axis of the QRS complex moves from a vertical toward a horizontal position, as shown at the top of Figure 3.13.[8] Therefore, during childhood, the T-wave axis is more horizontal than that of the QRS complex, but during adulthood, the T-wave axis becomes more vertical than that of the QRS complex. Despite these changes, the QRS–T angle in the frontal plane does not normally exceed 45 degrees.[10]

In the normal young child, the T-wave axis in the transverse plane may be so posterior that the T waves may be negative in even the most leftward precordial leads V5 and V6 (see Fig. 3.13, bottom). During childhood, the T-wave axis moves anteriorly, toward the positive pole of lead V5, and the QRS axis moves posteriorly, toward the negative pole of lead V1, where these two axes typically remain throughout life. The QRS–T angle in the transverse plane normally does not exceed 60 degrees in the adult.[10]

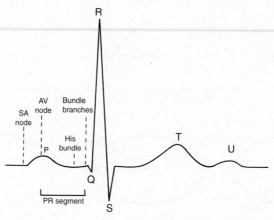

Wave forms. P, atrial activation; Q, R, and S, ventricular activation; T and U, ventricular recovery. AV, atrioventricular; SA, sinoatrial.

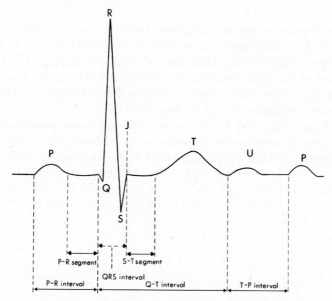

Magnified cardiac long-axis viewpoint of ECG segments and time intervals.

The U wave is normally either absent from the ECG or present as a small, rounded wave following the T wave (see Figs. 1.9 and 1.12, repeated here). It is normally oriented in the same direction as the T wave, has approximately 10% of the amplitude of the latter, and is usually most prominent in leads V2 or V3. The U wave is larger at slower heart rates, and both the U wave and the T wave diminish in size and merge with the following P wave at faster heart rates. The U wave is usually separated from the T wave, with the *TU junction* occurring along the baseline of the ECG. However, there may be fusion of the T and U waves, making measurement of the QT interval more difficult. The source of the U wave is uncertain. Three possible theories regarding its origin are (a) tardy repolarization of the subendocardial Purkinje fibers, (b) prolonged repolarization of the midmyocardium ("M cells"), and (c) after-potentials resulting from mechanical forces in the ventricular wall.[11]

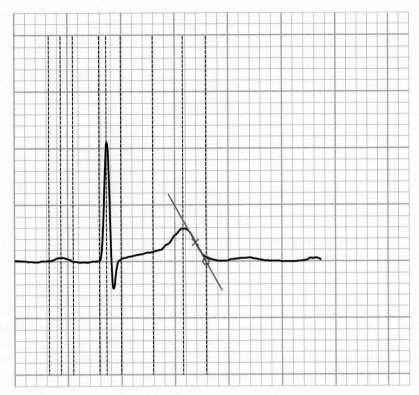

FIGURE 3.14. Tangential method used for determining end of the T wave.

The QT interval measures the duration of electrical activation and recovery of the ventricular myocardium. Currently used in determining the end of the T wave for QT interval measuring is the tangential method. This is defined as a tangent line that is drawn at the end of the T wave's steepest portion of its terminal point crossing the isoelectric line[12] (Fig. 3.14). In addition, the QT interval varies inversely with the cardiac rate. To ensure complete recovery from one cardiac cycle before the next cycle begins, the duration of recovery must decrease as the rate of activation increases. Therefore, the "normality" of the QT interval can be determined only by correcting for the cardiac rate. The corrected QT interval (QTc interval) rather than the measured QT interval is included in routine ECG analysis. Bazett[13] developed the following formula for performing this correction:

$$QTc = QT/\sqrt{RR}$$

RR is defined as the interval duration between two consecutive R waves measured in seconds. The modification of Bazett's formula by Hodges and coworkers,[14,15] as follows, corrects more completely for high and low heart rates: $QTc = QT + 0.00175$ (ventricular rate -60). The upper limit of QTc interval duration is approximately 0.46 second (460 milliseconds). The QTc interval is slightly longer in adult females than males and increases slightly with age. Adjustment of the duration of electrical recovery to the rate of electrical activation does not occur immediately, but it requires several cardiac cycles. Thus, an accurate measurement of the QTc interval can be made only after a series of regular, equal cardiac cycles.

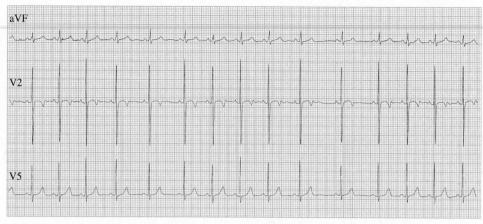

FIGURE 3.15. Sinus arrhythmia.

Assessment of the final electrocardiographic feature named at the beginning of this chapter, the cardiac rhythm, requires consideration of all eight other electrocardiographic features. Certain irregularities of cardiac rate and regularity, P-wave morphology, and the PR interval may in themselves indicate abnormalities in cardiac rhythm, and certain irregularities of the remaining five electrocardiographic features may indicate the potential for development of abnormalities in cardiac rhythm.

Cardiac Rate and Regularity

The normal cardiac rhythm is called *sinus rhythm* because it is produced by electrical impulses formed within the SA node. The rate of sinus rhythm is normally between 60 and 100 beats per minute during wakefulness and at rest. When <60 beats per minute, the rhythm is called *sinus bradycardia*, and when >100 beats per minute it is called *sinus tachycardia*. However, the designation of "normal" requires consideration of the individual's activity level: Sinus bradycardia with a rate as low as 40 beats per minute may be normal during sleep, and sinus tachycardia with a rate as rapid as 200 beats per minute may be normal during exercise. Indeed, a rate of 90 beats per minute would be "abnormal" during either sleep or vigorous exercise. Sinus rates in the bradycardic range may occur normally during wakefulness, especially in well-trained athletes whose resting heart rates range at 30 beats per minute and often <60 beats per minute even with moderate exertion.

As indicated, normal sinus rhythm is essentially but not absolutely regular because of continual variation of the balance between the sympathetic and parasympathetic divisions of the autonomic nervous system. Loss of this normal *heart rate variability* may be associated with significant underlying autonomic or cardiac abnormalities.[16] The term *sinus arrhythmia* describes the normal variation in cardiac rate that cycles with the phases of respiration; sinus rate accelerates with inspiration and slows with expiration (Fig. 3.15). Occasionally, sinus arrhythmia produces such marked irregularity that it can be confused with clinically important arrhythmias.

P-Wave Axis

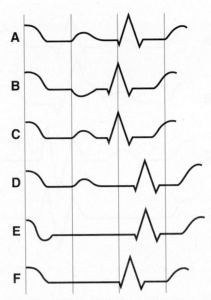

FIGURE 3.16. *Vertical grid lines*, 0.2-second time intervals. Note that in **A,** the PR interval is 0.2 second (the upper limit of normal). See Animation 3.1.

The normal frontal plane axis of the P wave was discussed in the section on "P-Wave Morphology". Alteration of this axis to either <+30 degrees *or* >+75 degrees may indicate that the cardiac rhythm is being initiated from a site low in the right atrium, AV node, or left atrium.

PR Interval

The normal relationship between the P wave and QRS complex (the *PR interval*) is presented schematically in Figure 3.16A, and various abnormal relationships between the P wave and QRS complex are illustrated in Figure 3.16B–F. An abnormal P-wave axis is often accompanied by an abnormally short PR interval, because the site of impulse formation has moved from the SA node to a position closer to the AV node (see Fig. 3.16B). However, a short PR interval in the presence of a normal P-wave axis (see Fig. 3.16C) suggests either an abnormally rapid conduction pathway within the AV node or the presence of an abnormal bundle of cardiac muscle connecting the atria to the Bundle of His (an unusual source of *ventricular preexcitation*; see Chapter 7). This is not in itself an abnormality of the cardiac rhythm; however, the pathway either within or bypassing the AV node that is responsible for the preexcitation creates the potential for electrical *reactivation* or *reentry* into the atria, thereby producing a tachyarrhythmia.

An abnormally long PR interval in the presence of a normal P-wave axis indicates delay of impulse transmission at some point along the normal pathway between the atrial and ventricular myocardium (see Fig. 3.16D). When a prolonged PR interval is accompanied by an abnormal P-wave contour, it should be considered that the P wave may actually be associated with the preceding rather than with the following QRS complex because of reverse activation from the ventricles to the atria (see Fig. 3.16E). This occurs when the cardiac impulse originates from the ventricles rather than the atria. In this case, the P wave might only be identified as a distortion of the T wave. When the PR interval cannot be determined because of the absence of any visible P wave, there is obvious abnormality of the cardiac rhythm (see Fig. 3.16F).

Animation 3.1

Morphology of the QRS Complex

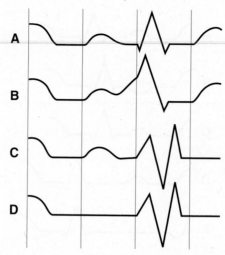

FIGURE 3.17. **A.** Normal. **B–D.** Abnormal. *Vertical grid lines*, 0.2-second time intervals. See Animation 3.2.

Figure 3.16A is presented again as Figure 3.17A for reference to atypical, normally appearing QRS complex with Q, R, and S waves present. Various causes of abnormal QRS-complex morphology are presented in Figure 3.17B–D.

A normal P-wave axis with an abnormally short PR interval is accompanied by a normal morphology of the QRS complex when there is no AV nodal bypass directly into the ventricular myocardium (see Fig. 3.16C). When such a bypass directly enters the ventricular myocardium, it creates abnormality in the morphology of the QRS complex (see Fig. 3.17B). This ventricular "pre-excitation" eliminates the isoelectric PR segment and creates a fusion between the P wave and the QRS complex. The initial Q or R wave begins slowly (in what is termed a *delta wave*), prolonging the duration of the QRS complex.

Abnormally slow impulse conduction within the normal intraventricular conduction pathways also produces abnormalities of QRS complex morphology (see Fig. 3.17C). The cardiac rhythm remains normal when the conduction abnormality is confined to either the right or left bundle branch. However, if the process responsible for the slow conduction spreads to the other bundle branch, the serious rhythm abnormality of partial or even total failure of AV conduction could suddenly occur.

An abnormally prolonged QRS duration in the absence of a preceding P wave suggests that the cardiac rhythm is originating from the ventricles rather than from the atria (see Fig. 3.17D).

Animation 3.2

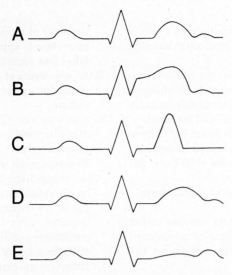

FIGURE 3.18. QRS-to-T relationship. **A.** Normal. **B–E.** Abnormal. See Animation 3.3.

Marked elevation of the ST segment (Fig. 3.18B), an increase or decrease in T-wave amplitude (see Fig. 3.18C, E), prolongation of the QTc interval (see Fig. 3.18D), or an increase in U-wave amplitude (see Fig. 3.18E) may be indications of underlying cardiac conditions that may produce serious abnormalities of cardiac rhythm.[17] Each example begins with the completion of a TP segment and ends with the initiation of the following TP segment. These abnormal QRS-to-T relationships are discussed in Chapters 11 (Fig. 3.18B, C) and 13 (Fig. 3.18C–E).

Animation 3.3

Amplitude: the vertical magnitude of a waveform extending from the isoelectric baseline to the waveform peak.

Autonomic nervous system: the nervous system that spontaneously controls involuntary bodily functions; it innervates glands, smooth-muscle tissue, blood vessels, and the heart.

Axis: direction of an ECG waveform in the frontal or horizontal plane, measured in degrees.

Bradycardia: a slow heart rate, <60 beats per minute.

Contour: the general shape of a waveform—peaked or flat.

Deflections: ECG waveforms moving either upward (positive deflection) or downward (negative deflection) with respect to the baseline.

Duration: the interval in milliseconds between the onset and offset of a waveform. Because the apparent duration may vary in an individual lead because either the initial or terminal portion of the wave is perpendicular to that lead and is therefore isoelectric, the true waveform duration extends from the earliest onset to the latest offset in multiple simultaneously recorded ECG leads.

Extreme axis deviation: deviation of the frontal-plane QRS axis from normal, with the axis located between −90 degrees and ±180 degrees.

Fusion: merging together of waveforms (i.e., P and T waves).

Heart rate variability: the normal range of variability of heart rates observed while an individual is in the resting state.

Intrinsicoid deflection: the time interval between the beginning of the QRS complex and the peak of the R wave; this represents the time required for the electrical impulse to travel from the endocardial to the epicardial surfaces of the ventricular myocardium.

Left-axis deviation: Deviation of the frontal plane QRS axis from normal, with the axis located between −30 degrees and −90 degrees.

QRS–T angle: the number of degrees between the QRS complex and T-wave axes in the frontal and horizontal planes.

QTc interval: the corrected QT interval; it represents the duration of activation and recovery of the ventricular myocardium; the correction is applied by using a formula that takes into consideration the ventricular rate.

Rate: a measure of the frequency of occurrence of cardiac cycles; it is expressed in beats per minute.

Reentry or reactivation: passage of the cardiac electrical impulse for a second time or an even greater number of times through a structure such as the AV node or the atrial or ventricular myocardium, as the result of a conduction abnormality in that area of the heart. Normally, the cardiac electrical impulse, after its initiation in specialized pacemaking cells, spreads through each area of the heart only once.

Regularity: an expression for the consistency of the cardiac rate over a period of time.

Right-axis deviation: deviation of the frontal plane QRS axis from normal, with the axis located between +90 degrees and ±180 degrees.

Sinus arrhythmia: the normal variation in sinus rhythm that occurs during the inspiratory and expiratory phases of respiration.

Sinus rhythm: the normal cardiac rhythm originating via impulse formation in the SA or sinus node.

Tachycardia: a rapid heart rate of >100 beats per minute.

Transitional lead: the lead in which the positive and negative components of an ECG waveform are of almost equal amplitude, indicating that that lead is perpendicular to the direction of the waveform.

TP junction: the merging point of the T and P waves that occurs at faster heart rates.

TU junction: the point of merging of the T and U waves; it is sometimes on and sometimes off of the isoelectric line.

Ventricular preexcitation: an event that occurs when a cardiac activating impulse bypasses the AV node and Purkinje system owing to an abnormal bundle of muscle fibers connecting the atria and ventricles. Normally, the electrical impulse must spread through the slowly conducting AV node and rapidly conducting Purkinje system to travel from the atrial to the ventricular myocardium.

REFERENCES

1. Grant RP. *Clinical Electrocardiography: The Spatial Vector Approach*. New York, NY: McGraw-Hill; 1957.

2. Beckwith JR. *Grant's Clinical Electrocardiography*. New York, NY: McGraw-Hill; 1970:50.

3. Wagner GS, Freye CJ, Palmeri ST, et al. Evaluation of a QRS scoring system for estimating myocardial infarct size. I. Specificity and observer agreement. *Circulation*. 1982; 65:342–347.

4. Macfarlane PW, Lawrie TDV, eds. *Comprehensive Electrocardiology*. Vol 3. New York, NY: Pergamon Press; 1989:1442.

5. Beckwith JR. *Basic Electrocardiography and Vectorcardiography*. New York, NY: Raven Press; 1982:46.

6. Macfarlane PW, Lawrie TDV, eds. *Comprehensive Electrocardiology*. Vol 1. New York: Pergamon Press; 1989:296–305.

7. Anderson ST, Pahlm O, Selvester RH, et al. A panoramic display of the orderly sequenced 12 lead electrocardiogram. *J Electrocardiol*. 1994;27:347–352.

8. Macfarlane PW, Lawrie TDV, eds. *Comprehensive Electrocardiology*. Vol III. New York, NY: Pergamon Press; 1989:1459.

9. Surawicz B. STT abnormalities. In: Macfarlane PW, Lawrie TDV, eds. *Comprehensive Electrocardiology*. Vol 1. New York, NY: Pergamon Press; 1989:515.

10. Beckwith JR. *Grant's Clinical Electrocardiography*. New York, NY: McGraw-Hill; 1970:59–63.

11. Ritsema van Eck HJ, Kors JA, van Herpen G. The U wave in the electrocardiogram: a solution for a 100-year-old riddle. *Cardiovasc Res*. 2005;67:256–262.

12. Castellanos A, Inerian A Jr, Myerburg RJ. The resting electrocardiogram. In: Fuster V, Alexander RW, O Rourke RA, eds. *Hurst's The Heart*. 11th ed. New York, NY: McGraw-Hill; 2004:299–300.

13. Bazett HC. An analysis of the time relations of electrocardiograms. *Heart*. 1920;7: 353–370.

14. Hodges M, Salerno D, Erlien D. Bazett's QT correction reviewed. Evidence that a linear QT correction for heart is better. *J Am Coll Cardiol*. 1983;1:69.

15. Macfarlane PW, Lawrie TDV. The normal electrocardiogram and vectorcardiogram. In: Macfarlane PW, Lawrie TDV, eds. *Comprehensive Electrocardiology*. Vol 1. New York: Pergamon Press; 1989: 451–452.

16. Kleiger RE, Miller JP, Bigger JT, et al. The MultiCenter PostInfarction Research Group. Decreased heart rate variability and its association with increased mortality after acute myocardial infarction. *Am J Cardiol*. 1987;59:256–262.

17. Antzelevitch C, Sicouri S. Clinical relevance of cardiac arrhythmias generated by after depolarizations. Role of M cells in the generation of U waves, triggered activity and Torsade de pointes. *J Am Coll Cardiol*. 1994;23:259–277.

4

The Three-Dimensional Electrocardiogram

CHARLES W. OLSON, E. HARVEY ESTES, JR., VIVIAN PAOLA KAMPHUIS, ESBEN A. CARLSEN, DAVID G. STRAUSS, AND GALEN S. WAGNER

PERSPECTIVE

The initial four chapters are intended for the student of electrocardiography to learn to read a standard 12-lead electrocardiogram (ECG) and to decide whether or not it is normal. Increasingly, the ECG is obtained by an instrument capable of electronically determining measurements, applying diagnostic algorithms and delivering a diagnostic statement. However, these automated ECG analysis systems are not infallible and require expert human interpretation to provide optimal clinical decision support.

The human ECG reader is no longer required to measure intervals, plot axes, and so forth. The availability of this automated analysis has led to diminished attention to ECG interpretation in medical education and medical practice, but its availability also presents the opportunity to explore new information and new methods of presenting old information. The purpose of this final chapter in this introductory section is to introduce the student to three-dimensional presentations of the cardiac electrical information, and because this information is closely related to that seen in the standard ECG, it can be transformed from one to the other. This chapter also shows that the fundamental electrical process at the myocardial cellular level is the basis for all of the electrical information transmitted to the body surface. The three-dimensional vectorcardiogram (VCG) is closely related to and easily derived from the cellular activity making the diagnosis more intuitive and accurate. Having the additional three-dimensional rendering of real time electrical cardiac information to assist the decision-making process is invaluable.

In this chapter, the electrical forces generated by the heart and their transmission to the body surface are presented in more detail than in Chapter 1 using a three-dimensional approach. The VCG is introduced as a different three-dimensional form of recording, with some advantages over the standard ECG.

THREE-DIMENSIONAL ELECTROCARDIOGRAPHY

The three-dimensional approach provides a better understanding of the electrical forces producing the ECG by linking these forces (a) to depolarization and repolarization of myocardial cells, (b) to the spread of these forces through the layers of myocardium, and (c) to recording techniques such as the spatial VCG. This approach is not new and can be traced back to Waller in the 19th century. It is based on the concept that the forces recorded by the ECG can be represented at any point in time by a single vector, whose magnitude and direction can be represented by a vector originating at the center of the heart.[1] The change in the magnitude and direction of this vector during each heart cycle can be visualized as a loop, one for each of the ECG waveforms. Although the P and T loops are also recorded, most attention is directed to the QRS loop, and it is this loop that is used in this chapter to demonstrate the relationships between the spatial VCG and the conventional 12-lead ECG.

In the mid-20th century, this perspective was described and formalized as "spatial vector electrocardiography" by Grant,[2] who demonstrated that this method could lead to a better understanding of the forces generating the ECG and the changes in its waveforms induced by disease. This will also enable the reader to understand the changes that are produced by disease states in each of the 12 standard ECG leads and predict those which would occur in the VCG. An added benefit of using the vector loop instead of the 12-lead ECG is that the memorization of normal and abnormal waveforms in each of the 12 leads is no longer necessary.

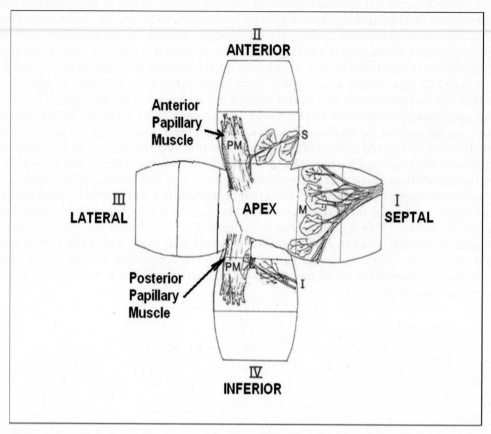

FIGURE 4.1. This shows the four quadrants of the left ventricle folded out from the apex at the center. The anterior and posterior papillary muscles are shown as well as the initial excitation points of the Purkinje fibers. LBB Fascicles: S, Superior also Anterior; M, Middle; I, Inferior also Posterior. (From Wagner NB, White RD, Wagner GS, et al. The 12 lead ECG and the extent of myocardium at risk of acute infarction. In: Califf RM, Mark DB, Wagner, GS, eds. *Acute Coronary Care in the Thrombolytic Era.* Chicago, IL: Yearbook; 1988:22, with permission.)

Chapter 1 considers the normal activation of the ventricles, beginning from the atrioventricular node and continuing through the common bundle (His), the left and right bundle branches, and the peripheral Purkinje fibers. Figure 4.1 shows the distribution and termination of the left bundle and its branches and the transition to Purkinje fibers in the endocardial layers near the apex of the left ventricle (LV).[3] The important points to note are the wide, fanlike branching of the left bundle and the wide distribution of these fibers to the area at the top of the apex, the base of both papillary muscles, and the septal wall of the LV. The early arrival of activation in these locations is thought to ensure the early tension of the papillary muscles and the mitral valve and the early contraction of the apex, directing blood to the outflow track at the base of the heart.

Activation of the bundle branches and Purkinje fibers also generates electrical forces, but these are too small to be detected by conventional ECG recording devices, hence the isoelectric line between the P wave and QRS complex. The earliest forces are those spreading in a semicircular ring in the endocardial septal surface between the papillary muscles. The early excitation

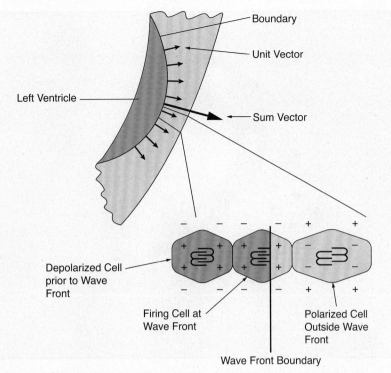

FIGURE 4.2. On the left, in a segment of the left-ventricular wall, there is endocardial to epicardial spread of the activation front. The depolarized cells are shown in dark pink and the polarized cells in light pink. On the right, the activation front is seen proceeding through three individual cells. Firing Cell means Depolarizing Cell. (Modified from Olson CW, Warner RA, Wagner GS, et al. A dynamic three dimensional display of ventricular excitation and the generation of the vector and electrocardiogram. *J Electrocardiol.* 2001;34(suppl):7–16, with permission.)

of the papillary muscles provides an initial vector superiorly along the long axis of the LV. As the activation process spreads through the ventricular wall, more cells are recruited, and a visible record can be detected on the body surface, the beginning of the QRS complex.

The electrical stimulus then spreads into a wider area of endocardial layers of the myocardium by the Purkinje cell network and continues to spread from the endocardium outward toward the epicardial surface. Figure 4.2 shows this activation front in a segment of the left-ventricular wall as it is moving from its endocardial location across the wall.[4] The boundary marking the activation front is seen as a curved black line, with the cells already depolarized on the left (dark pink) and the still polarized cells on the right (light pink). The expanded diagrammatic view on the right shows the process as it proceeds from cell to cell, with the boundary seen as a vertical line. At the activation front, ions are rapidly moving across the cell wall. It is this ionic movement that induces the potential difference we record in the VCG and ECG. The electrical forces in each cell undergoing this process can be represented by a small vector (the unit vector). The sum vector is the vectoral sum of all unit vectors at a given instant.

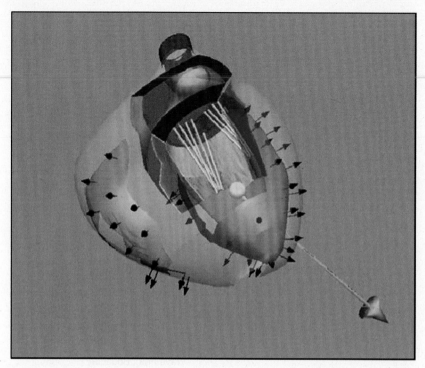

FIGURE 4.3. A 3-D model of the ventricles presented at one instant in the depolarization phase (between 20 and 40 milliseconds). The *black arrows* represent the unit vectors from which the sum vector (*blue arrow*) is determined. The sum vector originates at the electrical center of the heart (*yellow dot*). The length of the *arrows* represents the magnitude and the *arrowhead* indicates the positive pole. (Modified from Loring Z, Olson CW, Maynard C, et al. Modeling vectorcardiograms based on left ventricle papillary muscle position. *J Electrocardiol.* 2011;44:584–589, with permission.)[5]

Figure 4.3 shows these same forces in a form more closely resembling the process seen in the heart. As the activation boundary moves from endocardium to epicardium, there are many cells undergoing depolarization at any instant in time. Each cell contributes a small unit vector, directed perpendicular to the wave front. Again, the sum of all unit vectors acting at that instant can be represented as a single sum vector. As seen in Figure 4.3, not all unit vectors have the same direction as the overall sum vector. These opposing unit vectors pointing in the opposite direction reduce the magnitude of the sum vector; this phenomenon is referred to as cancellation.

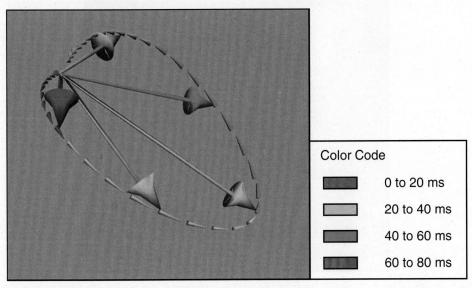

FIGURE 4.4. Five sum vectors at selected time intervals during the depolarization phase of the cardiac cycle indicated by a color code. (Modified from Olson CW, Lange DM, Chan JK, et al. 3D heart: a new visual training method for electrocardiographic analysis. *J Electrocardiol.* 2007;40:457.e1–457.e7, with permission.)[6]

Figure 4.4 shows the sum vectors at five selected time intervals during the depolarization phase of the cardiac cycle. Note that this cycle could have been divided into 50 intervals, and each would have a sum vector indicating the magnitude and direction of the sum vector at that instant. As you can see, connecting the tips of these sum vectors forms a loop-shaped figure, which returns to the point of origin at the end of the cycle (80 milliseconds). Like the 12-lead ECG, this loop can be directly recorded from conventional points on the body surface. Note that the loop is located in space and does not have a fixed relationship with body anatomy. The VCG is recorded as the projection of the loop on three defined leads: the X, Y, and Z leads. These leads are shown in Figure 4.5.

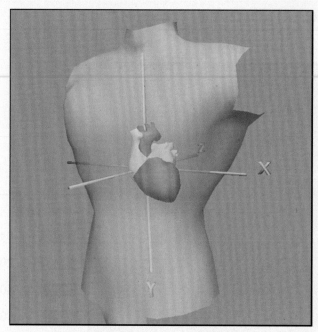

FIGURE 4.5. The X, Y, and Z leads of the vectorcardiogram. The X lead is similar to both leads I and V5, the Y lead is similar to lead aVF, and the Z lead is similar to lead V2 (Image from Viewpoint Data Labs International, Inc, with permission.)

The transmission of these forces to the body surface was studied in detail by Frank,[7,8] whose experimental work with a current dipole in the center of anatomic models of the human torso made it possible to design new leads (X, Y, and Z leads) that are used to record the VCG from the body surface, which are at right angles to each other (orthogonal) and intersect at the center of the heart, as shown in Figure 4.5. These and similar studies also show us how to transform signals from one lead to another, including those in the conventional 12-lead ECG.

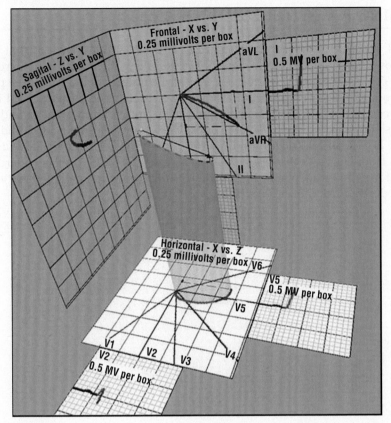

FIGURE 4.6. The projection of the QRS vector loop can be considered as a shadow cast by the loop onto each of the three orthogonal planes (frontal, sagittal, horizontal), as shown for the horizontal plane (X versus Z lead) in this figure. (Modified from Olson CW, Wagner GS, Selvester RH, et al. A model for simulating bundle branch and fascicular block. *Computers in Cardiology.* 2007:333–336, with permission.) See Video 4.1.

The QRS loop in a single cardiac cycle can be represented as a projection onto each of the three orthogonal planes as shown in Figure 4.6. This projection can be considered as a shadow cast by the vector loop onto each of the planes. Only the initial half of the vector loop to the point of the overall sum vector at 40 milliseconds is included in this figure. The relationships between depolarization events in the ventricle and the inscription of the loop are available to the reader in video form, in which the vector loop will be seen in motion and described in more detail.

Video 4.1

RECORDING A VECTORCARDIOGRAM

The VCG is usually recorded from a special set of electrodes, such as that designed by Frank[7,8] (above), which enable us to measure forces along three axes which are at right angles to each other (orthogonal), with the center at the intersection of the three planes in the center of the heart. The design of the Frank[7,8] and similar lead systems used in recording the VCG is complex and will not be discussed here, but it is important to understand that the relationships between the X, Y, and Z leads used in recording a VCG and each of the 12 standard ECG leads is known, and mathematical transformations allow us to convert information from lead systems designed for recording the VCG to the standard 12 leads of the ECG. Information from one can be predicted from the other, and information about the loop can be derived from the 12-lead ECG.

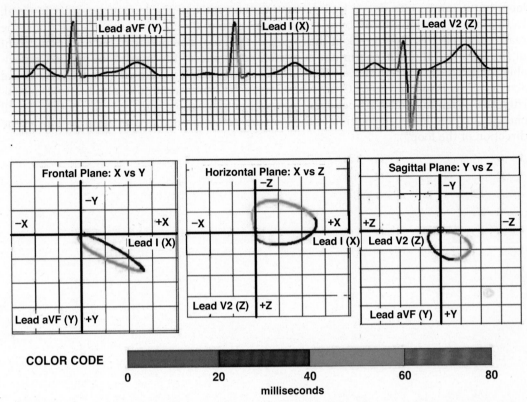

FIGURE 4.7. The relationship between ECG **(top)** and VCG **(bottom)** recordings. The red, blue, green, and purple colors indicate the four successive 20-millisecond intervals during the 80-millisecond duration of this example QRS complex on both the ECG and VCG recordings, as indicated by the color code bar. Each of the three orthogonal leads has both ECG and VCG names: right to left, I and X; superior to inferior, aVF and Y; and anterior to posterior, V2 or Z. Each of the VCG loops is a plot of two of these three orthogonal leads: frontal plane, X versus Y, horizontal plane, X versus Z; and sagittal plane, Y versus Z.

Understanding the relationship between the VCG and the ECG provided the basis for Grant's spatial vector method of interpretation of the ECG. He pointed out that the ECG reader can gain information, not only about the mean forces represented by the P, QRS, and T waves but also that these waves can be broken into early, mid, and late components with each of these forces visualized as segments of loops. The QRS complex can be visualized in its loop or vector form in the frontal plane using the six limb leads and in the horizontal plane using the six chest leads. As illustrated in Figure 4.7, the right- to left-oriented X lead is approximated by frontal plane lead I, as shown in Figure 4.7, and horizontal plane V5. The anterior-posterior–oriented Z lead is approximated by horizontal plane lead V2, and the superior-inferior–oriented Y lead is approximated by frontal plane lead aVF. The frontal plane loop is seen when a Frank "X" lead is plotted against a Frank "Y" lead. The frontal plane loop can also be seen by plotting their "equivalents," leads I and aVF (with some mathematical corrections) against each other at right angles.

Note that the vector loop is a plot of electrical force in one axis against electrical force in another axis at a 90-degree angle, whereas the ECG is a plot of electrical force (voltage) in the vertical axis against time in the horizontal axis. Time is not a component of the vector loop, but it can be introduced by interrupting the course of the loop at a regular interval. In this figure it is introduced by using different colors. By counting the interruptions, the reader can gain information about the timing of the loop. The timing of the maximum point in the loop and the half maximum points on each side of the maximum is quite repeatable for the normal heart and a practical way of recognizing the normal cardiac electrical activity. This is lost in the ECG presentation. A VCG presentation is also better at visualizing the phase relationships between forces in one direction and those in another. Small changes in direction or in rotation of the loop are better appreciated as perturbations in the direction of the loop.

VISUALIZING VECTOR LOOPS FROM THE ELECTROCARDIOGRAM

Reading an ECG using spatial techniques begins with the determination of the mean axis of the three major waves of the ECG in the frontal plane, which is described in Chapter 3. As a brief review, the broad principle is to identify the frontal plane lead (limb lead) in which the area under the contour of the ECG wave is closest to zero. The mean axis vector direction for that wave is perpendicular to that lead. This direction is thus narrowed to one of the two possible directions at right angles to that lead. Inspection of any lead parallel to that vector quickly establishes which of the two possibilities fits with the true vector. This method is used for the frontal plane direction of P, QRS, and T vectors.

The anterior–posterior direction of these vectors is determined using the same general method, utilizing the precordial leads to identify the wave in which the area under the curve most closely approaches zero. The chest is visualized as a cylinder, with the heart vector located at its center. The presence of an electrical force, represented by the heart vector at that instant of time, divides the torso into two electrical fields: one in which the surface recording generates a positive wave on the recording instrument and the other in which it generates a negative wave. These are separated by a plane in which the recorded wave is a net zero. This plane is at right angles to the direction of the vector at the center of the heart. The frontal plane direction is known (from the above process using the limb leads). The reader must now visualize the anterior or posterior tilt which must be added to make this plane fit the null complex as seen in the precordial leads as they are arrayed across the left anterior chest.

It is emphasized that this chapter is not intended to prepare the reader of ECGs to interpret VCGs, but it is intended as an introduction to the concept of three-dimensional information which can be obtained from the ECG and how this relates to the electrical events within the heart. The application of vector methods to the conduction defects of the heart is analyzed in Olson et al.[9]

GLOSSARY

Null Plane: the plane which separates the positive and negative fields within a volume conductor (the torso). This plane generally lies perpendicular to the vector loop at the center of the volume conductor.

Vector: a representation of the magnitude and direction in three-dimensional space. The electrical cardiac vectors are typically displayed on orthogonal frontal, horizontal and left sagittal planar views as arrows with their lengths indicating magnitude and their spatial orientations indicating direction. A tilt of the arrowhead can be added to indicate direction in the third dimension.

Vector loop: a line connecting the tips of the arrowheads of the electrical vectors at sequential specified time intervals during each wave in a cardiac cycle.

Vectorcardiogram: display of the vector loops generated by depolarization of the atria and ventricles and repolarization of the ventricles onto the orthogonal frontal, horizontal, and left sagittal planes.

REFERENCES

1. Grant RP. An approach to the spatial electrocardiogram. *Am Heart J*. 1950;39:17.
2. Grant RP. Spatial vector electrocardiography—a method for calculating the spatial electrical vectors of the heart from conventional leads. *Circulation*. 1950;2:676.
3. Wagner NB, White RD, Wagner GS, et al. The 12 lead ECG and the extent of myocardium at risk of acute infarction. In: Califf RM, Mark DB, Wagner, GS, eds. *Acute Coronary Care in the Thrombolytic Era*. Chicago, IL: Yearbook; 1988:22.
4. Olson CW, Warner RA, Wagner GS, et al. A dynamic three dimensional display of ventricular excitation and the generation of the vector and electrocardiogram. *J Electrocardiol*. 2001;34:Supp 7–16.
5. Loring Z, Olson CW, Maynard C, et al. Modeling vectorcardiograms based on left ventricle papillary muscle position. *J Electrocardiol*. 2011;44:584–589.
6. Olson CW, Lange DM, Chan JK, et al. 3D heart: a new visual training method for electrocardiographic analysis. *J Electrocardiol*. 2007;40:457.e1–457.e7.
7. Frank E. The image surface of a homogeneous torso. *Am Heart J*. 1954;47:757.
8. Frank E, Kay CF. Frontal plane studies of homogeneous torso models. *Circulation*. 1954;9:724–740.
9. Olson CW, Wagner GS, Selvester RH, et al. A model for simulating bundle branch and fascicular block. *Computers in Cardiology*. 2007:333–336.

Abnormal Wave Morphology

5

Chamber Enlargement

DAVID G. STRAUSS, LJUBA BACHAROVA,
GALEN S. WAGNER, AND TOBIN H. LIM

CHAMBER ENLARGEMENT

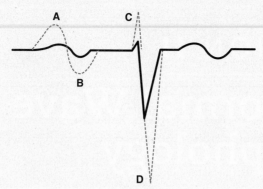

FIGURE 5.1. *Dashed* lines indicate chamber enlargements.

Cardiac chamber enlargement may occur because of either an increase in the volume of blood within the chamber or an increase in the resistance to blood flow out of it. The former condition is termed *volume overload* or *diastolic overload* and the latter is termed *pressure overload* or *systolic overload*.[1] The increase in blood volume causes *dilation* of the chamber, and the increase in resistance causes thickening of the myocardial wall of the chamber (*hypertrophy*).

The short-axis–oriented recording (see Fig. 1.14) provides the key electrocardiographic view for identifying enlargement of one of the four cardiac chambers and localizing the site of a delay in ventricular activation (Fig. 5.1). Right-atrial enlargement produces an abnormally prominent initial part of the P wave (see Fig. 5.1A), whereas left-atrial enlargement produces an abnormally prominent terminal part of the P wave (see Fig. 5.1B). Right-ventricular enlargement produces an abnormally prominent R wave (see Fig. 5.1C), whereas left-ventricular enlargement produces an abnormally prominent S wave (see Fig. 5.1D).

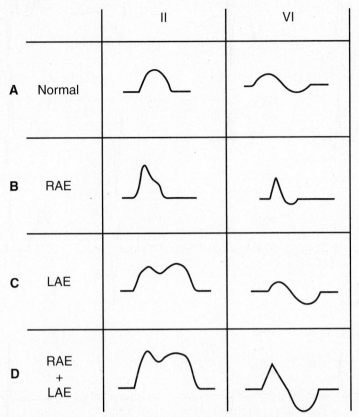

FIGURE 5.2. P-wave morphology typical of atrial enlargement in leads II and V1. LAE, left-atrial enlargement; RAE, right-atrial enlargement; RAE + LAE, biatrial enlargement.

The thinner-walled atrial chambers generally respond to both of these overloads with characteristic changes in the electrocardiogram (ECG). The usual terms for enlargement of the atria are *right-atrial enlargement* (RAE) and *left-atrial enlargement* (*LAE*). Indeed, "overload" rather than "enlargement" might be a more accurate general term for the ECG changes seen with enlargement because electrical effects may occur before measurable dilation or hypertrophy of the affected chamber (as can be seen by echocardiography).

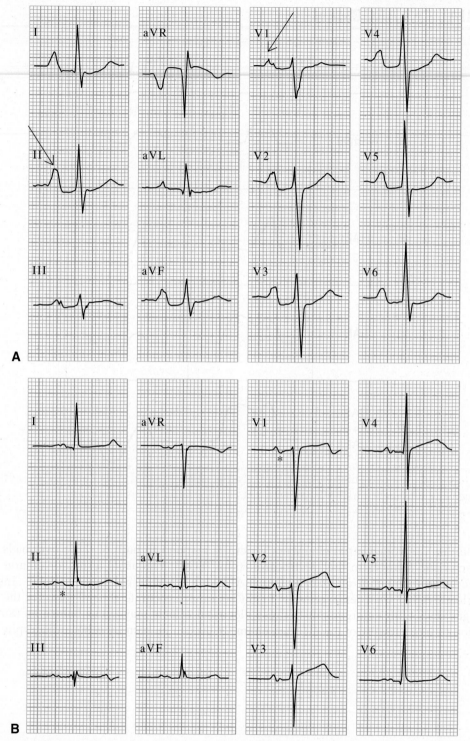

FIGURE 5.3. **A–C.** ECGs of patients with atrial enlargement. Note the prolonged PR interval (0.28 second) in **A.** *Arrows*, P-wave changes in right atrial enlargement; *asterisks*, left-atrial enlargement.

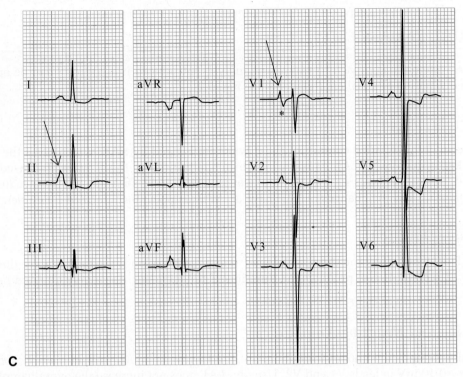

FIGURE 5.3. *(continued)*

The ECG evaluation of RAE and LAE is facilitated by the differing times of initiating activation of the two atria and by the differing directional spread of activation in each. As indicated in Figure 2.5, the optimal lead for differentiating left versus right cardiac activity is V1, with its positive electrode in the fourth intercostal space at the right sternal border (see Fig. 2.6). Right-atrial activation begins first. It proceeds from the sinoatrial (SA) node in an inferior and anterior direction and produces the initial deflection of the P wave, which has a positive direction in all leads except aVR (Fig. 5.2). Left-atrial activation begins later. It proceeds from high in the interatrial septum in a left, inferior, and posterior direction. This produces the final deflection of the P wave, which is positive in long-axis lead II but negative in short-axis lead V1 (see Fig. 5.2). Therefore, RAE is characterized by an increase in the initial deflection (see Figs. 5.2B and 5.3A) and LAE by an increase in the final deflection of the P wave (see Figs. 5.2C and 5.3B). In most of the other standard leads, both the right- and left-atrial components of the P wave appear as similarly directed deflections. An increase in both the initial and final aspects of the P wave suggests biatrial enlargement (see Figs. 5.2D and 5.3C).

SYSTEMATIC APPROACH TO THE EVALUATION OF ATRIAL ENLARGEMENT

The systematic approach to waveform analysis introduced in Chapter 3 can be applied to the evaluation of atrial enlargement (see Fig. 5.2).

General Contour

The smooth, rounded contour of the P wave is changed by RAE, which gives the wave a peaked appearance. LAE causes a notch in the middle of the P wave, followed by a second "hump." In leads such as II, the P waves of RAE have an A-like appearance (termed *P pulmonale*), and the changes of LAE have an M-like appearance (termed *P mitrale*).

P-Wave Duration

RAE does not affect the duration of the P wave. LAE prolongs the total P-wave duration to >0.12 second. It also prolongs the duration of the terminal, negatively directed portion of the P wave in lead V1 to >0.04 second.

Positive and Negative Amplitudes

RAE increases the maximal amplitude of the P wave to >0.20 mV in leads II and aVF and to >0.10 mV in leads V1 and V2. Usually, LAE does not increase the overall amplitude of the P wave but increases only the amplitude of the terminal, negatively directed portion of the wave in lead V1 to >0.10 mV.

Axis in the Frontal and Transverse Planes

Estimate the axes of the P wave in the two electrocardiographic planes. RAE may cause a slight rightward shift and LAE may cause a slight leftward shift in the P-wave axis in the frontal plane. However, the axis usually remains within the normal limits of 0 degrees to +75 degrees.

With extreme RAE, the P wave may be inverted in lead V1, creating the illusion of LAE. With extreme LAE, the P-wave amplitude may increase and the terminal portion of the wave may become negative in leads II, III, and aVF. *Biatrial enlargement* produces characteristics of RAE and LAE (see Figs. 5.2D and 5.3C).

Table 5.1.

Echocardiographic Evaluation of Electrocardiographic (ECG) Criteria for Left-Atrial Enlargement

ECG Criteria	% True Positive[a]	% True Negative[b]
Duration of terminal negative P-wave deflection in lead V1 >0.04 s	83	80
Amplitude of terminal negative P-wave deflection in lead V1 >0.10 mV	60	93
Duration between peaks of P-wave notches >0.04 s	15	100
Maximal P-wave duration >0.11 s	33	88
Ratio of P-wave duration to PR-segment duration >1:1.6	31	64

[a]Percentage of patients with LAE by echocardiogram who meet the ECG criterion for LAE.
[b]Percentage of patients without LAE by echocardiogram who do not meet the ECG criterion for LAE.
Modified from Munuswamy K, Alpert MA, Martin RH, Whiting RB, Mechlin NJ. Sensitivity and specificity of commonly used electrocardiographic criteria for left atrial enlargement determined by M-mode echocardiography. *Am J Cardiol.* 1984;53(6):829–832, with permission.

Munuswamy and colleagues,[2] using echocardiography as the standard for determining LAE, have evaluated the percentage of patients with truly positive and truly negative ECG criteria for LAE (Table 5.1). They found that the most *sensitive* criterion for LAE is an increased duration (>0.04 second) of the terminal, negative portion of the P wave in lead V1, whereas the most *specific* criterion for LAE is a wide, notched P wave that resembles the P wave seen in the case of an *intra-atrial block*.

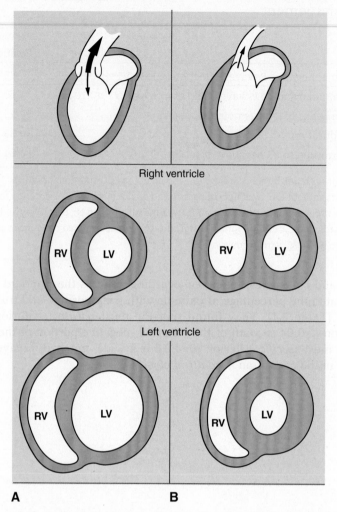

FIGURE 5.4. **A.** Volume load. *Thick upward arrow*, direction of blood flow; *thin downward arrow*, regurgitant blood. **B.** Pressure load. *Thin upward arrow*, direction of blood flow through narrowed outflow valve. (Adapted from Rushmer RF. Cardiac compensation, hypertrophy, myopathy and congestive heart failure. In: Rushmer RF, ed. *Cardiovascular Dynamics*. 4th ed. Philadelphia, PA: WB Saunders; 1976:532–565, with permission.)

The thick-walled ventricles dilate in response to receiving an excess volume of blood during diastole, and they become hypertrophied in response to exerting excess pressure in ejecting the blood during systole (Fig. 5.4). Volume overload in the ventricles may be caused by regurgitation of blood through a leaking outflow valve back into the partially emptied ventricle (see Fig. 5.4A). Pressure overload caused by obstruction to ejection through a narrowed outflow valve is displayed in Figure 5.4B. Enlargement of the right or left ventricle is commonly accompanied by enlargement of its corresponding atrium. Therefore, ECG findings that meet the criteria for atrial enlargement should be considered suggestive of ventricular enlargement.

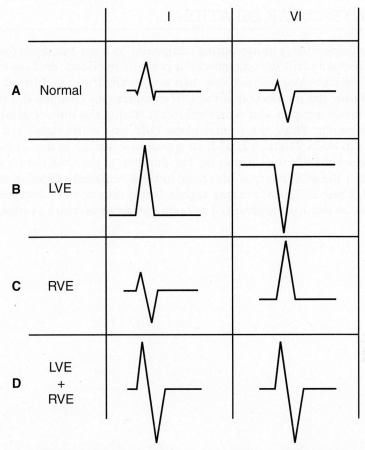

FIGURE 5.5. QRS complex typical of ventricular enlargement in leads I and V1. LVE, left-ventricular enlargement; RVE, right-ventricular enlargement; RVE + LVE, biventricular enlargement.

Figure 5.5 illustrates the typical changes in the QRS waveforms that occur with enlargement of the ventricles. In the absence of either right- or left-ventricular enlargement, a predominantly positive QRS complex appears in lead I and a predominantly negative QRS complex appears in lead V1 (see Fig 5.5A). These QRS complexes increase in amplitude but do not change in direction with left-ventricular enlargement (see Fig. 5.5B). With right-ventricular enlargement, however, the directions of the overall QRS waveform reverse to predominantly negative in lead I and predominantly positive in lead V1 (see Fig. 5.5C). With combined right- and left-ventricular enlargement, a hybrid of these waveform abnormalities results (see Fig. 5.5D).

RIGHT-VENTRICULAR DILATION

The right ventricle dilates either during compensation for volume overload or after its hypertrophy eventually fails to compensate for pressure overload. Because of this dilation, the right ventricle takes longer to activate than is normally the case. Instead of completing its activation during the midportion of the QRS complex (see Chapter 1), the dilated right ventricle contributes anterior and rightward forces during the time of completion of left-ventricular activation. Thus, the frontal plane QRS axis shifts rightward and an RSR' pattern appears in leads V1 and V2, with an appearance similar to that in *incomplete right-bundle-branch block* (RBBB; see Chapter 6). The duration of the QRS complex may become so prolonged that the ECG changes occurring in right-ventricular dilation mimic those in *complete RBBB*. These ECG changes may appear during the early or compensatory phase of volume overload or during the advanced or failing phase of pressure overload.[3]

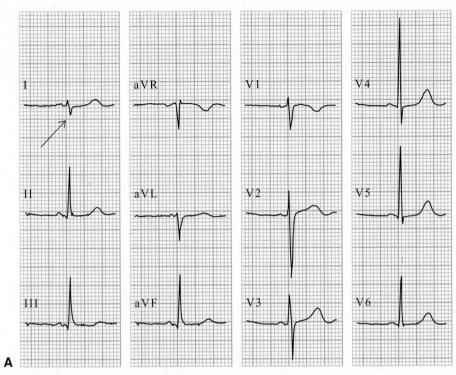

FIGURE 5.6. **A–C.** ECGs of patients with RVH. *Arrows*, RVH in the QRS complex; *asterisk:* ST- and T-wave in right-ventricular strain.

The right ventricle hypertrophies because of compensation for pressure overload. The final third of the QRS complex is normally produced solely by activation of the thicker walled left ventricle and interventricular septum. As the right ventricle hypertrophies, it provides an increasing contribution to the early portion of the QRS complex and also begins to contribute to the later portion of the complex.

Lead V1, with its left-to-right orientation, provides the optimal view of the competition between the two ventricles for electrical predominance. As shown in Figure 5.5A, the normal QRS complex in the adult is predominantly negative in lead V1, with a small R wave followed by a prominent S wave. When the right ventricle hypertrophies in response to pressure overload, this negative predominance may be lost, producing a prominent R wave and a small S wave (see Fig. 5.5C). In mild right-ventricular hypertrophy (RVH), the left ventricle retains predominance, and there is either no ECG change or the QRS axis moves rightward (Fig. 5.6A). Note the S > R amplitude in lead I, indicating that the frontal plane axis is slightly >+90 degrees, meeting the threshold presented in Chapter 3 for right-axis deviation (RAD). With moderate RVH, the initial QRS forces are predominantly anterior (with an increased R wave in lead V1), and the terminal QRS forces may or may not be predominantly rightward (see Fig. 5.6B). These changes could also be indicative of myocardial infarction in the lateral wall of the left ventricle (see Chapter 12). With severe RVH, the QRS complex typically becomes predominantly negative in lead I and positive in lead V1, and the delayed repolarization of the right-ventricular myocardium may produce negativity of the ST segment and a T-wave pattern indicative of so-called right-ventricular *strain* in leads such as V1 to V3 (see Fig. 5.6C).[4]

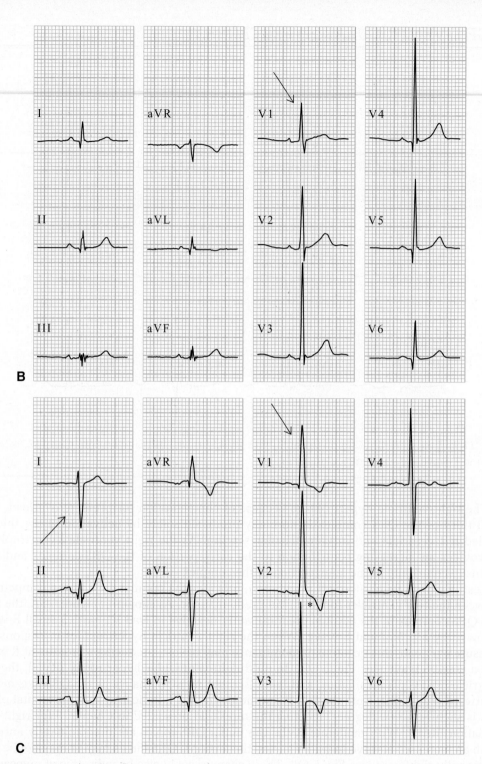

FIGURE 5.6. (continued)

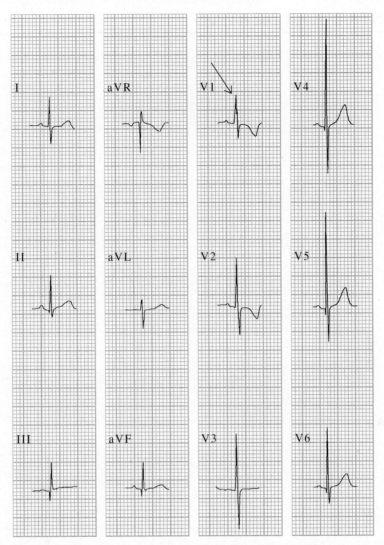

FIGURE 5.7. Healthy neonatal ECG. *Arrow,* normal RV predominance.

In the neonate, the right ventricle is more hypertrophied than the left because there is greater resistance in the pulmonary circulation than in the systemic circulation during fetal development (Fig. 5.7). Right-sided resistance is greatly diminished when the lungs fill with air, and left-sided resistance is greatly increased when the placenta is removed.[5] From this time onward, the ECG evidence of right-ventricular predominance is gradually lost as the left ventricle becomes hypertrophied in relation to the right. Therefore, hypertrophy, like dilation, may be a compensatory rather than a pathologic condition.[6] A pressure overload of the right ventricle may recur in later years because of increased resistance to blood flow through the pulmonary valve, the pulmonary circulation, or the left side of the heart.

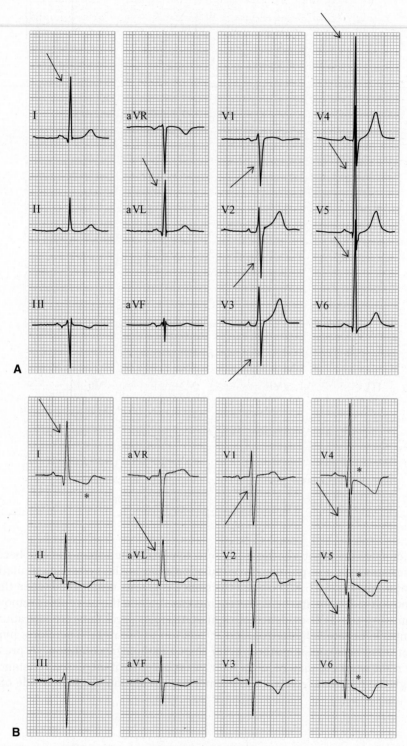

FIGURE 5.8.   **A and B.** ECGs of patients with left-ventricular dilation. *Arrows*, increased leftward posterior and upward QRS waveforms; *asterisks*, ST-segment and T-wave changes in left-ventricular strain.

The left ventricle dilates for the same reasons indicated previously for the right ventricle. Two factors affect the resultant ECG patterns in left-ventricular dilation: the change in size and anatomic shape of the left ventricle and the alteration in the impulse propagation velocity in the left ventricle.[3,4] The longer time required for the spread of an electrical impulse across the dilated left ventricle may produce an ECG pattern similar to that of *incomplete left-bundle-branch block* (LBBB; see Chapter 6). The duration of the QRS complex may become so prolonged that the ECG changes in left-ventricular dilation mimic those in complete LBBB.

Dilation enlarges the area of the activation front in the left ventricle, which increases the amplitudes of leftward and posteriorly directed QRS waveforms[5] (Fig. 5.8). The S-wave amplitudes are increased in leads V2 and V3, and the R-wave amplitudes are increased in leads I, aVL, V5, and V6 (see Fig. 5.5B). The T-wave amplitudes may also be increased in the same direction as the amplitudes of the QRS complex (see Fig. 5.8A), or the T waves may be directed away from the QRS complex, indicating left-ventricular "strain" (see Fig. 5.8B). Figure 5.8A illustrates ECG changes indicating mild to moderate left-ventricular dilation, and Figure 5.8B shows more severe changes, including abnormally prominent Q waves in many leads and *left-ventricular strain*.

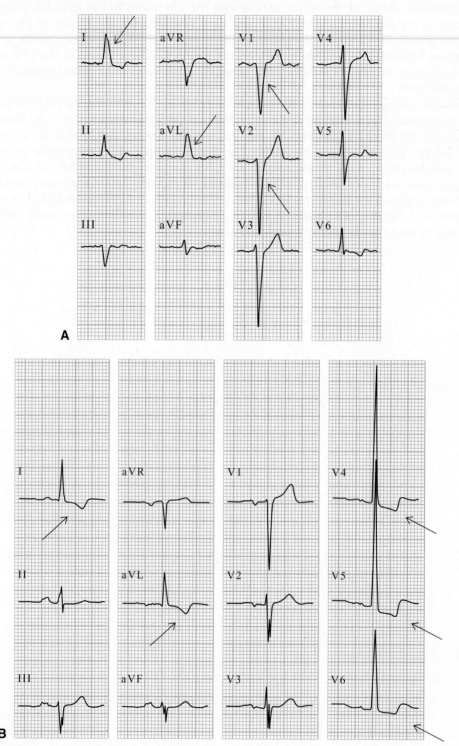

FIGURE 5.9. **A and B**. ECGs of patients with left-ventricular hypertrophy. **A**. *Arrows*, intraventricular conduction delay. **B**. *Arrows*, ST-segment depression and T-wave inversion.

As discussed, the left ventricle normally becomes larger than the right ventricle after the neonatal period. Abnormal hypertrophy, which occurs in response to a pressure overload, produces exaggeration of the normal ECG pattern of left-ventricular predominance. Like dilation, hypertrophy enlarges the area of the activation front in the left ventricle, which increases the voltages of leftward and posteriorly directed QRS waveforms, thereby causing similar shifts in the frontal and transverse plane axes.

As in left-ventricular dilation, two factors affect the resultant ECG patterns: the change in size and anatomic shape of the left ventricle and the alteration in the impulse propagation velocity in the left ventricle.[3,4] Thus, with left-ventricular hypertrophy (LVH), a longer period is required for spread of electrical activation from the endocardial to the epicardial surfaces of the hypertrophied myocardium, prolonging the intrinsicoid deflection (time to peak R wave) (see Fig. 3.9), as well as for total left-ventricular activation. Because of the disproportion between the activation of the left and right ventricles, an interventricular conduction delay mimicking incomplete or even complete LBBB may occur with LVH as with left-ventricular dilation (Fig. 5.9A).

Pressure overload causes sustained delayed repolarization of the left ventricle, producing a negative ST segment and T wave in leads with leftward orientation (i.e., V5 to V6); this condition is termed *left-ventricular strain* (see Fig. 5.9B).[6] The epicardial cells no longer repolarize early, reversing the spread of recovery so that it proceeds from endocardium to epicardium. The mechanism responsible for the strain is uncertain, but it is related to the increased pressure (overload) in the left-ventricular cavity. The development of strain has been shown to correlate with increasing left-ventricular mass as determined with echocardiography.[7] Computer simulation studies show that the delayed depolarization of the left ventricle can also contribute to the changes in ST segment and T wave.[4]

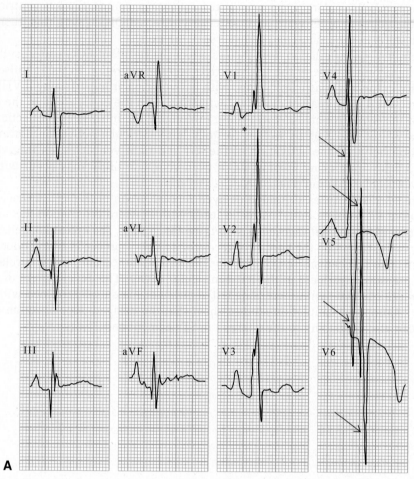

FIGURE 5.10. **A–D.** ECGs of patients with biventricular hypertrophy. **A.** *Arrows,* high-voltage biphasic RS complexes. **B and C.** *Arrows,* S > R in lead I, prominent R in lead V1, and increased S in lead V3. **D.** *Arrows,* prominent R precordial leads. **A and B.** *Asterisks,* typical P-wave abnormalities of RAE and LAE. **C.** *Asterisks,* typical P-wave abnormalities of RAE. Note that waveforms for lead V6, shown in **A,** are displaced rightward only for illustrative purposes.

Although the two varieties of right- and left-ventricular enlargement—dilation and hypertrophy—have somewhat different effects on ECG waveforms as discussed, no specific sets of criteria for dilation versus hypertrophy have been developed. The term *enlargement* has currently been accepted with regard to the atria, but the term *hypertrophy* is still used instead of "enlargement" with regard to the ventricles. Therefore, the systematic approach to waveform analysis introduced in Chapter 3 is applied here to "ventricular hypertrophy."

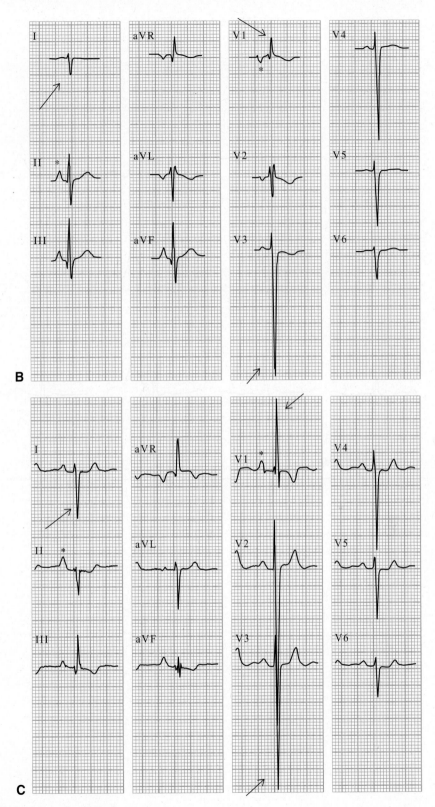

FIGURE 5.10. *(continued)*

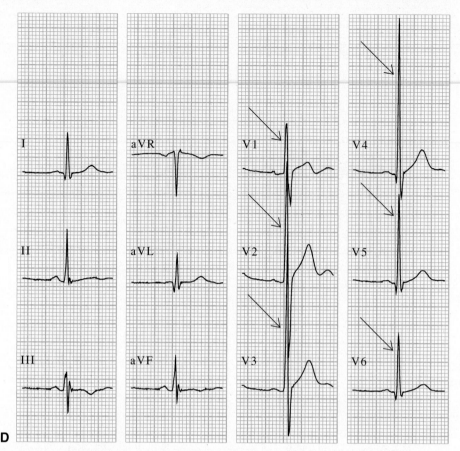

FIGURE 5.10. *(continued)*

General Contour

Prolongation of the intrinsicoid deflection by the hypertrophied ventricular myocardium diminishes the slope of the initial waveforms of the QRS complex. As activation of the ventricular myocardium spreads, the smooth contour of the mid-QRS waveforms may be disrupted by indentations or notches (Fig. 5.10A). The terminal portions of the prolonged QRS complexes have low-frequency, smooth waveforms.

The contour of the ECG baseline may be altered. Ventricular hypertrophy shifts the J point off the horizontal baseline formed by the PR and TP segments and causes the ST segment to slope in the direction of the T wave (see Figs. 5.6C and 5.9B). When this occurs in the rightward precordial leads, it is referred to as right-ventricular strain; in the left precordial leads, it is referred to as left-ventricular strain.

QRS Complex Duration

Hypertrophy of the left ventricle may cause prolongation of the QRS complex beyond its normal limit of 0.07 to 0.11 second, but hypertrophy of the right ventricle usually does not prolong the duration of the QRS complex. RVH can cause slight prolongation of the QRS complex when there is marked right-ventricular dilation. However, hypertrophy of the left ventricle, even without dilation, may prolong the duration of the QRS complex to 0.13 or 0.14 second.

Figure 5.11 shows ECGs from a patient who developed progressive LVH with corresponding QRS prolongation at a rate of 6.2 milliseconds per year over a period of 6.5 years. It is important to note that the ECG at 6.5 years with a QRS duration of 0.142 second would meet conventional ECG criteria for LBBB (discussed in Chapter 6); however, this progressive QRS prolongation is characteristic of hypertrophy rather than bundle-branch block (where there should be a sudden onset in QRS prolongation). A key distinguishing factor between left-ventricular hypertrophy and LBBB block is that LBBB block ECGs should have mid-QRS notching/slurring (discussed in Chapter 6), which is not present in the ECGs in Figure 5.11. When complete LBBB is present in a patient with LVH, QRS duration may even extend to 0.20 second.

Positive and Negative Amplitudes

The amplitude of the QRS complex is normally maximal in the left posterior downward direction. The left posterior direction is accentuated by LVH and opposed by RVH, and the electrical axis of the heart in frontal plane is shifted to the left (i.e., upward). The criteria for LVH reflect these changes. The Sokolow–Lyon criteria[8] consider transverse plane leads (V1, V5/6), that is, the left and posterior waveform amplitudes, whereas the Cornell criteria[9] and the Romhilt–Estes criteria[10] consider both transverse plane leads and frontal plane leads (aVL, electrical axis), that is, the left- (upward) axis deviation.

The Sokolow–Lyon criteria for RVH contain thresholds for rightward and anterior amplitudes in the transverse plane leads.[11] Butler–Leggett criteria[12] require that the combination of maximal anterior and maximal rightward amplitudes exceeds the maximal leftward posterior amplitude by a threshold voltage difference.

Axis in the Frontal and Transverse Planes

RVH shifts the frontal plane QRS axis rightward, to a vertical or rightward position, and shifts the transverse plane QRS axis anteriorly (see Fig. 5.6C). LVH shifts the frontal plane QRS axis leftward and the transverse plane QRS axis posteriorly (see Fig. 5.3C).

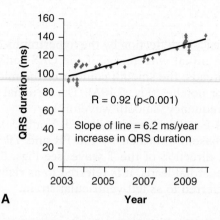

A

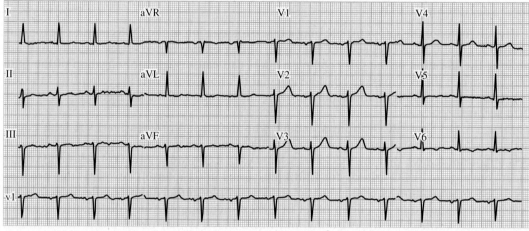

B

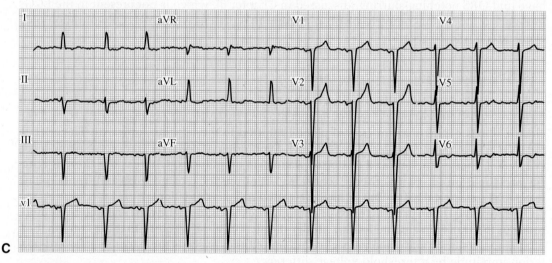

C

FIGURE 5.11. ECGs from a patient who developed progressive LVH. The scatterplot
(A) shows QRS duration measurements over time from 42 ECGs from the same patient. The
patient's QRS duration increased linearly at a rate of 6.2 milliseconds per year. ECGs are shown
at baseline **(B)** and after 1.5 years **(C)**, 5 years **(D)**, and 6.5 years **(E)**. Although later ECGs **(D and
E)** meet conventional ECG criteria for LBBB (QRS duration ≥0.12 second with an LV conduction
delay), review of the serial ECGs shows that QRS morphology did not change as the QRS prolonged.

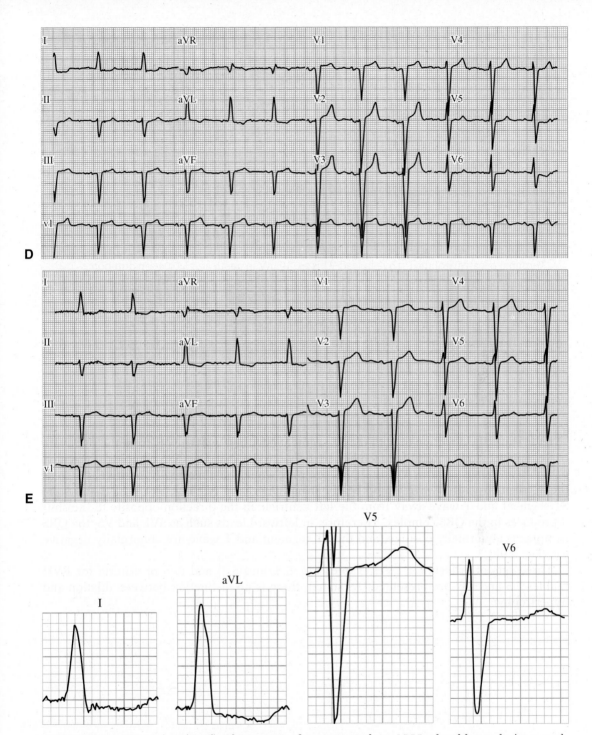

FIGURE 5.11. *(continued)* The onset of true complete LBBB should result in a sudden increase in QRS duration of ≥60 milliseconds along with a change in QRS morphology. The ECG in **(E)** (QRS duration 142 milliseconds) contains very similar QRS morphology to the previous ECGs. The gradual increase in QRS duration over time strongly suggests the development of intraventricular conduction delay due to hypertrophy rather than the onset of bundle-branch block. The final ECG meets both Cornell (Table 5.4) and Romhilt–Estes (Table 5.2) criteria for LVH. Reproduced from Strauss DG, Selvester RH, Wagner GS. Defining left bundle branch block in the era of cardiac resynchronization therapy. Am J Cardiol. 2011;107(6):927–934, with permission.

Table 5.2.

Romhilt–Estes Scoring System for Left-Ventricular Hypertrophy[a]

	Points
1. R or S wave in any limb ≥2 mV	3
or S in lead V1 or V2	
or R in lead V5 or V6 ≥3 mV	
2. Left-ventricular strain	
ST segment and T wave in opposite direction to QRS complex	
without digitalis	3
with digitalis	1
3. Left-atrial enlargement	
Terminal negativity of the P wave in lead V1 is ≥0.10 mV in depth and ≥0.04 s in duration	3
4. Left-axis deviation ≥−30 degrees	2
5. QRS duration ≥0.09 s	1
6. Intrinsicoid detection in lead V5 or V6 ≥0.05 s	1
Maximally attainable	13

[a]LVH, 5 points; probably LVH, 4 points.
Modified from Romhilt DW, Bove KE, Norris RJ, et al. A critical appraisal of the electrocardiographic criteria for the diagnosis of left ventricular hypertrophy. *Circulation.* 1969;40(2):185–195, with permission.

RVH shifts the direction of both the ST segment and the T wave away from the right ventricle, opposite to the shift that such hypertrophy produces in the QRS complex. Typically, in rightward leads such as V1, the QRS complex would be abnormally positive, whereas the ST segment and T wave would be abnormally negative (see Fig. 5.6C). LVH shifts the ST segment and T wave away from the left ventricle in the direction opposite to the shift it produces in the QRS complex. Therefore, in leftward leads such as aVL and V5, the QRS complex is abnormally positive, and the ST segment and T wave are abnormally negative (see Fig. 5.9B).

Three sets of criteria for LVH (Tables 5.2, 5.3, and 5.4) and two of criteria for RVH (Tables 5.5 and 5.6) are presented. As stated, there is no distinction between dilation and hypertrophy.

Table 5.3.

Sokolow–Lyon Criteria for Left-Ventricular Hypertrophy

S wave in lead V1 + R wave in lead V5 or V6 ≥3.50 mV

or

R wave in lead V5 or V6 >2.60 mV

Modified from Sokolow M, Lyon TP. The ventricular complex in left ventricular hypertrophy as obtained by unipolar precordial and limb leads. *Am Heart J.* 1949;37(2):161–186, with permission.

Table 5.4.

Cornell Voltage Criteria for Left-Ventricular Hypertrophy

| Females | R wave in lead aVL + S wave in lead V3 >2.00 mV |
| Males | R wave in lead aVL + S wave in lead V3 >2.80 mV |

Modified from Casale PN, Devereux RB, Alonso DR, et al. Improved sex-specific criteria of left ventricular hypertrophy for clinical and computer interpretation of electrocardiograms: validation with autopsy findings. *Circulation.* 1987;75(3):565–572, with permission.

Table 5.5.

Butler–Leggett Formula for Right-Ventricular Hypertrophy (RVH)

Directions	Anterior	Rightward	Posterior Leftward
Amplitude	Tallest R or R′ in lead V1 or V2	Deepest S in lead 1 or V6	S in lead V1
RVH formula	A + R − PL ≥0.70 mV		

Modified from Butler PM, Leggett SI, Howe CM, et al. Identification of electrocardiographic criteria for diagnosis of right ventricular hypertrophy due to mitral stenosis. *Am J Cardiol.* 1986;57(8):639–643, with permission.

Table 5.6.

Sokolow–Lyon Criteria for Right-Ventricular Hypertrophy

R wave in lead V1 + S wave in lead V5 or V6 ≥1.10 mV

Modified from Sokolow M, Lyon TP. The ventricular complex in right ventricular hypertrophy as obtained by unipolar precordial and limb leads. *Am Heart J.* 1949;38(2):273–294, with permission.

GLOSSARY

Biatrial enlargement: enlargement of both the right and left atria.

Complete bundle-branch block: total failure of conduction in the right or left bundle branch.

Dilation: stretching of the myocardium beyond its normal dimensions.

Enlargement: dilation or hypertrophy of a cardiac chamber.

Hypertrophy: (noun) an increase in bulk of a cardiac chamber, caused by the thickening of myocardial fibers; (verb) to increase in bulk.

Incomplete bundle-branch block: partial failure of conduction in the right or left bundle branch.

Intra-atrial block: a conduction delay within the atria.

Left-atrial enlargement (LAE): dilation of the left atrium to accommodate an increase in blood volume or resistance to outflow.

Left-bundle-branch block (LBBB): failure of conduction in the left bundle branch of the ventricular Tawara's system.

Left-ventricular strain: an ECG pattern characteristic of marked left-ventricular hypertrophy, which is accompanied by ST-segment and T-wave changes (negativity of the ST segment and T wave) in addition to changes in the QRS complex.

P mitrale: appearance of the P wave in LAE; named for its common occurrence in mitral valve disease.

P pulmonale: appearance of the P wave in RAE; named for its common occurrence in chronic pulmonary disease.

Pressure or systolic overload: a condition in which a ventricle is forced to pump against an increased resistance during systole.

Right-atrial enlargement (RAE): dilation of the right atrium to accommodate an increase in blood volume or resistance to outflow.

Right-bundle-branch block (RBBB): failure of conduction in the right branch of the ventricular Tawara's system.

Sensitive: a term referring to the ability (sensitivity) of a test to indicate the presence of a condition (i.e., if the test is positive in every subject with the condition, it attains 100% sensitivity).

Specific: a term referring to the ability (specificity) of a test to indicate the absence of a condition (i.e., if the test is negative in every control subject without the condition, it attains 100% specificity).

Strain: an ECG pattern characteristic of marked hypertrophy that is accompanied by ST-segment and T-wave changes in addition to changes in the QRS complex.

Volume or diastolic overload: a condition in which a ventricle becomes filled with an increased amount of blood during diastole.

REFERENCES

1. Rushmer RF. Cardiac compensation, hypertrophy, myopathy and congestive heart failure. In: Rushmer RF, ed. *Cardiovascular Dynamics*. 4th ed. Philadelphia, PA: WB Saunders; 1976:532–565.

2. Munuswamy K, Alpert MA, Martin RH, et al. Sensitivity and specificity of commonly used electrocardiographic criteria for left atrial enlargement determined by M-mode echocardiography. *Am J Cardiol.* 1984;53(6):829–832.

3. Bacharova L, Szathmary V, Kovalcik M, et al. Effect of changes in left ventricular anatomy and conduction velocity on the QRS voltage and morphology in left ventricular hypertrophy: a model study. *J Electrocardiol.* 2010;43(3):200–208.

4. Bacharova L, Szathmary V, Mateasik A. Primary and secondary T wave changes in LVH: a model study. *J Electrocardiol.* 2010;43(6):624–633.

5. Cabrera E, Monroy JR. Systolic and diastolic loading of the heart. II. Electrocardiographic data. *Am Heart J* 1952;43(5):669–686.

6. Devereux RB, Reichek N. Repolarization abnormalities of left ventricular hypertrophy. Clinical, echocardiographic and hemodynamic correlates. *J Electrocardiol.* 1982;15(1):47–53.

7. Palmeiri V, Dahlof B, DeQuattro V, et al. Reliability of echocardiographic assess-

ment of left ventricular structure and function: the PRESERVE study. Prospective randomized study evaluating regression of ventricular enlargement. *J Am Coll Cardiol.* 1999;34(5):1625–1632.

8. Sokolow M, Lyon TP. The ventricular complex in left ventricular hypertrophy as obtained by unipolar precordial and limb leads. *Am Heart J.* 1949;37(2):161–186.

9. Casale PN, Devereux RB, Alonso DR, et al. Improved sex-specific criteria of left ventricular hypertrophy for clinical and computer interpretation of electrocardiograms: validation with autopsy findings. *Circulation.* 1987;75(3):565–572.

10. Romhilt DW, Bove KE, Norris RJ, et al. A critical appraisal of the electrocardiographic criteria for the diagnosis of left ventricular hypertrophy. *Circulation.* 1969;40(2):185–195.

11. Sokolow M, Lyon TP. The ventricular complex in right ventricular hypertrophy as obtained by unipolar precordial and limb leads. *Am Heart J.* 1949;38(2):273–294.

12. Butler PM, Leggett SI, Howe CM, et al. Identification of electrocardiographic criteria for diagnosis of right ventricular hypertrophy due to mitral stenosis. *Am J Cardiol.* 1986;57(8):639–643.

13. Strauss DG, Selvester RH, Wagner GS. Defining left bundle branch block in the era of cardiac resynchronization therapy. *Am J Cardiol.* 2011;107(6):927–934.

6

Intraventricular Conduction Abnormalities

DAVID G. STRAUSS, TOBIN H. LIM, AND GALEN S. WAGNER

NORMAL CONDUCTION

Many cardiac conditions cause electrical impulses to be conducted abnormally through the ventricular myocardium, producing changes in QRS complexes and T waves. Therefore, it is important to understand the conditions that can mimic or complicate the diagnosis of bundle-branch block (BBB) or fascicular block (intraventricular conduction abnormalities). These are as follows:

1. The left and right ventricles are not in an enlarged state that would prolong the time required for their activation and recovery (see Chapter 5).
2. Myocardial ischemia or infarction is not present or is of insufficient magnitude to disrupt the spread of the activation and recovery waves (see Chapter 9).
3. There is rapid impulse conduction through the right- and left-ventricular Purkinje networks so that the endocardial surfaces are activated almost simultaneously (as discussed later in this chapter).
4. There are no accessory pathways for conduction from the atria to the ventricles (see Chapter 7).

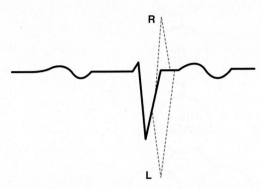

FIGURE 6.1. *Dashed lines* indicate right-sided (R) and left-sided (L) intraventricular conduction delays in this schematic recording from lead V1 that provides the short-axis viewpoint.

Because the activation of the ventricular Purkinje system is not represented on the surface electrocardiogram (ECG), abnormalities of its conduction must be detected indirectly by their effects on myocardial activation and recovery. ECG waveforms (see Fig. 1.14) are reproduced with the addition of specific QRS complex abnormalities in Figure 6.1. A conduction disturbance within the right bundle branch (RBB) causes right-ventricular activation to occur after left-ventricular activation is completed, producing an R′ deflection in lead V1 (see Fig. 6.1). A delay in conduction through the left bundle branch (LBB) markedly postpones left-ventricular activation, resulting in an abnormally prominent S wave in lead V1 (see Fig. 6.1).

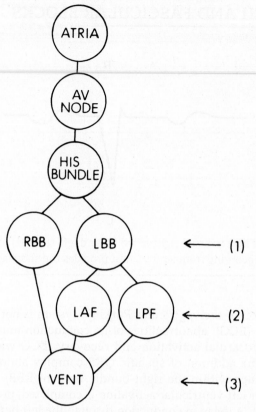

FIGURE 6.2. Possible locations of intraventricular conduction abnormalities causing QRS complex and T-wave alterations are indicated by numbers 1, 2, and 3. AV, atrioventricular; LAF, left anterior fascicle; LBB, left-bundle-branch block; LPF, left posterior fascicle; RBB, right-bundle-branch block; VENT, ventricle. (Modified from Wagner GS, Waugh RA, Ramo BW. *Cardiac Arrhythmias.* New York, NY: Churchill Livingstone; 1983:18, with permission.)

Conduction delays in the left-bundle *fascicles* or between the Purkinje fibers and the adjacent myocardium may alter the QRS complex and T wave (Fig. 6.2). A conduction disturbance in the common bundle (Bundle of His) has similar effects on the entire distal Purkinje system and therefore does not alter the appearance of the QRS complex or T wave.

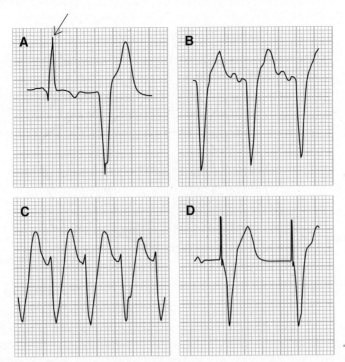

FIGURE 6.3. Comparison of patterns of QRS morphology in lead V1 when the two ventricles are activated successively rather than simultaneously. **A.** Ventricular beat. **B.** Bundle-branch block. **C.** Ventricular tachycardia. **D.** Artificially paced ventricular rhythm.

Block of an entire bundle branch requires that its ventricle be activated by myocardial spread of electrical activity from the other ventricle, with prolongation of the overall QRS complex. Block of the entire RBB is termed "complete right-bundle-branch block" (RBBB), and block of the entire LBB is termed "complete left-bundle-branch block" (LBBB). In both of these conditions, the ventricles are activated successively instead of simultaneously. The other conditions in which the ventricles are activated successively occur when one ventricle is preexcited via an accessory atrioventricular (AV) pathway (see Chapter 7) and when there are independent ventricular rhythms (see Chapters 15 and 19). Under these conditions, there is a fundamental similarity in the distortions of the ECG waveforms: the duration of the QRS complex is prolonged and the ST segment slopes into the T wave in the direction away from the ventricle in which the abnormality is located. Figure 6.3 compares QRS morphologies in lead V1 when the two ventricles are activated successively rather than simultaneously.

A ventricular conduction delay with only slight prolongation of the QRS complex due to slowed conduction through the bundle branches could be termed incomplete RBBB or incomplete LBBB. However, it is important to remember from Chapter 5 that enlargement of the right ventricle may produce a distortion of the QRS complex that mimics incomplete RBBB (see Fig. 5.10B), whereas enlargement of the left ventricle may produce a prolongation of the QRS complex that mimics incomplete LBBB (see Fig. 5.9A). Because the LBB has multiple fascicles, another form of incomplete LBBB could be produced by a disturbance in one of its major fascicles.

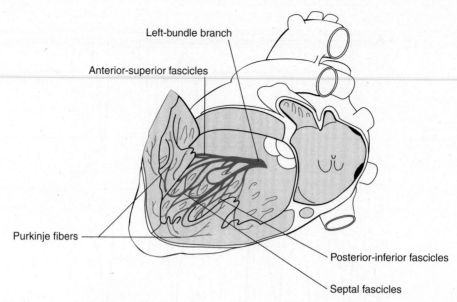

Left-bundle branch

Anterior-superior fascicles

Purkinje fibers

Posterior-inferior fascicles

Septal fascicles

FIGURE 6.4. The left ventricle has been opened to reveal the LBB and its fascicles as originally presented in Figure 1.7C. Note that the anterior and posterior fascicles to the LBB are also designated superior and inferior, respectively, because these terms indicate their true anatomic positions. (From Netter FH. *The CIBA Collection of Medical Illustrations. Vol 5. Heart* Summit, NJ: Ciba-Geigy; 1978:13, with permission.)

The ventricular Purkinje system is considered trifascicular. It consists of the RBB and the anterior and posterior portions of the LBB. The proximal RBB is small and compact and may therefore be considered either a bundle branch or a fascicle. The proximal LBB is also compact but is too large to be considered a fascicle. It remains compact for 1 to 2 cm and then fans into its two fascicles.[1] As Demoulin and Kulbertus[2] have shown in humans, there are multiple anatomic variations in these fascicles among individuals. The left ventricle has been opened (Fig. 6.4) to reveal the LBB and its fascicles as originally presented in Figure 1.7C. Note the anterior and posterior fascicles of the LBB are also designated superior and inferior, respectively, because these terms indicate their true anatomic positions. Based on their anatomic locations, the two fascicles are termed the left anterior fascicle (LAF) and left posterior fascicle (LPF; see Fig. 6.4). The LAF of the LBB courses toward the anterosuperior papillary muscle, and the LPF of the LBB courses toward the posteroinferior papillary muscle. There are also Purkinje fibers that emerge from the LBB that proceed along the surface of the interventricular septum (sometimes termed the left septal fascicle) and initiate left-to-right spread of activation through the interventricular septum.

Rosenbaum and coworkers[3] described the concept of blocks in the fascicles of the LBB, which they termed "left anterior and left posterior hemiblock." However, these two kinds of block are more appropriately termed *left anterior fascicular block* (LAFB) and *left posterior fascicular block* (LPFB). Isolated LAFB, LPFB, or RBBB is considered *unifascicular* block. Complete LBBB or combinations of RBBB with LAFB or with LPFB are *bifascicular blocks,* and the combination of RBBB with both LAFB and LPFB is considered *trifascicular block.*

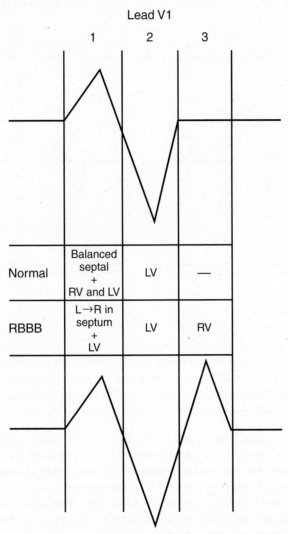

FIGURE 6.5. The contributions from activation of the interventricular septum and the right- and left-ventricular free walls to the appearance of the QRS complex in lead V1, with normal intraventricular conduction **(top)** and with RBBB **(bottom)**. The numbers refer to the first, second, and third sequential 0.04-second periods of time. Only two 0.04-second periods are required for normal conduction, but a third is required when RBBB is present. LV, left ventricle; RBBB, right bundle branch block; RV, right ventricle..

The term *unifascicular block* is used when there is ECG evidence of blockage of only the RBB, LAF, or LPF. Isolated RBBB or LAFB occur commonly, whereas isolated LPFB is rare. Rosenbaum and coworkers[3] identified only 30 patients with LPFB, as compared with 900 patients with LAFB.

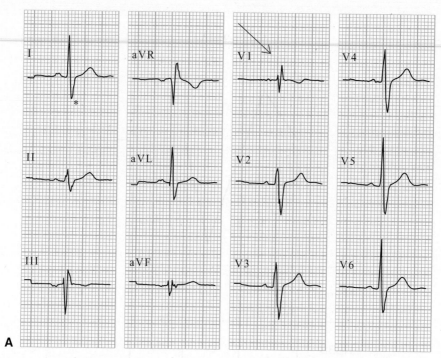

A

FIGURE 6.6. Twelve-lead ECGs from a 17-year-old girl with an ostium secundum atrial septal defect **(A)**, an 81-year-old woman with fibrosis of the RBB **(B)**, and an 82-year-old man with fibrosis of both the RBB and the anterior fascicle of the LBB **(C)**. *Arrows* in **A**, **B**, and **C** indicate the prominent terminal R′ wave in V1, and asterisks in **A** and **C** indicate the rightward and leftward axis shifts, respectively.

Because the right ventricle contributes minimally to the normal QRS complex, RBBB produces little distortion of the QRS complex during the time required for left-ventricular activation. Figure 6.5 illustrates the minimal distortion of the early portion and marked distortion of the late portion of the QRS complex (in lead V1) that typically occurs with RBBB. The activation sequence of the interventricular septum and the right- and left-ventricular free walls contribute to the appearance of the QRS complex in lead V1 (see Fig. 6.5). Normal intraventricular conduction requires only two sequential 0.04-second periods, whereas a third is required when RBBB is present. The minimal contribution of the normal right-ventricular myocardium is completely subtracted from the early portion of the QRS complex and then added later, when the right ventricle is activated after the spread of impulses from the left ventricle through the interventricular septum to the right ventricle. This produces a late prominent positive wave in lead V1 termed R′ because it follows the earlier positive R wave produced by the normal left-to-right spread of activation through the interventricular septum (see Fig. 6.5; Table 6.1).

Table 6.1.

Criteria for Right-Bundle-Branch Block

QRS duration ≥ 0.12 s	
Lead V1	Late intrinsicoid (R′ peak or late R peak), M-shaped QRS (RSR′); sometimes wide R or qR
Lead V6	Early intrinsicoid (R peak), wide S wave
Lead I	Wide S wave

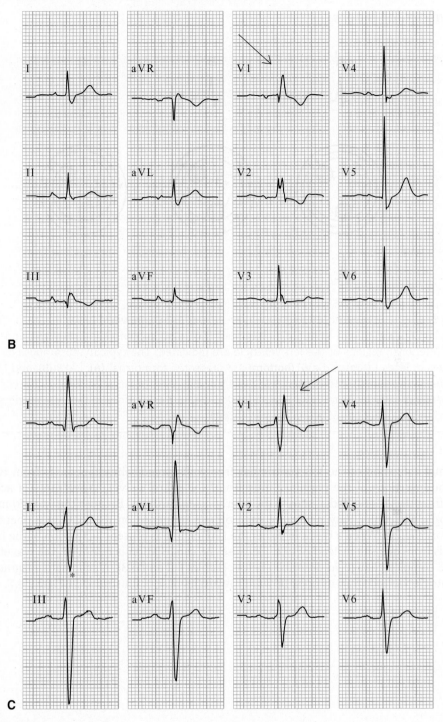

FIGURE 6.6. *(continued)*

RBBB has many variations in its ECG appearance (Fig. 6.6A–C). In Figure 6.6A, the RBBB is considered "incomplete" because the duration of the QRS complex is only 0.10 second; but in Figure 6.6B and C, the RBBB is considered "complete" because the duration of the QRS complex is ≥0.12 second.

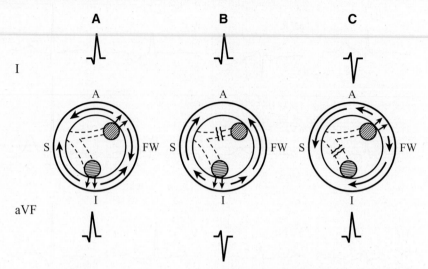

FIGURE 6.7. Schematic left ventricle viewed from its apex upward toward its base. The interventricular septum (S), left-ventricular free wall (FW; also known as lateral wall), and anterior (A) and inferior (I) regions of the left ventricle are indicated. The typical appearances of the QRS complexes in leads I **(top)** and aVF **(bottom)** are presented for normal **(A)**, LAFB **(B)**, and LPFB left-ventricular activation **(C)**. *Dashed lines*, fascicles; *wavy lines*, sites of fascicular block; *small crosshatched circles*, papillary muscles; *outer rings*, endocardial and epicardial surface of the left-ventricular myocardium; *arrows*, directions of activation wavefronts.

Normal activation of the left-ventricular free wall spreads simultaneously from two sites (near the insertions of the papillary muscles of the mitral valve). Wavefronts of activation spread from these endocardial sites to the overlying epicardium. Because the wavefronts travel in opposite directions, they neutralize each other's influence on the ECG in a phenomenon called *cancellation*. When a block in either the LAF or LPF is present, activation of the free wall proceeds from one site instead of two. Because the cancellation is removed, the waveforms of the QRS complex change, as described below (Tables 6.2 and 6.3). A schematic diagram of the left ventricle viewed from its apex upward toward its base is illustrated in Figure 6.7.

Table 6.2.

Criteria for Left Anterior Fascicular Block

1. Left-axis deviation (usually ≥–60 degrees)
2. Small Q in leads I and aVL; small R in II, III, and aVF
3. Minimal QRS prolongation (0.020 s) from baseline
4. Late intrinsicoid (R wave peak) deflection in aVL (>0.045 s)
5. Increased QRS voltage in limb leads

Table 6.3.

Criteria for Left Posterior Fascicular Block

1. Right-axis deviation (usually ≥+120 degrees)
2. Small R in leads I and aVL; small Q in II, III, and aVF
3. Usually normal QRS duration
4. Late intrinsicoid deflection in aVF (>0.045 s)
5. Increased QRS voltage in limb leads
6. No evidence of RVH

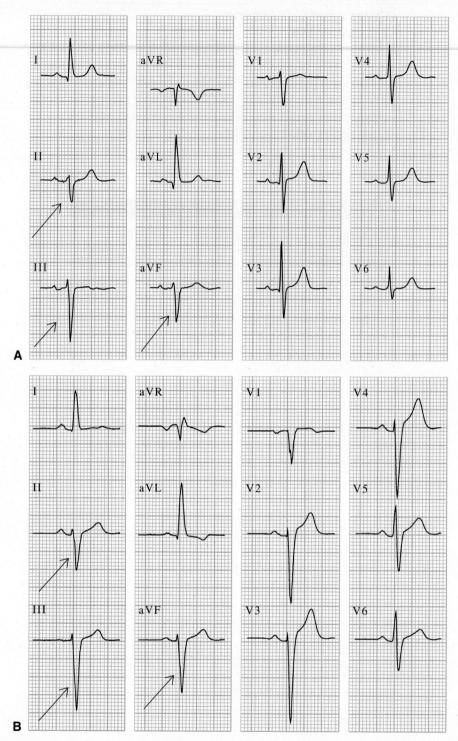

FIGURE 6.8. Twelve-lead ECGs from a 53-year-old woman with no medical problems **(A)** and a 75-year-old man with a long history of poorly treated hypertension **(B)**. *Arrows* indicate the deep S waves in leads II, III, and aVF that reflect extreme left-axis deviation.

If the LAF of the LBB is blocked (see Fig. 6.7B), the initial activation of the left-ventricular free wall occurs via the LPF. Activation spreading from endocardium to the epicardium in this region is directed inferiorly and rightward. Because the block in the LAF has removed the initial superior and leftward activation, a Q wave appears in leads that have their positive electrodes in a superior-leftward position (i.e., lead I) and an R wave appears in leads that have their positive electrodes in an inferior-rightward position (i.e., lead aVF) (see Fig. 6.8). Following this initial period, the activation wave spreads over the remainder of the left-ventricular free wall in a superior-leftward direction, producing a prominent R wave in lead I and a prominent S wave in lead aVF. This change in the left-ventricular activation sequence produces a leftward shift of the axis of the QRS complex to at least −45 degrees. The overall duration of the QRS complex may be within the normal range but is usually prolonged by 0.02 second from the patient's baseline.[4]

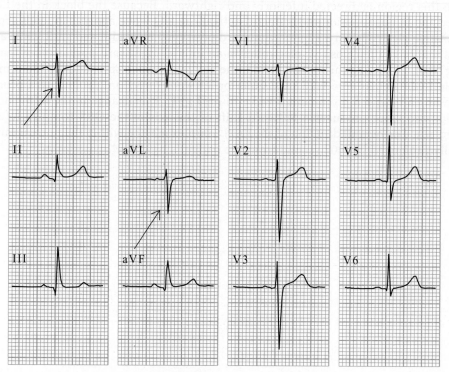

FIGURE 6.9. ECG of an asymptomatic individual shows deep S waves in leads I and aVL, typical of both LPFB and RVH (*arrows*).

If the LPF of the LBB is blocked (see Fig. 6.7C), the situation is reversed from that in LAF block, and the initial activation of the left-ventricular free wall occurs via the LAF. Activation spreading from the endocardium to the epicardium in this region is directed superiorly and leftward. Because the block in the LPF has removed the initial inferior and rightward activation, a Q wave appears in leads with their positive electrodes in an inferior-rightward position (i.e., lead aVF) and an R wave appears in leads with their positive electrodes in a superior-leftward direction (i.e., lead I). Following this initial period, the activation spreads over the remainder of the left-ventricular free wall in an inferior/ rightward direction, producing a prominent R wave in lead aVF and a prominent S wave in lead I. This change in the left-ventricular activation sequence produces a rightward shift of the axis of the QRS complex to $\geq +90$ degrees.[5] The duration of the QRS complex may be normal or slightly prolonged (Fig. 6.9).

The consideration that LPFB may be present requires that there be no evidence of right-ventricular hypertrophy (RVH) from either the precordial leads (see Fig. 6.9) or from other clinical data. However, even the absence of RVH does not allow diagnosis of LPFB because RVH can produce the same pattern as LPFB in the limb leads and RVH is much more common than LPFB.

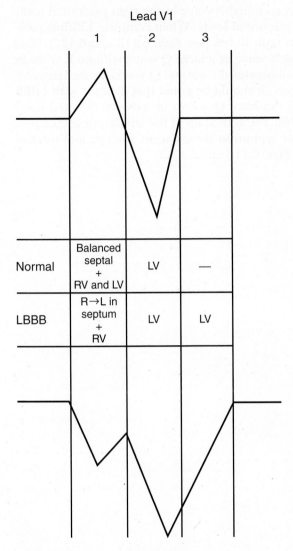

FIGURE 6.10. Contributors to the QRS complex in lead V1. **Top**. Normal intraventricular conduction. **Bottom**. LBBB. The numbers refer to the first, second, and third sequential 0.04-second periods of time. LBBB, left-bundle-branch block; LV, left ventricle; RV, right ventricle.

The term *bifascicular block* is used when there is ECG evidence of involvement of any two of the RBBB, LAF, or LPF. Such evidence may appear at different times or may coexist on the same ECG. Bifascicular block is sometimes applied to complete LBBB and is commonly applied to the combination of RBBB with either LAFB or LPFB. The combination of RBBB with LAFB can be caused by a large anteroseptal infarct. The term *bilateral bundle-branch block* is also appropriate when RBBB and either LAFB or LPFB are present.[6] When there is bifascicular block, the duration of the QRS complex is prolonged to ≥0.12 second.

Left-Bundle-Branch Block

Figure 6.10 illustrates the QRS complex distortion produced by LBBB in lead V1. It also identifies the various contributions from ventricular myocardium to the appearances of the QRS complex. Complete LBBB may be caused by disease in either the main LBB (*predivisional*) or in both of its fascicles (*postdivisional*). When the impulse cannot progress along the LBB, electrical activation must first occur in the right ventricle and then travel through the interventricular septum to the left ventricle.

Figure 6.11 shows the electrical activation in normal activation (A) and in the presence of LBBB (B). In normal activation, the interventricular septum is activated from left to right (see Figs. 6.11A and 6.12A), producing an initial R wave in the right precordial leads and a Q wave in leads I, aVL, and the left precordial leads. When complete LBBB is present, however, the septum is activated from right to left (see Figs. 6.11B and 6.12C). This produces a small R wave followed by a large S wave or a large Q wave with no R wave in the right precordial leads (V1 and V2) and eliminates the normal Q waves in the leftward-oriented leads (leads V5-V6, I, aVL). However, it should be noted that patients with LBBB and an anterior myocardial infarction (MI) can have Q waves in leftward-oriented leads even with LBBB (see Chapter 12, Fig. 12.17B). The activation of the left ventricle then proceeds sequentially from the interventricular septum to the adjacent anterior and inferior walls, and then to the lateral free wall (see Figs. 6.11B and 6.12C).

A **Normal Conduction**

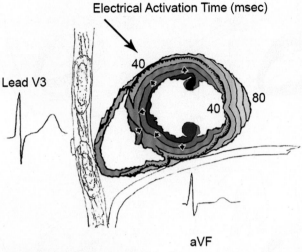

B **Left Bundle Branch Block**

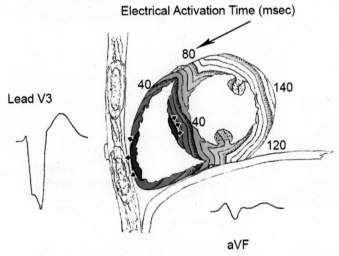

FIGURE 6.11.   Ventricular activation in normal **(A)** and complete LBBB **(B)** activation. For reference, 2 QRS-T waveforms are shown in their anatomic locations in each image. Electrical activation starts at the *small arrows* and spreads in a wave front, with each *colored line* representing successive 0.01 second. Comparing **A** and **B** reveals the difference between normal and complete LBBB activation. In normal activation **(A)**, activation begins within the left- and right-ventricular endocardium. In complete LBBB **(B)**, activation only begins in the right ventricle and must proceed through the septum for 0.04 to 0.05 second before reaching the LV endocardium. It then requires another 0.05 second for reentry into the left-ventricular Purkinje network and to propagate to the endocardium of the lateral wall. It then requires another 0.05 second to activate the lateral wall, producing a total QRS duration of 0.14 to 0.15 second. Any increase in septal or lateral wall thickness or left-ventricular endocardial surface area further increases QRS duration. Because the propagation velocity in human myocardium is 3 to 4 mm per 0.1 second, a circumferential increase in left-ventricular wall thickness by 3 mm will increase total QRS duration by 0.02 second in LBBB (0.1 seconds for the septum and 0.1 second for the lateral wall). Reprinted with permission from Strauss et al. ECG quantification of myocardial scar in cardiomyopathy patients with or without conduction defects: correlation with cardiac magnetic resonance and arrhythmogenesis. *Circ Arrhythm Electrophysiol.* 2008;1:327–336.

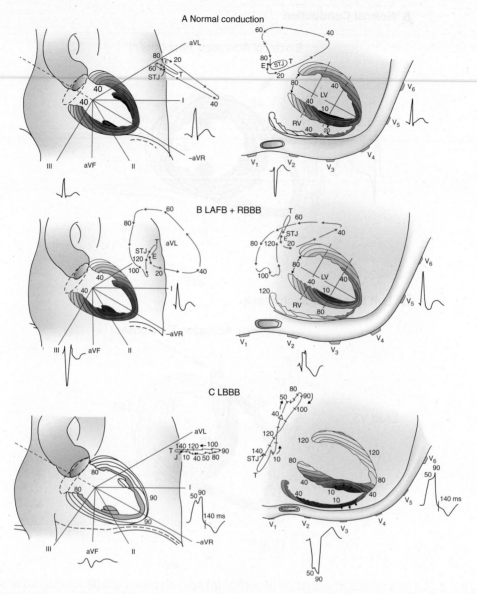

FIGURE 6.12. Ventricular activation sequence, vector loops, and ECG waveforms in the frontal and transverse planes. The frontal and transverse planes are shown in normal conduction **(A)**, left anterior fascicular block (LAFB) and right-bundle-branch block (RBBB) **(B)**, and left-bundle-branch block (LBBB) **(C)**. *Colored lines* represent areas of myocardium activated within the same 10-millisecond period *(isochrones)*. *Numbers* represent milliseconds since beginning of activation. (Modified from Strauss DG, Selvester RH. The QRS complex—a biomarker that "images" the heart: QRS scores to quantify myocardial scar in the presence of normal and abnormal ventricular conduction. *J Electrocardiol.* 2009;42:85–96, with permission. Copyright 2009, Elsevier.)

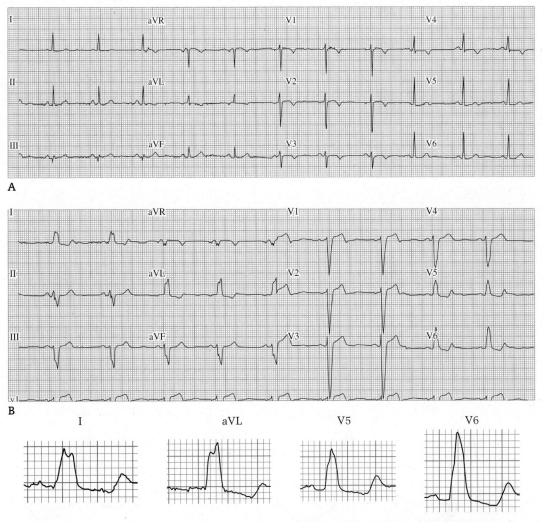

FIGURE 6.13. ECGs from an 82-year-old woman with a sudden increase in QRS duration from 0.076 seconds **(A)** to 0.148 seconds **(B)** 1 year later (a 95% increase) with the development of complete LBBB. In addition to the increase in QRS duration, notice the change in QRS morphology that includes distinctive mid-QRS notching in leads I and aVL, along with mid-QRS slurring in leads V5 and V6. Reproduced with permission from Strauss et al. *Am J Cardiol.* 2011;107(6):927–934.

A critical component of diagnosing LBBB on the ECG is the presence of mid-QRS notching/slurring in frontward-backward leads (V1 and V2) or leftward-rightward leads (V5, V6, I, and aVL) as shown in activation sequence Figures 6.11B and 6.12C. Figure 6.13 shows ECGs from an 82-year-old woman before (A) and after (B) the development of LBBB. Notice that QRS duration increases from 0.76 to 0.148 second with the development of LBBB. In addition to the increase in QRS duration, notice the change in QRS morphology that includes distinctive mid-QRS notching in leads I and aVL, along with mid-QRS slurring in leads V5 and V6. Figure 6.14 shows another example of a patient who has a sudden QRS prolongation due to LBBB with the appearance of clear mid-QRS notching/slurring. This is in contrast to the ECGs in Figure 5.11 where the patient developed progressive left-ventricular hypertrophy with QRS duration of 0.142 second, but no mid-QRS notching/slurring.

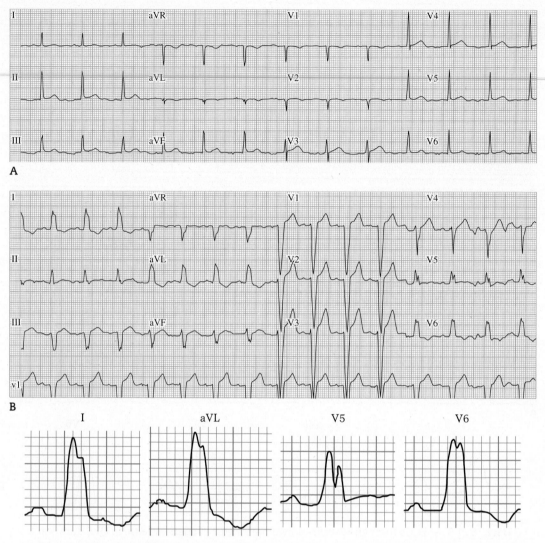

FIGURE 6.14. ECGs from a 75-year-old woman with a sudden increase in QRS duration from 0.092 second **(A)** to 0.156 second **(B)** in 6 months (a 70% increase) with the development of complete LBBB. The patient developed distinctive mid-QRS notching in leads I, aVL, V5, and V6. (Reproduced from Strauss DG, Selvester RH, Wagner GS. Defining left bundle branch block in the era of cardiac resynchronization therapy. Am J Cardiol. 2011;107(6):927–934, with permission.)

Table 6.4 contains "conventional" criteria for LBBB that consists primarily of a QRS duration ≥0.12 second and a leftward conduction delay (QS or rS) in lead V1. However, simulation and endocardial mapping research has demonstrated that approximately 1 of 3 patients diagnosed with LBBB by conventional criteria do not have activation consistent with LBBB.[7] Table 6.5 contains "strict" criteria for LBBB that requires QRS duration ≥0.13 second in women and QRS duration ≥0.14 seconds in men; a QS or rS in V1; and mid-QRS notching/slurring in two of the leads I, aVL, V1, V2, V5, or V6.[7]

Table 6.4.

Conventional Criteria for Left-Bundle-Branch Block

Lead V1	QS or rS
Lead V6	Late intrinsicoid (R or R′ peak), no Q waves, monophasic R
Lead I	Monophasic R wave, no Q

Table 6.5.

Strict Criteria for Left-Bundle-Branch Block

QRS duration	≥0.13 s in women or ≥0.14 s in men
Lead V1	QS or rS
Mid-QRS notching/slurring in two of the leads I, aVL, V1, V2, V5, or V6	

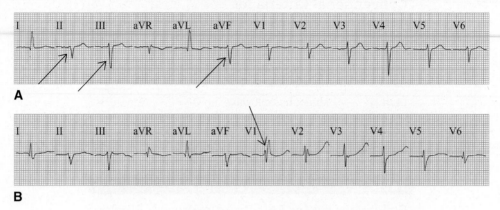

A

B

FIGURE 6.15. **A.** Deep S waves characteristic of LAFB *(arrows)*. **B.** Prominent R' wave characteristic of RBBB *(arrow)*.

Just as LAFB appears as a unifascicular block much more commonly than does LPFB, it more commonly accompanies RBBB as a bifascicular block. The combination of RBBB and LAFB is commonly a sign of a large anteroseptal infarct because the RBB and LAF are perfused by the same coronary artery (see Chapter 12).[8] Figure 6.12B shows the ventricular activation sequence and corresponding QRST waveforms in the presence of RBBB plus LAFB. The diagnosis of LAFB plus RBBB is made by observing the late prominent R or R' wave in precordial lead V1 of RBBB, and the initial R waves and prominent S waves in limb leads II, III, and aVF of LAFB. The duration of the QRS complex should be ≥0.12 second and the frontal plane axis of the complex should be between −45 degrees and −120 degrees (Fig. 6.15). In a 12-lead ECG from a 1-year previous examination (see Fig. 6.15A), only LAFB (deep S waves in II, III, and aVF) is present. In a current ECG evaluation of the same patient (see Fig. 6.15B), the presence of RBBB (prominent R' wave in V1) indicates that a second fascicle has been blocked.

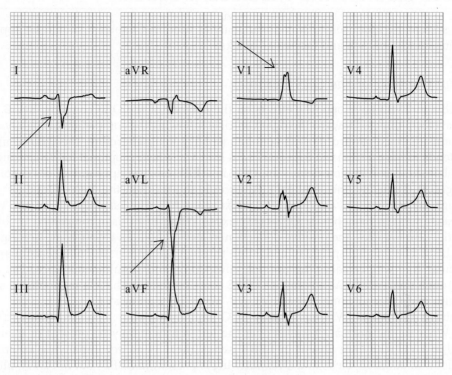

FIGURE 6.16. Right-bundle-branch block with LPFB. *Arrows,* prominent S waves (I and aVL) and RR′ complex (V1).

The example of bifascicular block consisting of RBBB with LPFB rarely occurs. Even when changes in the ECG are entirely typical of this combination, the diagnosis should be considered only if there is no clinical evidence of RVH. The diagnosis of RBBB with LPFB should be considered when precordial lead V1 shows changes typical of RBBB and limb leads I and aVL show the initial R waves and prominent S waves typical of LPFB. The duration of the QRS complex should be ≥0.12 second, and the frontal plane axis of the complex should be ≥+90 degrees (Fig. 6.16).[9]

SYSTEMATIC APPROACH TO THE ANALYSIS OF BUNDLE-BRANCH AND FASCICULAR BLOCKS

The systematic approach to waveform analysis used in Chapter 3 should be applied in analyzing bundle-branch and fascicular blocks.

General Contour of the QRS Complex

RBBB and LBBB have opposite effects on the contour of the QRS complex. RBBB adds a new waveform directed toward the right ventricle following the completion of slightly altered waveforms directed toward the left ventricle (see Fig. 6.5). Therefore, the QRS complex in RBBB tends to have a triphasic appearance. In lead V1, which is optimal for visualizing right-versus left-sided conduction delay, the QRS in RBBB has the appearance of "rabbit ears" (see Fig. 6.6). Typically, the "first ear" (R wave) is shorter than the "second ear" (R' wave). (Although the term "rabbit ears" in this context refers to a triphasic QRS, it can also refer to two peaks found in monophasic QRS complexes.) When RBBB is accompanied by block in one of the LBB fascicles, the positive deflection in lead V1 is often monophasic (see Fig. 6.16).

In LBBB, a sequential spread of activation through the interventricular septum and left-ventricular free wall replaces the normal, competing, and simultaneous spread of activation through these areas. As a result, the QRS complex tends to have a monophasic appearance with mid-QRS notching in leads V1, V2, V5, V6, I, and/or aVL.

Although LBBB and LVH have many ECG similarities, they also show marked differences. Whereas the normal Q waves over the left ventricle may be present or even exaggerated in LVH, they are absent in LBBB (when there is no accompanying anteroapical infarction). In addition, clear mid-QRS notching is present in LBBB, but not LVH, although LVH and apical MI could cause mid-QRS notching, mimicking LBBB.

QRS Complex Duration

Complete RBBB usually increases the duration of the QRS complex by ≥ 0.04 second, and complete LBBB increases the duration of the complex by ≥ 0.06 second. Block within the LAF or LPF of the LBB usually prolongs the duration of the QRS complex by approximately 0.02 second (see Figs. 6.8B and 6.9).[4]

Positive and Negative Amplitudes

BBB produces QRS waveforms with lower voltage and more definite notching than those that occur with ventricular hypertrophy. However, the amplitude of the QRS complex does increase in LBBB because of the relatively unopposed spread of activation over the left ventricle.

One general rule for differentiating between LBBB and LVH is that the greater the amplitude of the QRS complex, the more likely is LVH to be the cause of this. Similarly, the more prolonged is the duration of the QRS complex, the more likely is LBBB to be the cause of this effect. Klein and colleagues[10] have suggested that in the presence of LBBB, either of the following criteria are associated with LVH:

1. S wave in V2 + R wave in V6 >45 mm.
2. Evidence of left-atrial enlargement with a QRS complex duration >0.16 second.

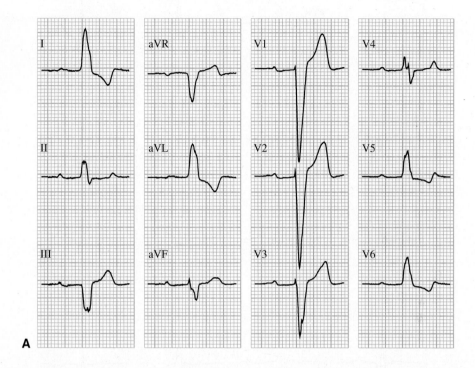

FIGURE 6.17. **A.** An 89-year-old woman during a routine health evaluation. **B.** A 45-year-old pilot during an annual health evaluation. **C.** A 64-year-old woman on the first day after coronary bypass surgery. *Arrows,* concordant directions of the terminal QRS complex and T wave in leads V2 to V4.

Because complete RBBB and complete LBBB alter conduction to entire ventricles, they might not be expected to produce much net alteration of the frontal plane QRS axis. However, Rosenbaum et al[3] studied patients with intermittent LBBB in which blocked and unblocked complexes could be examined side by side. LBBB was often observed to produce a significant left-axis shift and sometimes even a right-axis shift. The axis was unchanged in only a minority of patients.

However, block in either the LAF or LPF of the LBB alone produces marked axis deviation. The initial 0.20 second of the QRS complex is directed away from the blocked fascicles, and the middle and late portions are directed toward the blocked fascicles, causing the overall direction of the QRS complex to be shifted toward the site of the block (see Figs. 6.8 and 6.9).[2] When block in either of these LBB fascicles is accompanied by RBBB, an even later waveform is added to the QRS complex, thereby further prolonging its duration. The direction of this final waveform in the frontal plane is in the vicinity of 180 degrees, as a result of the RBBB (see Fig. 6.6C).[2]

In BBB, the T wave is usually directed opposite to the latter portion of the QRS complex (e.g., in Fig. 6.17A, the T wave in lead I is inverted and the latter part of the QRS complex is upright; in Fig. 6.17B, the T wave is upright and the latter part of the QRS complex is negative). This opposite polarity is the natural result of the depolarization–repolarization disturbance produced by the BBB and is therefore termed *"secondary."* Indeed, if the direction of the T wave is similar to that of the terminal part of the QRS complex (see Fig. 6.17C), it should be considered abnormal. Such T-wave changes are *primary* and imply myocardial disease. The diagnosis of MI in the presence of BBB is considered in Chapter 12.

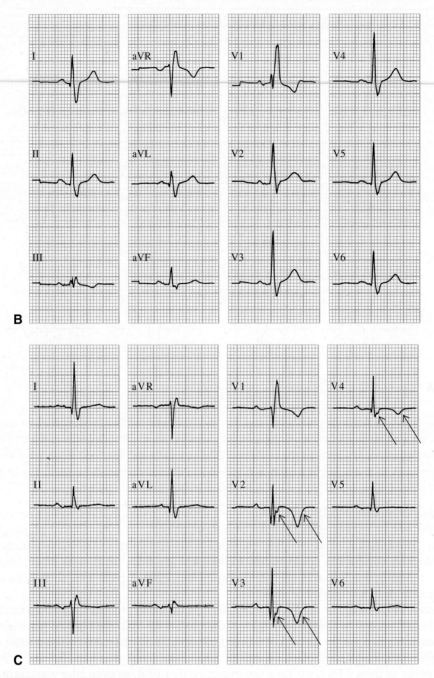

FIGURE 6.17. *(continued)*

One method of determining the clinical significance of T-wave changes in BBB is to measure the angle between the axis of the T wave and that of the terminal part of the QRS complex. Obviously, if the two are oppositely directed (as they are with secondary T-wave changes), the angle between them is wide and may approach 180 degrees. It has been proposed that if this angle is <110 degrees, myocardial disease is present. In Figure 6.17B, the angle is about 150 degrees, whereas in Figure 6.17C it is only a few degrees.

CLINICAL PERSPECTIVE ON INTRAVENTRICULAR-CONDUCTION DISTURBANCES

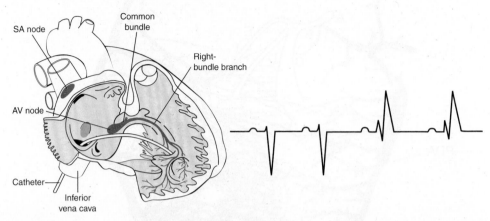

FIGURE 6.18. RBBB is induced by trauma to the RBB. A catheter has been advanced from the leg via the inferior vena cava, and its tip lies against the right-ventricular endocardium in the vicinity of the RBB. The resultant RBBB is illustrated in the third and fourth beats of the schematic lead V1 ECG recording. AV, atrioventricular; SA, sinoatrial. (*The CIBA Collection of Medical Illustrations. Vol 5. Heart.* Summit, NJ: CIBA-Geigy; 1978:13, with permission.)

Both RBBB and LBBB are often seen in apparently normal individuals.[11] The cause of this is *fibrosis* of the Purkinje fibers, which has been described as *Lenegre disease*[12] or *Lev disease*.[13] The process of Purkinje fibrosis progresses slowly: a 10-year follow-up study of healthy aviators with BBB revealed no incidence of complete *AV block, syncope,* or sudden death.[14] The pathologic process may be accelerated by systemic hypertension; it preceded the appearance of BBB in 60% of the individuals in the Framingham study. The mean age of onset of the BBB was 61 years.[15]

Insight into the long-term prognosis for individuals with chronic BBB but no other evidence of cardiac disease comes from studies of the ECG changes preceding the development of transient or permanent complete AV block. Lasser and associates[16] documented the common presence of some combination of bundle-branch or fascicular block immediately before onset of the AV block. The most common combination was RBBB with LAFB.

The combined results of these studies suggest that Lenegre or Lev disease is a slowly developing process of fibrosis of the Purkinje fibers that has the ultimate potential of causing complete AV block because of bilateral bundle branch involvement. Because the Purkinje cells lack the physiologic capacity of the AV nodal cells to conduct at varying speeds, a sudden progression from no AV block to complete AV block may occur.[17] When this does occur, ventricular activation can result only from impulse formation within a Purkinje cell beyond the site of the block. Several clinical conditions may result, including syncope and sudden death.

Bundle-branch or fascicular block may also be the result of other serious cardiac diseases. In Central and South America, *Chagas disease*, produced by infection with *Trypanosoma cruzi*, is almost endemic and is a common cause of RBBB with LAFB.[18] As indicated in Chapter 5, RBBB is commonly produced by the distention of the right ventricle that occurs with volume overloading. Transient RBBB may be produced during right heart catheterization as a result of catheter-tip–induced trauma (Fig. 6.18). The resultant RBBB is displayed in the third and fourth beats of the schematic lead V1 recording.

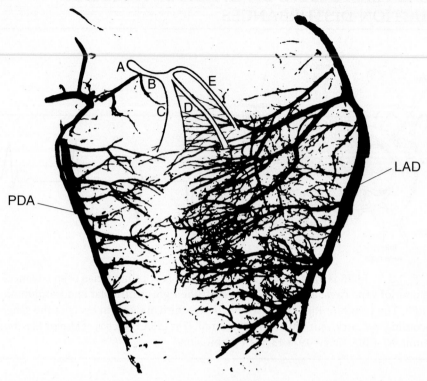

FIGURE 6.19. The proximal portion of specialized conduction system is shown in relation to its blood supply from a right anterior oblique view: **(A)**, AV node; **(B)**, Common bundle; **(C)**, LPF; **(D)**, LAF; **(E)**, RBB. LAD, left anterior descending artery; PDA, posterior descending artery. (From Rotman M, Wagner GS, Wallace AG. Bradyarrhythmias in acute myocardial infarction. *Circulation.* 1972;45:703–722, with permission. Copyright 1972, American Heart Association.)

Conventional teaching prescribes that new-onset LBBB or RBBB that occurs with acute MI is associated with massive MIs.[19] However, pathology studies have demonstrated that the proximal left anterior descending coronary artery septal perforators perfuse the RBB and left anterior fascicle of the LBB in 90% of cases, whereas the right coronary artery (via the AV nodal artery) perfuses the posterior fascicle of the LBB in 90% of cases, and there is dual blood supply to each of these fascicles in 40% to 50% of cases.[8] Thus, proximal LAD occlusions could cause RBBB and/or LAFB; however, both proximal LAD and right coronary artery occlusions would be required for MIs to be the direct cause of LBBB in 90% of patients. See Figure 6.19 for a schematic of the relationship between the fascicles and coronary arteries. Of note, histopathology studies have found that interruption of the LBB almost always occurs at its junction with the main bundle where the LBB can be compressed between connective tissue at the base of the ventricular septum.[20-22] This likely occurs more frequently when the ventricles are subjected to mechanical strain from hypertrophy or dilatation.

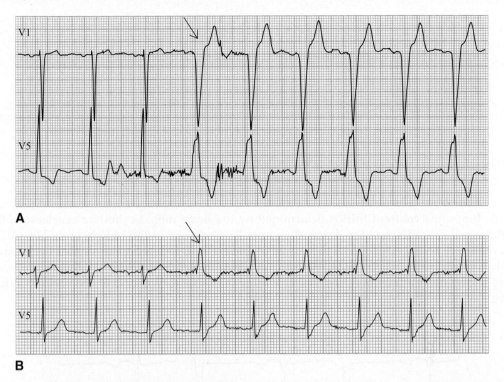

FIGURE 6.20. Precordial leads V1 and V5 are shown from a 62-year-old woman during routine ECG monitoring after uncomplicated abdominal surgery **(A)** and a 54-year-old man during 24-hour ECG monitoring for a complaint of dizziness **(B)**. *Arrows* indicate the onsets in the V1 leads of typically appearing LBBB in **A** and RBBB in **B**.

Intermittent BBB (prolonged QRS complexes present at some times but not at others) usually represents a transition stage before permanent block is established. Figure 6.20 shows an example of sudden onset LBBB from a 62-year-old woman during routine ECG monitoring after uncomplicated abdominal surgery (see Fig. 6.20A) and sudden onset RBBB from a 54-year-old man during 24-hour ECG monitoring for a complaint of dizziness (see Fig. 6.20B).

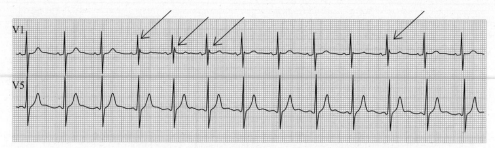

FIGURE 6.21. Appearance of tachycardia-dependent incomplete RBBB *(arrows)*.

At times, intermittent BBB is determined by the heart rate. As the rate accelerates, the *RR interval* shortens, and the descending impulse finds one of the bundle branches still in its *refractory period*. The appearance of incomplete RBBB following the shorter cycle intervals is illustrated in Figure 6.21. With this *tachycardia-dependent BBB*, slowing of the heart rate allows descending impulses to arrive after the refractory period of the entire conduction system, and normal conduction is resumed.

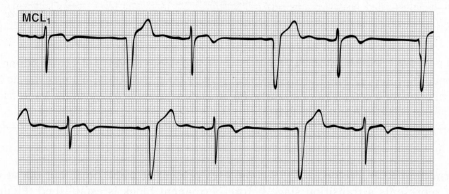

FIGURE 6.22. Bradycardia-dependent BBB.

A rarer form of intermittent BBB, which develops only when the cardiac cycle lengthens rather than shortens, is termed *bradycardia-dependent BBB*. All beats are conducted sinus beats grouped in pairs. Those ending the shorter cycles are conducted normally, whereas those ending the longer cycles are conducted with LBBB (Fig. 6.22). Intermittent BBB is a form of intermittent aberrant conduction of electrical impulses through the ventricular myocardium.

GLOSSARY

Atherosclerosis: a thickening of the inner arterial wall caused by the deposition of fatty substances.

AV block: a block in the cardiac conduction system that causes a disruption of atrial-to-ventricular electrical conduction.

Bifascicular block: an intraventricular conduction abnormality involving any two of the RBB, the anterior division of the LBB, and the posterior division of the LBB.

Bilateral bundle-branch block: an intraventricular conduction abnormality involving both the right and left bundle branches, as indicated either by the presence of some conducted beats with RBBB and others with LBBB, or by AV block located distal to the common bundle.

Bradycardia-dependent BBB: RBBB or LBBB that is intermittent, appearing only with a slowing of the atrial rate.

Cancellation: elimination of an abnormality produced by a particular cardiac problem by a similar abnormality in another part of the heart or by a different abnormality in the same part of the heart, because the ECG waveforms represent the summation of the wavefronts of activation and recovery within the heart.

Chagas disease: a tropical disease caused by the flagellate organism *Trypanosoma cruzi,* which is marked by prolonged high fever, edema, and enlargement of the spleen, liver, and lymph nodes and is complicated by cardiac involvement.

Fascicle: a group of Purkinje fibers too small to be called a "branch."

Fibrosis: a condition in which Purkinje fibers are transformed into nonconducting interstitial fibrous tissue.

Left anterior fascicular block: a conduction abnormality in the anterior fascicle of the LBB.

Left posterior fascicular block: a conduction abnormality in the posterior fascicle of the LBB.

Lenegre (Lev) disease: both Lenegre and Lev described variations of fibrosis of the intraventricular Purkinje fibers in the absence of other significant cardiac disease.

Predivisional and postdivisional: terms referring to block within the LBB either "pre-" or proximal to its division into fascicles, or "post-" and involving both the anterior and posterior fascicles.

Primary and secondary T-wave changes: in the presence of RBBB or LBBB, the term *primary T-wave changes* refers to abnormal T waves that are directed similarly to the latter portion of the QRS complex, and *secondary T-wave changes* refers to normal T waves that are directed opposite to the latter portion of the QRS complex.

Refractory period: the period following electrical activation during which a cardiac cell cannot be reactivated.

RR interval: the period between successive QRS complexes.

Septal Q wave: a normal, initially negative QRS waveform that appears in leftward-oriented ECG leads because of earliest activation of the interventricular septum via the septal fascicles of the LBB.

Syncope: a brief loss of consciousness associated with transient lack of cerebral blood flow.

Tachycardia-dependent BBB: RBBB or LBBB that is intermittent, appearing only with an acceleration of the atrial rate.

Trifascicular block: an intraventricular conduction abnormality involving the RBB and both the anterior and posterior fascicles of the LBB.

Unifascicular block: an intraventricular conduction abnormality involving only one of the three principal fascicles of the intraventricular Purkinje system.

References

1. Wellens HJJ, Lie KI, Janse MJ, eds. *The Conduction System of the Heart: Structure, Function and Clinical Implications.* The Hague, The Netherlands: Martinus Nijhoff; 1978.
2. Demoulin JC, Kulbertus HE. Histopathological examination of concept of left hemiblock. *Br Heart J.* 1972;34:807–814.
3. Rosenbaum MB, Elizari MV, Lazzari JO. *The Hemiblocks.* Oldsmar, FL: Tampa Tracings; 1970.
4. Loring Z, Chelliah S, Selvester RH, et al. A detailed guide for quantification of myocardial scar with the selvester qrs score in the presence of electrocardiogram

confounders. *J Electrocardiol*. 2011;44: 544–554.

5. Eriksson P, Hansson PO, Eriksson H, et al. Bundle-branch block in a general male population: the study of men born 1913. *Circulation*. 1998;98:2494–2500.

6. Hindman MC, Wagner GS, JaRo M, et al. The clinical significance of bundle branch block complicating acute myocardial infarction. 2. Indications for temporary and permanent pacemaker insertion. *Circulation*. 1978;58:689–699.

7. Strauss DG, Selvester RH, Wagner GS. Defining left bundle branch block in the era of cardiac resynchronization therapy. *Am J Cardiol*. 2011;107(6):927–934.

8. Frink RJ, James TN. Normal blood supply to the human his bundle and proximal bundle branches. *Circulation*. 1973;47:8–18.

9. Willems JL, Robles de Medina EO, Bernard R, et al. Criteria for intraventricular conduction disturbances and pre-excitation. World Health Organization/International Society and Federation for Cardiology Task Force Ad Hoc *J Am Coll Cardiol*. 1985;5:1261–1275.

10. Klein RC, Vera Z, DeMaria AN, et al. Electrocardiographic diagnosis of left ventricular hypertrophy in the presence of left bundle branch block. *Am Heart J*. 1984;108:502–506.

11. Hiss RG, Lamb LE. Electrocardiographic findings in 122,043 individuals. *Circulation*. 1962;25:947–961.

12. Lenegre J. Etiology and pathology of bilateral bundle branch block in relation to complete heart block. *Prog Cardiovasc Dis*. 1964;6:409–444.

13. Lev M. Anatomic basis for atrioventricular block. *Am J Med*. 1964;37:742–748.

14. Rotman M, Triebwasser JH. A clinical and follow-up study of right and left bundle branch block. *Circulation*. 1975;51: 477–484.

15. Schneider JF, Thomas HE Jr, McNamara PM, et al. Clinical-electrocardiographic correlates of newly acquired left bundle branch block: the framingham study. *Am J Cardiol*. 1985;55: 1332–1338.

16. Lasser RP, Haft JI, Friedberg CK. Relationship of right bundle-branch block and marked left axis deviation (with left parietal or peri-infarction block) to complete heart block and syncope. *Circulation*. 1968;37:429–437.

17. Pick A, Langendorf R. *Interpretation of Complex Arrhythmias*. Philadelphia, PA: Lea & Febiger; 1979.

18. Acquatella H, Catalioti F, Gomez-Mancebo JR, et al. Long-term control of Chagas disease in Venezuela: effects on serologic findings, electrocardiographic abnormalities, and clinical outcome. *Circulation*. 1987;76:556–562.

19. Neeland IJ, Kontos MC, de Lemos JA. Evolving considerations in the management of patients with left bundle branch block and suspected myocardial infarction. *J Am Coll Cardiol*. 2012;60:96–105.

20. Lenegre J. *Contribution à l'etude des blocs de branche*. Paris, France: JB Bailliere et Fils; 1958.

21. Lev M, Unger PN, Rosen KM, et al. The anatomic substrate of complete left bundle branch block. *Circulation*. 1974;50: 479–486.

22. Sugiura M, Okada R, Okawa S, et al. Pathohistological studies on the conduction system in 8 cases of complete left bundle branch block. *Jpn Heart J*. 1970;11:5–16.

7

Ventricular Preexcitation

GALEN S. WAGNER

HISTORICAL PERSPECTIVE

In the normal heart, there are no muscular connections between the atria and ventricles. In 1893, Kent[1] described the rare occurrence of such connections but wrongly assumed that they represented pathways of normal conduction. Mines suggested in 1914 that this accessory atrioventricular (AV) connection (*bundle of Kent*) might cause tachyarrhythmias. In 1930, Wolff and White in Boston and Parkinson in London reported their combined series of 11 patients with bizarre ventricular complexes and short PR intervals.[2] Then, in 1944, Segers introduced the triad of short PR interval, preexcitation of the ventricles characterized by a prolonged upstroke of the QRS complex (*delta wave*), and tachyarrhythmia that characterize the *Wolff–Parkinson–White* (WPW) *syndrome*.

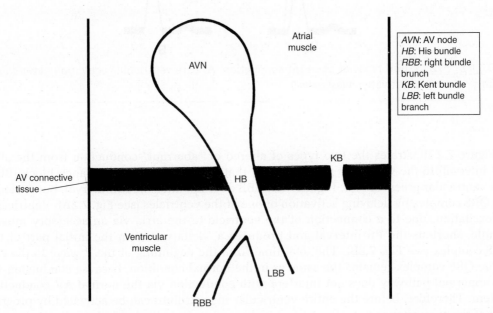

FIGURE 7.1. Normal and accessory AV conduction system. *Solid bar,* nonconducting structures. AV, atrioventricular.

Ventricular preexcitation refers to a congenital cardiac abnormality where part of the ventricular myocardium receives electrical activation from the atria before the impulse arrives via the normal AV conduction system. A schematic illustration of the anatomic relationship between the normal AV conduction system and the accessory AV conduction pathway provided by the bundle of Kent is displayed in Figure 7.1. Nonconducting structures, which include the coronary arteries and veins, valves, and fibrous and fatty connective tissues, prevent conduction of electrical impulses from the atrial myocardium to the ventricular myocardium. AV myocardial bundles commonly exist during fetal life but then disappear by the time of birth.[3] When even a single myocardial connection persists, there is the potential for ventricular preexcitation. In some individuals, evidence of preexcitation may not appear until late in life; whereas in others with lifelong evidence of ventricular preexcitation on the electrocardiogram (ECG), the WPW syndrome may not occur until late in life. Conversely, infants with the WPW syndrome may outgrow any or all evidence of this abnormality within a few years.[4]

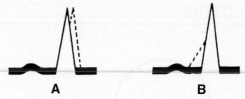

FIGURE 7.2. Two types of aberrant conduction. **A.** Late ventricular activation (*dashed line*). **B.** Early ventricular activation (*dashed line*).

Figure 7.2 illustrates the two types of altered or "aberrant" conduction from the atria (PR interval) to the ventricles (QRS interval) that results from bundle-branch block (BBB) and ventricular preexcitation. Right or left BBB does not alter the PR interval, but prolongs the QRS complex by delaying activation of one of the ventricles (see Fig. 7.2A). Ventricular preexcitation, due to a connection of the ventricle to the atria via an accessory muscle bundle, shortens the PR interval and produces a "delta wave" in the initial part of the QRS complex (see Fig. 7.2B). The total time from the beginning of the P wave to the end of the QRS complex remains the same as in the normal condition, because conduction via the abnormal pathway does not interfere with conduction via the normal AV conduction system. Therefore, before the entire ventricular myocardium can be activated by progression of the preexcitation wavefront, electrical impulses from the normal conduction system arrive to activate the remainder of the ventricular myocardium.

PATHOPHYSIOLOGY

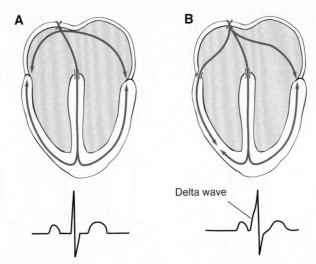

FIGURE 7.3. Anatomic basis for preexcitation. **A.** Normal condition. **B.** Abnormal congenital anomaly. *Pink X,* sinoatrial node; *pink lines,* direction of electrical impulses; *open channel,* conductive pathway between atria and ventricles. (Modified from Wagner GS, Waugh RA, Ramo BW. *Cardiac Arrhythmias.* New York, NY: Churchill Livingstone; 1983:13, with permission.)

The combination of the following has been termed the WPW syndrome.

1. PR interval duration of <0.12 second.
2. A delta wave at the beginning of the QRS complex.
3. A rapid, regular tachyarrhythmia.

The PR interval is short because the electrical impulse bypasses the normal AV nodal conduction delay. The delta wave is produced by slow intramyocardial conduction that results when the impulse, instead of being delivered to the ventricular myocardium via the normal conduction system, is delivered directly into the ventricular myocardium via an abnormal or "anomalous" muscle bundle. The duration of the QRS complex is prolonged because it begins "too early," in contrast with the situations presented in Chapters 5 and 6, in which the duration of the QRS complex is prolonged because it ends too late. The ventricles are activated successively rather than simultaneously; the preexcited ventricle is activated via the bundle of Kent, and the other ventricle is then activated via the normal AV node and His–Purkinje system (Fig. 7.3).

The relationship between an anatomic bundle of Kent and physiologic preexcitation of the ventricular myocardium, and the typical ECG changes of ventricular preexcitation, are illustrated on top and on bottom, respectively (see Fig. 7.3). Figure 7.3A illustrates the normal cardiac anatomy that permits AV conduction only via the AV node (the open channel at the crest of the interventricular septum). Thus, there is normally a delay in the activation of the ventricular myocardium (PR segment), as noted in the ECG recording shown in the figure. When the congenital abnormality responsible for the WPW syndrome is present, the ventricular myocardium is activated from two sources via: (a) the preexcitation pathway (the open channel between the right atrium and right ventricle shown in Fig. 7.3B) and (b) the normal AV conduction pathway. The resultant abnormal QRS complex (termed a *fusion beat*) is composed of the abnormal preexcitation wave and normal mid- and terminal-QRS waveforms.

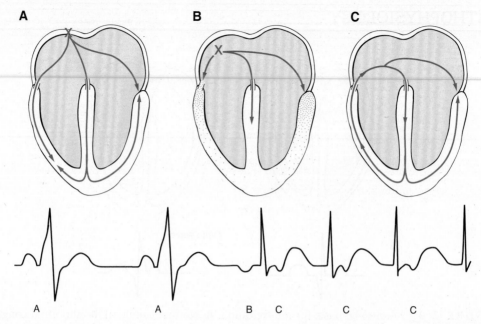

FIGURE 7.4. **A.** Typical ventricular preexcitation. **B.** Atrial premature beat. **C.** Retrograde atrial excitation. *Pink X,* origin of electrical impulse (**A.** Sinoatrial node. **B.** Ectopic origin.); *pink lines,* direction of electrical impulses; *open channel,* conductive pathway between atria and ventricles; *stippling,* persistent refractoriness of myocardium. (Modified from Wagner GS, Waugh RA, Ramo BW. *Cardiac Arrhythmias.* New York, NY: Churchill Livingstone; 1983:13, with permission.)

The abnormal AV muscular connection completes a circuit by providing a pathway for electrical reactivation of the atria from the ventricles. This circuit provides a continuous loop for the electrical activating current, which may result in a single premature beat or a prolonged, regular, rapid atrial and ventricular rate called a *tachyarrhythmia* (Fig. 7.4). In Figure 7.4B, an atrial premature beat has occurred and sends a wave of depolarization through the atria and toward the bundle of Kent. Because this beat originated in such close proximity to the bundle of Kent, the bundle has not had sufficient time to repolarize. As a result, the premature wave of depolarization cannot continue through this accessory AV conduction pathway to preexcite the ventricles. However, the premature wave is able to progress to the ventricles via the normal AV conduction pathway in the AV node and interventricular septum. This depolarization wave then travels through the ventricles, and because it does not collide with an opposing wave (as occurs with ventricular preexcitation in Fig. 7.4A), it reenters the atrium through the bundle of Kent, creating a retrograde atrial excitation (see Fig. 7.4C).

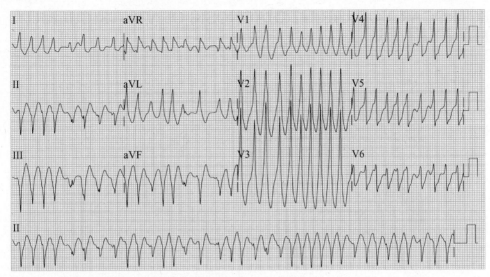

FIGURE 7.5. Ventricular preexcitation during atrial fibrillation.

Ventricular preexcitation, induced by an accessory pathway, influences the ventricular rate to become rapid in the presence of an atrial tachyarrhythmia such as atrial flutter/fibrillation (see Chapter 17). During such an episode, the ventricles are no longer "protected" by the slowly conducting AV node. A 12-lead ECG recording with a lead II rhythm strip of a 24-year-old woman with ventricular preexcitation during atrial fibrillation is displayed in Figure 7.5. The irregularities of both the ventricular rate and QRS complex morphology are apparent, especially on the 10-second lead II rhythm strip at the bottom of the figure.

ELECTROCARDIOGRAPHIC DIAGNOSIS OF VENTRICULAR PREEXCITATION

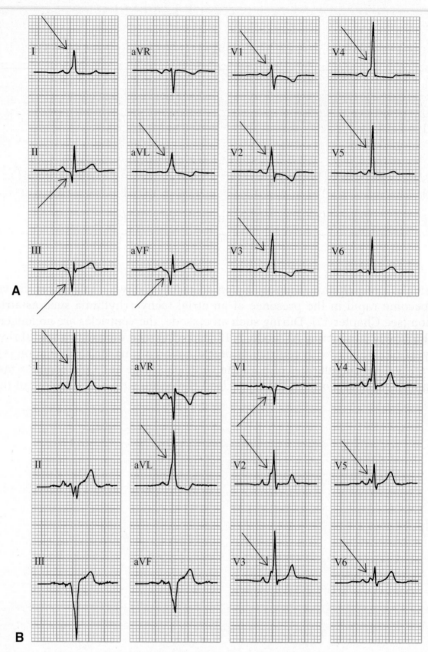

FIGURE 7.6. Positive and negative delta waves (*arrows*) in two patients.

Typically, with ventricular preexcitation, the PR interval is <0.12 second in duration and the QRS complex is >0.10 second. Ventricular preexcitation produces a prolonged upstroke of the QRS complex, which has been termed a "delta wave." Positive delta (V1 to V5, I and aVL) and negative delta (II, III, and aVF) waves are illustrated in Figure 7.6.

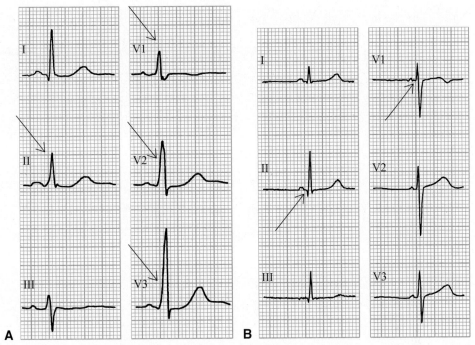

FIGURE 7.7. **A.** Slow onset of the QRS complex following a normal PR interval (*arrows*). **B.** Short PR interval preceding a normal QRS complex duration (*arrows*).

However, the PR interval is not always abnormally short and the QRS complex is not always abnormally prolonged. Figure 7.7A illustrates an abnormally slow onset of the QRS complex following a normal PR interval (0.16 second). Figure 7.7B illustrates an abnormally short PR interval preceding a QRS complex of normal duration (0.08 second). Conduction through the bundle of Kent may be relatively slow, or the bundle of Kent may directly enter the His bundle. Among almost 600 patients with documented ventricular preexcitation, 25% had PR intervals of ≥0.12 second and 25% had a QRS complex duration of ≤0.10 second.[5]

When ventricular preexcitation is suspected in a patient with tachyarrhythmia but no ECG evidence of preexcitation, the following diagnostic procedures may be helpful:

1. Pace the atria electronically at increasingly rapid rates to induce conduction via any existing accessory pathway.
2. Produce vagal nerve stimulation to impair normal conduction through the AV node so as to induce conduction via any existing accessory pathway.
3. Infuse digoxin intravenously for the same purpose as in procedure 2.

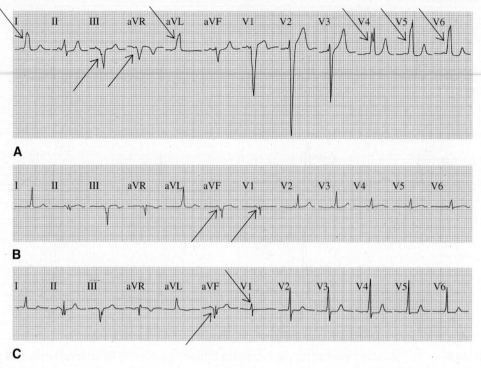

FIGURE 7.8. **A.** Delta waves (*arrows*). **B and C.** Delta waves mimicking myocardial infarction (*arrows*).

Ventricular preexcitation may mimic a number of other cardiac abnormalities. When there is a wide, positive QRS complex in leads V1 and V2, it may simulate right-bundle-branch block, right-ventricular hypertrophy, or a posterior myocardial infarction. When there is a wide, negative QRS complex in lead V1 or V2, preexcitation may be mistaken for left-bundle-branch block (LBBB; Fig. 7.8A) or left-ventricular hypertrophy. A negative delta wave, producing Q waves in the appropriate leads, may imitate anterior, lateral, or inferior infarction. The prominent Q waves in leads aVF and V1 in Figure 7.8B could be mistaken for inferior or anterior infarction, respectively (see Chapter 12). Similarly, the deep, wide Q wave in lead aVF and broad initial R wave in lead V1 in Figure 7.8C could be mistaken for inferior or posterior infarction, respectively.

ELECTROCARDIOGRAPHIC LOCALIZATION OF THE PATHWAY OF VENTRICULAR PREEXCITATION

Table 7.1.

Relationship between Pathway Location and Electrocardiographic (ECG) Changes

ECG Appearance	Location of Abnormal Pathway
Group A: QRS mainly positive in leads V1 and V2	LA-LV
Group B: QRS mainly negative in leads V1 and V2	RA-RV

LA, left atrium; LV, left ventricle; RA, right atrium; RV, right ventricle.

Many attempts have been made to determine the myocardial location of ventricular preexcitation according to the direction of the delta waves in the various ECG leads. Rosenbaum and colleagues[6] divided patients into two groups (groups A and B) on the basis of the direction of the "main deflection of the QRS complex" in transverse plane leads V1 and V2 (Table 7.1).

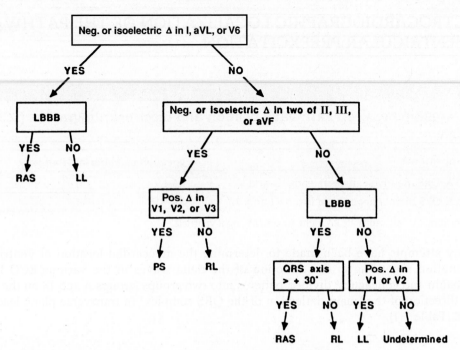

FIGURE 7.9.   Milstein's algorithm for accessory pathway localization. LBBB, left-bundle-branch block; LL, left lateral; Neg., negative; Pos., positive; PS, posteroseptal; RAS, right anteroseptal; RL, right lateral. (Modified from Milstein S, Sharma AD, Guiraudon GM, et al. An algorithm for the electrocardiographic localization of accessory pathways in the Wolff-Parkinson-White syndrome. *Pacing Clin Electrophysiol.* 1987;10:555–563, with permission.)

Other classification systems consider the direction only of the abnormal delta wave in attempting to better localize the pathway of ventricular preexcitation. Because curative surgical and catheter ablation techniques for eliminating it have become available, more precise localization of the accessory pathway is clinically important,[7] and many additional ECG criteria have therefore been proposed for achieving this. However, precise localization of an accessory AV pathway is made difficult by several factors, including minor degrees of preexcitation, the presence of more than one accessory pathway, distortions of the QRS complex caused by superimposed myocardial infarction, or ventricular hypertrophy. Nevertheless, Milstein and associates[8] devised an algorithm that enabled them to correctly identify the location of 90% of >140 accessory pathways (Fig. 7.9). For purposes of this schema (see Fig. 7.9), LBBB indicates a positive QRS complex in lead I with a duration of ≥0.09 second and rS complexes in leads V1 and V2.

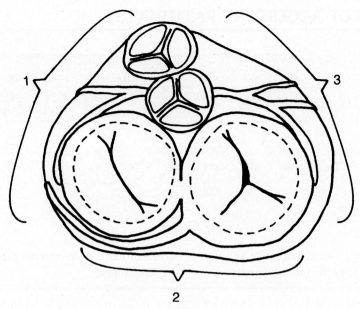

FIGURE 7.10. Bundle of Kent general locations. 1, LA-LV free wall; 2, posterior septal; 3, RA-RV free wall, a combination of Milstein and colleagues' right anteroseptal and right lateral locations. (Modified from Tonkin AM, Wagner GS, Gallagher JJ, et al. Initial forces of ventricular depolarization in the Wolff-Parkinson-White syndrome. Analysis based upon localization of the accessory pathway by epicardial mapping. *Circulation.* 1975;52:1030–1036, with permission.)

Although accessory pathways may be found anywhere in the connective tissue between the atria and ventricles, nearly all are found in three general locations, as follows:

1. Left laterally, between the left-atrial and left-ventricular free walls (50%).
2. Posteriorly, between the atrial and ventricular septa (30%).
3. Right laterally or anteriorly, between the right-atrial and right-ventricular free walls (20%).

The three general locations are illustrated as a schematic view (from above) of a cross-section of the heart at the junction between the atria and the ventricles in Figure 7.10. The ventricular outflow aortic and pulmonary valves are located anteriorly, and the ventricular inflow mitral (bicuspid) and tricuspid valves are located posteriorly.

Tonkin and associates[9] presented a simple method for localizing accessory pathways to one of the foregoing areas on the basis of the direction of the delta wave (Table 7.2). They considered a point 20 milliseconds after the onset of the delta wave in the QRS complex as their reference.

Table 7.2.

Consideration of Delta Wave at QRS Onset + 0.02 s

Direction of Preexcitation	Location of Pathway	Incidence Correct
Rightward	LA-LV free wall	10 of 10
Leftward and superior	Posterior septal	9 of 10
Leftward and inferior	RA-RV free wall	6 of 7

LA, left atrial; LV, left ventricular; RA, right atrial; RV, right ventricular.

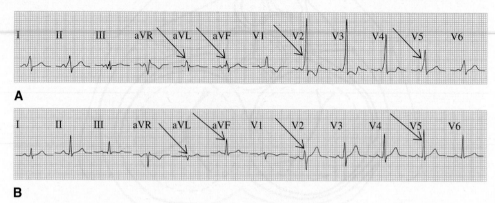

FIGURE 7.11. Radiofrequency ablation of bundle of Kent. **A.** Before the procedure (*arrows*, delta waves). **B.** After the procedure (*arrows*, normal QRS complex).

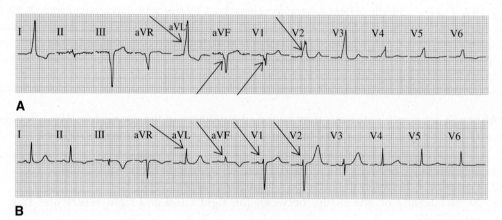

FIGURE 7.12. Radiofrequency ablation of bundle of Kent. **A.** Before the procedure (*arrows*, delta waves). **B.** After the procedure (*arrows*, normal QRS complex).

Ablation may be performed by surgical dissection or by percutaneous catheter techniques, in conjunction with a diagnostic electrophysiology test in localizing the accessory pathway. Figures 7.11A and 7.12A illustrate the typical ECG appearances of preexcitation of the right ventricular free wall and the interventricular septum, respectively. Successful ablation of the accessory pathways (see Figs. 7.11B and 7.12B) revealed the underlying presence of normal QRS complexes.

GLOSSARY

Bundle of Kent: a congenital abnormality in which a bundle of myocardial fibers connects the atria and the ventricles.

Delta wave: a slowing of the initial aspect of the QRS complex caused by premature excitation (preexcitation) of the ventricles via a bundle of Kent.

Fusion beat: activation of the ventricles by two different wavefronts, resulting in an abnormal appearance of the QRS complexes on the ECG.

Preexcitation premature activation of the ventricular myocardium via an abnormal AV pathway called a "bundle of Kent."

Tachyarrhythmia: an abnormal cardiac rhythm with a ventricular rate ≥100 beats per minute.

Wolff–Parkinson–White syndrome: the clinical combination of a short PR interval, an increased duration of the QRS complex caused by an initial slow deflection (delta wave), and supraventricular tachyarrhythmias.

REFERENCES

1. Kent AFS. Research on the structure and function of the mammalian heart. *J Physiol.* 1893;14:233.
2. Wolff L. Syndrome of short P-R interval with abnormal QRS complexes and paroxysmal tachycardia (Wolff-Parkinson-White syndrome). *Circulation.* 1954;10: 282.
3. Becker AE, Anderson RH, Durrer D, et al. The anatomical substrates of Wolff-Parkinson-White syndrome. *Circulation.* 1978;57:870–879.
4. Giardina ACV, Ehlers KH, Engle MA. Wolff-Parkinson-White syndrome in infants and children: a long term follow up study. *Br Heart J.* 1972;34:839–846.
5. Goudevenos JA, Katsouras CS, Graeklas G, et al. Ventricular preexcitation in the general population: a study on the mode of presentation and clinical course. *Heart.* 2000;83:29–34.
6. Rosenbaum FF, Hecht HH, Wilson FN, et al. Potential variations of thorax and esophagus in anomalous atrioventricular excitation (Wolff-Parkinson-White syndrome). *Am Heart J.* 1945;29:281–326.
7. Gallagher JJ, Gilbert M, Svenson RH, et al. Wolff-Parkinson-White syndrome: the problem, evaluation, and surgical correction. *Circulation.* 1975;51:767–785.
8. Milstein S, Sharma AD, Guiraudon GM, et al. An algorithm for the electrocardiographic localization of accessory pathways in the Wolff-Parkinson-White syndrome. *Pacing Clin Electrophysiol.* 1987;10:555–563.
9. Tonkin AM, Wagner GS, Gallagher JJ, et al. Initial forces of ventricular depolarization in the Wolff-Parkinson-White syndrome: analysis based upon localization of the accessory pathway by epicardial mapping. *Circulation.* 1975;52:1030–1036.

8

Inherited Arrhythmia Disorders

ALBERT Y. SUN AND GALEN S. WAGNER

Subtle differences in QRS-, ST-, or T-wave morphologies on electrocardiogram (ECG) most commonly represent benign variations on a population basis; however, in some instances, these changes represent diagnostic clues to identify rare inherited disorders associated with an increased risk of sudden cardiac death (SCD). This group of inherited arrhythmia disorders are heterogeneous in regard to underlying mechanism and presentation; however, they do share some important characteristics: (a) an increased risk of SCD; (b) result from functional mutations in ion channel, ion channel accessory proteins, or myocardial structural genes; (c) mostly appear in the absence of overt structural heart disease; and (d) have characteristic ECG patterns. The identification of these ECG patterns that include prolonged or shortened QT intervals, low amplitude notching in QRS complexes, or unusual-appearing bundle branch patterns is extremely important in the proper identification of these rare syndromes. This chapter explores this group of inherited arrhythmia disorders, their accompanying ECG patterns, and some of their defining clinical features.

THE LONG QT SYNDROME

The *long QT syndrome* (LQTS) is a disorder of abnormal myocardial repolarization characterized by a prolonged QT interval (Chapter 3) on ECG and an increased risk of SCD.[1] This abnormal repolarization can lead to the development of fatal ventricular arrhythmias such as torsades de pointes (Chapter 19). It can either be an inherited condition, often involving a mutation in an ion channel–associated gene, or an acquired condition resulting from medication exposure, electrolyte derangements, or myocardial ischemia.[2]

ELECTROCARDIOGRAPHIC CHARACTERISTICS

QT Interval

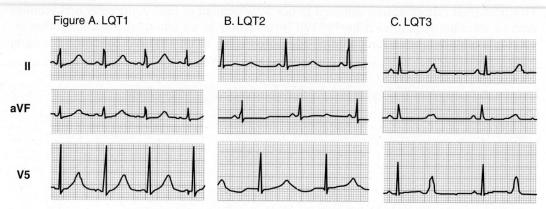

FIGURE 8.1. Genotype specific ECG patterns in long QT syndrome. **A.** LQT1 – early onset broad-based T wave. **B.** LQT2 - low amplitude and bifid T wave. **C.** LQT3 - long isoelectric ST segment with a late-appearing T wave. (Modified from Moss AJ, Zareba W, Benhorin J, et al. ECG T-wave patterns in genetically distinct forms of the hereditary long QT syndrome. *Circulation.* 1995;92:2929–2934, with permission.)

A prolonged QTc interval (Chapter 3) is the hallmark of LQTS. However, it should not be used as the sole diagnostic criteria because up to a quarter of genotype-positive LQTS patients may have a normal QTc. In addition, as QT intervals in a population follow a normal distribution, at least 2.5% of the general population will have a "prolonged QTc" (≥450 milliseconds in men and ≥460 milliseconds in women) per the guidelines.[3] *See the section on "ELECTROCARDIOGRAM AS USED IN DIAGNOSIS".*

In general, QTc intervals >500 milliseconds are associated with an increased risk of sudden death. Because the QTc interval is dynamic and changes under different physiologic conditions, the longest QTc interval should be used for risk stratification.[4]

T-Wave Morphology

Currently, there have been at least 13 genes identified as loci for congenital LQTS; however, three major genes (KCNQ1, KCNH2, and SCN5A) represent the majority of cases.[5] These three main subtypes of LQTS often have subtle characteristic differences in T-wave morphology that should be noted.[6]

LQT1 represents the most common loci of LQTS (30% to 25%) and results from a loss-of-function mutation in the KCNQ1 gene that encodes the alpha-subunit of Kv7.1, the slow-activating potassium channel responsible for the IKs current. The ECG in LQT1 is characterized by an early-onset broad-based T wave (Fig. 8.1A).

LQT2 is the second most common loci for LQTS (35% to 40%) and stems from mutations in the KCNH2 gene encoding the alpha (HERG) subunit of the potassium channel responsible for the IKr current. The T waves in LQT2 are usually low amplitude and bifid (see Fig. 8.1B).

LQT3 arises from gain of function mutations in the SCN5A that encodes for the rapidly inactivating sodium channels NaV1.5. The ECG in LQT3 shows long isoelectric ST segments with a late-appearing T wave (see Fig. 8.1C).

Table 8.1.

Schwartz Score

Characteristics	Points
Electrocardiographic findings	
• QTc (calculated with Bazett formula)	
≥480 ms	3
460–470 ms	2
450 ms and male gender	1
• QTc fourth minute of recovery from exercise stress test ≥480 ms	1
• Torsades de pointes	2
• T wave alternans	1
• Notched T wave in three leads	1
• Low heart rate for age (children), resting heart rate below second percentile for age	0.5
Clinical history	
• Syncope (one cannot receive points both for syncope and torsades de pointes)	
With stress	2
Without stress	1
• Congenital deafness	0.5
Family history	
• Other family members with definite LQTS	1
• Sudden death in immediate family members (before age 30 years)	0.5

SCORE: ≤1 point, low probability of LQTS; 1.5 to 3 points, intermediate probability of LQTS; ≥3.5 points, high probability.

It is important to remember that a prolonged QT interval alone is *not* sufficient to make the diagnosis of LQTS; an increased risk of SCD is necessary. To assist with the diagnosis of LQTS, a diagnostic score has been created, known as the International Long QT Score or "Schwartz score" (Table 8.1). Although a score ≥3.5 makes the diagnosis of LQTS more likely, it also is not diagnostic.[8]

THE SHORT QT SYNDROME

As with LQTS, *short QT syndrome* (SQTS) is a disorder of repolarization, in this case associated with more rapid repolarization and therefore a short QT interval. Again, like LQTS, this condition can be congenital or acquired. Acquired causes of short QT include hyperthermia, hyperkalemia, hypercalcemia, acidosis, and changes in autonomic tone. Congenital SQTS is much more rare than LQTS, with <100 cases reported worldwide. SQTS is defined by the presence of an abnormal QT interval (<300 milliseconds) and an increased risk of ventricular arrhythmias and SCD. Not surprisingly, the genes currently associated with SQTS are involved in the repolarization phase of the cardiac action potential. These functional mutations lead to a gain-of-function in the three voltage-gated potassium channel genes: KCNH2, KCNQ1, and KCNJ2. This gain of function results in an increased efflux of potassium from the cell during the repolarization phase and a shortening of the action potential.[9]

ELECTROCARDIOGRAPHIC CHARACTERISTICS

QT Interval

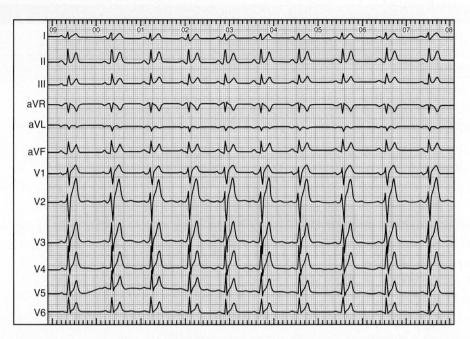

FIGURE 8.2. Short QT Syndrome. (From Moreno-Reviriego S, Merino JL. Short QT syndrome. *E-J ESC Counc Cardiol Prac.* 2010;9, with permission.)

Similar to LQTS, the QT interval in a population follows a normal distribution, thus there will be many "normal" patients in the general population with a short QT interval <360 milliseconds. However, patients with very short QT intervals (QTc <330 milliseconds in males and QTc <340 milliseconds in females) should be considered for SQTS even if they are asymptomatic because QT intervals this short are quite rare.

T-Wave Morphology

Most SQTS patients have an absent ST segment, with the T wave beginning immediately after the S wave. The T wave also often appears peaked and narrow (Fig. 8.2).

Table 8.2.	
Short QT Syndrome Diagnostic Criteria	
Characteristic	Points
Electrocardiographic findings	
• QTc (calculated with Bazett formula)	
<370 ms	1
<350 ms	2
<330 ms	3
• J-point–T-peak interval <120 ms	1
Clinical history	
• History of sudden cardiac arrest	2
• Documented polymorphic VT or VF	2
• Unexplained syncope	1
• Atrial fibrillation	1
Family history	
• First- or second-degree relative with high-probability SQTS	2
• First- or second-degree relative with autopsy-negative SCD	1
• Sudden infant death syndrome	1
Genotype	
• Genotype positive	2
• Mutation of undetermined significance in a culprit gene	1

SCORE: ≤2 points, low probability; 3 points, intermediate probability; ≥4 points, high probability of SQTS.

Similar to LQTS, a prolonged QT interval alone is not sufficient to make the diagnosis of SQTS; an increased risk of SCD is necessary. To assist with the diagnosis of SQTS, a diagnostic score has been created (Table 8.2).[9] Although a score ≥4 makes the diagnosis of SQTS more likely, it is not sufficient to make the diagnosis.

Table 8.3.

ST-Segment Abnormalities in Leads V1 to V3[10]

	Type I	Type II	Type III
J-wave amplitude	≥2 mm	≥2 mm	≥2 mm
T wave	Negative	Positive or biphasis	Positive
ST-T configuration	Coved type	Saddleback	Saddleback
ST segment (terminal portion)	Gradually descending	Elevated ≥1 mm	Elevated <1 mm

The Brugada pattern was first reported in 1953, but it was not until ECG pattern was associated with SCD in 1992 that it became a recognized clinical syndrome.

The *Brugada pattern* is the hallmark of the syndrome and has a characteristic pattern on ECG consisting of a pseudo–right-bundle-branch block (RBBB) and persistent ST-segment elevation in leads V1 to V3.[10]

Since the original description by Brugada et al,[11] there have been three main patterns described: (Table 8.3, Fig. 8.3)

1. Type 1: Prominent high take-off J-point elevation with a "coved-type" ST-segment elevation with amplitude of ≥2 mm leading to a negative T wave (Fig. 8.4).
2. Type 2: High take-off J-point elevation ≥2 mm with a gradually *descending* ST segment that remains ≥1 mm above the baseline leading to a positive or biphasic T wave. A "saddleback configuration."
3. Type 3: Right precordial ST-segment elevation of <1 mm with either coved- or saddleback-type morphology.

It is important to recognize that this pattern is often dynamic, and all three patterns can be observed in a single individual or even be completely concealed. Intravenous administration of certain drugs (mostly sodium channel blockers) may exaggerate the ST-segment elevation or unmask it if it is initially absent.

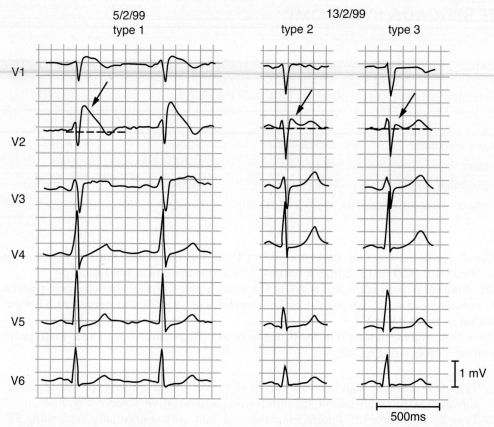

FIGURE 8.3. All three Brugada patterns demonstrated in the same patient. (From Wilde A, Antzelevitch C, Borggrefe M, et al. Proposed diagnostic criteria for the Brugada syndrome. *Circulation.* 2002;106:2514–2518.)

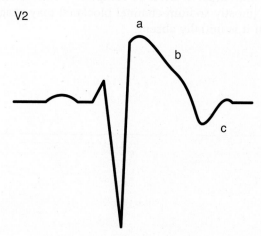

FIGURE 8.4. ECG characteristics of the type I Brugada pattern: a, J-point elevation >2.0 mm; b, coved downsloping ST segment; and c, T-wave inversion. (Modified from http://www.heartregistry. org.au/patients-families/genetic-heart-diseases/brugada-syndrome/)

ARRHYTHMOGENIC RIGHT-VENTRICULAR CARDIOMYOPATHY/DYSPLASIA

Table 8.4.

2010 Revised ECG Related Task Force Criteria for Diagnosis of Arrhythmogenic Right Ventricular Cardiomyopathy/Dysplasia

I. Repolarization abnormalities

Major

Inverted T waves in right precordial leads (V1, V2, and V3) or beyond in individuals .14 years of age (in the absence of complete right bundle-branch block QRS ≥ 120 ms) (Fig. 8.5)

Minor

Inverted T waves in leads V1 and V2 in individuals .14 years of age (in the absence of complete right bundle-branch block) or in V4, V5, or V6

Inverted T waves in leads V1, V2, V3, and V4 in individuals .14 years of age in the presence of complete right bundle-branch block

II. Depolarization/conduction abnormalities

Major

Epsilon wave (reproducible low-amplitude signals between end of QRS complex to onset of the T wave) in the right precordial leads (V1 to V3) (Fig. 8.6)

Minor

Late potentials by SAECG in ≥ 1 of 3 parameters in the absence of a QRS duration of ≥ 110 ms on the standard ECG

Filtered QRS duration (fQRS) ≥ 114 ms

Duration of terminal QRS ,40 mV (low-amplitude signal duration) ≥ 38 ms

Root-mean-square voltage of terminal 40 ms ≤ 20 mV

Terminal activation duration of QRS ≥ 55 ms measured from the nadir of the S wave to the end of the QRS, including R0, in V1, V2, or V3, in the absence of complete right bundle-branch block (Fig. 8.5)

III. Arrhythmias

Major

Nonsustained or sustained ventricular tachycardia of left bundle-branch morphology with superior axis (negative or indeterminate QRS in leads II, III, and aVF and positive in lead aVL) (Fig. 8.7)

Minor

Nonsustained or sustained ventricular tachycardia of RV outflow configuration, left bundle-branch block morphology with inferior axis (positive QRS in leads II, III, and aVF and negative in lead aVL) or of unknown axis

500 ventricular extrasystoles per 24 hours (Holter)

Arrhythmogenic right-ventricular cardiomyopathy/dysplasia (ARVC/D) is a predominantly genetic disorder of the heart muscle characterized pathologically by fibrofatty replacement of the right-ventricular (RV) and, occasionally, the left-ventricular (LV) myocardium. This myocardial disruption often leads to nonsustained or sustained ventricular arrhythmias and increased risk of SCD.[12]

Repolarization abnormalities present early and are sensitive markers of myocardial involvement. In conjunction with depolarization/conduction abnormalities and the presence of ventricular arrhythmias, these ECG findings are part of the diagnostic criteria for ARVC/D put forth by the European Society of Cardiology that also includes imaging, histology and family history (Table 8.4).[12]

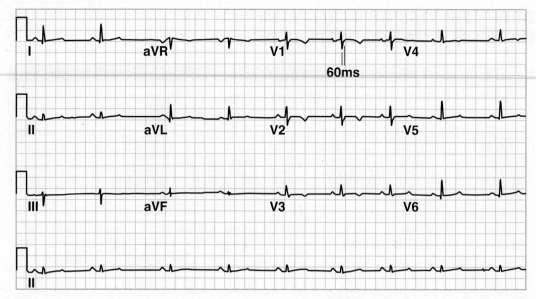

FIGURE 8.5. T-wave inversion in V1 through V4 and prolongation of the terminal activation duration ≥55 ms measured from the nadir of the S wave to the end of the QRS complex in V1. (From Marcus FI, McKenna WJ, Sherrill D, et al. Diagnosis of arrhythmogenic right ventricular cardiomyopathy/dysplasia: proposed modification of the Task Force Criteria. *Eur Heart J.* 2010;31:806–814. doi:10.1093/eurheartj/ehq025)

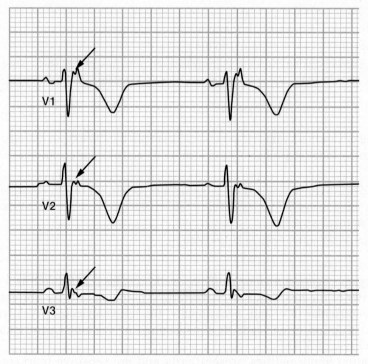

FIGURE 8.6. Epsilon wave (*arrow*) in leads V1–V3. (Modified from Kiès P, Bootsma M, Bax J, et al. Arrhythmogenic right ventricular dysplasia/cardiomyopathy: screening, diagnosis, and treatment. *Heart Rhythm.* 2006;3(2):225–234. http://dx.doi.org/10.1016/j.hrthm.2005.10.018)

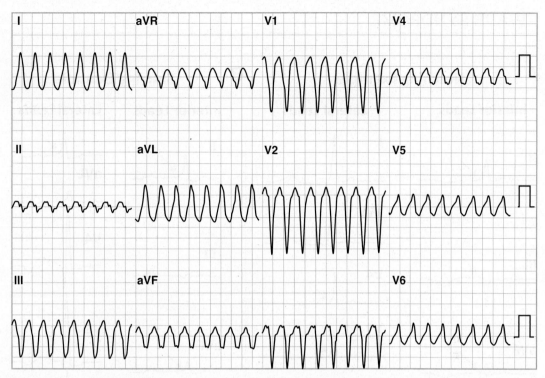

FIGURE 8.7. LBBB/superior axis VT from a patient with ARVD/C. (From Hoffmayer KS, Scheinman MM. Electrocardiographic patterns of ventricular arrhythmias in arrhythmogenic right ventricular dysplasia/cardiomyopathy. *Front Physiol.* 2012;3:23. doi: 10.3389/fphys.2012.00023)

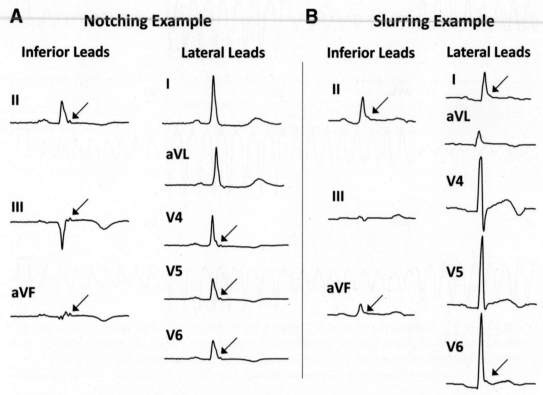

FIGURE 8.8. J Wave Patterns on ECG. **A.** example of notching pattern (*arrows*). **B.** example of slurring pattern (*arrows*). (From Patel RB, Ng J, Reddy V, et al. Early repolarization associated with ventricular arrhythmias in patients with chronic coronary artery disease. *Circ Arrhythm Electrophysiol.* 2010;3:489–495, with permission.)

The pattern on ECG characterized by accentuated J point elevation at the terminal portion of the QRS and beginning of the ST segment, previously described as early repolarization, is now referred to as the J wave pattern. This pattern is seen in approximately 6% of the general population, but it may be even more prevalent in younger patients, athletes, and persons of African descent. Recently, reports linking this supposedly benign pattern to an increased risk of SCD have garnered much attention.[16,17] Collectively, these studies have demonstrated an increased prevalence of this ECG pattern, defined as ≥0.1 mV J-point elevation in two adjacent inferior or lateral leads with a notching or slurring pattern (Fig. 8.8),[18] in patients who suffer from idiopathic ventricular fibrillation (VF). When this J wave pattern occurs with a resuscitated cardiac arrest event, documented VF or polymorphic ventricular tachycardia, or with a family history of a causative genetic mutation, the terminology J wave syndrome applies.[19]

Table 8.5.

Proposed Classification of J Wave Pattern

	Type 1	Type 2	Type 3
Anatomic location	Anterolateral left ventricle	Inferior left ventricle	Left and right ventricles
Leads displaying J-point or J-wave abnormalities	I, V4 to V6	II, III, aVF	Global

In J wave syndrome, the J point elevation and ST segment changes may be present in only a few ECG leads or globally, suggesting different anatomical locations responsible for each pattern. A classification system has been suggested by Antzelevitch and colleagues[20] (Table 8.5).

In addition to the location of the J point or J wave pattern, Tikkanen et al[21] suggest that including the magnitude of J-point elevation >0.2 mV further increases the risk of sudden death. The direction of the ST segment also appears to be a modifier, with a horizontal or downward direction of the ST segments carrying a 3 times higher risk of arrhythmic death.[22]

Despite these additional criteria, it is extremely important to note that J wave mediated SCD is extremely rare and thus the clinical implications of this finding in an asymptomatic individual are currently unclear.

GLOSSARY

Long QT Syndrome: The clinical syndrome of a prolonged QT interval and an increased risk of sudden cardiac death.

Short QT Syndrome: The clinical syndrome of a short QT interval and an increased risk of sudden cardiac death.

Brugada Pattern: pseudo-RBBB and persistent ST segment elevation in leads V1 to V3.

Brugada Syndrome: the clinical syndrome of a Brugada pattern and an increased risk of sudden cardiac death

Arrhythmogenic right-ventricular cardiomyopathy/dysplasia: disorder of the heart muscle characterized by fibrofatty replacement of the right or left ventricle

J wave pattern: ≥0.1 mV J-point elevation in two adjacent inferior or lateral leads with a notching or slurring pattern

J Wave Syndrome: the clinical syndrome of the J Wave Pattern and an increased risk of sudden cardiac death

References

1. Moss AJ. Long QT syndrome. *JAMA*. 2003;289:2041–2044.
2. Camm AJ, Janse MJ, Roden DM, et al. Congenital and acquired long QT syndrome. *Eur Heart J*. 2000;21:1232–1237.
3. Moss AJ. Measurement of the QT interval and the risk associated with qtc interval prolongation: a review. *Am J Cardiol*. 1993;72:23B–25B.
4. Priori SG, Schwartz PJ, Napolitano C, et al. Risk stratification in the long-qt syndrome. *New Engl J Med*. 2003;348:1866–1874.
5. Ackerman MJ, Priori SG, Willems S, et al. HRS/EHRA expert consensus statement on the state of genetic testing for the channelopathies and cardiomyopathies. This document was developed as a partnership between the Heart Rhythm Society (HRS) and the European Heart Rhythm Association (EHRA). *Europace*. 2011;13(8):1077–1109.
6. Zareba W. Genotype-specific ECG patterns in long QT syndrome. *J Electrocardiol*. 2006;39:S101–S106.
7. Moss AJ, Zareba W, Benhorin J, et al. ECG T-wave patterns in genetically distinct forms of the hereditary long QT syndrome. *Circulation*. 1995;92:2929–2934.
8. Schwartz PJ, Moss AJ, Vincent GM, et al. Diagnostic criteria for the long QT syndrome. An update. *Circulation*. 1993;88:782–784.
9. Gollob MH, Redpath CJ, Roberts JD. The short QT syndrome: proposed diagnostic criteria. *J Am Coll Cardiol*. 2011;57:802–812.
10. Wilde AA, Antzelevitch C, Borggrefe M, et al. Proposed diagnostic criteria for the Brugada syndrome. *Eur Heart J*. 2002;23:1648–1654.
11. Brugada P, Brugada J. Right bundle branch block, persistent ST segment elevation and sudden cardiac death: a distinct clinical and electrocardiographic syndrome. A multicenter report. *J Am Coll Cardiol*. 1992;20:1391–1396.
12. Marcus FI, McKenna WJ, Sherrill D, et al. Diagnosis of arrhythmogenic right ventricular cardiomyopathy/dysplasia: proposed modification of the task force criteria. *Eur Heart J*. 2010;31:806–814.
13. Marcus FI. Prevalence of T-wave inversion beyond V1 in young normal individuals and usefulness for the diagnosis of arrhythmogenic right ventricular cardiomyopathy/dysplasia. *Am J Cardiol*. 2005;95:1070–1071.
14. Marcus FI, Abidov A. Arrhythmogenic right ventricular cardiomyopathy 2012: diagnostic challenges and treatment. *J Cardiovasc Electrophysiol*. 2012;23:1149–1153.
15. Cox MG, Nelen MR, Wilde AA, et al. Activation delay and VT parameters in arrhythmogenic right ventricular dysplasia/cardiomyopathy: toward improvement of diagnostic ECG criteria. *J Cardiovasc Electrophysiol*. 2008;19:775–781.
16. Haissaguerre M, Derval N, Sacher F, et al. Sudden cardiac arrest associated with early repolarization. *New Engl J Med*. 2008;358:2016–2023.
17. Rosso R, Kogan E, Belhassen B, et al. J-point elevation in survivors of primary ventricu-

lar fibrillation and matched control subjects: incidence and clinical significance. *J Am Coll Cardiol*. 2008;52:1231–1238.

18. Patel RB, Ng J, Reddy V, et al. Early repolarization associated with ventricular arrhythmias in patients with chronic coronary artery disease. *Circ Arrhythm Electrophysiol*. 2010;3:489–495.

19. Huikuri HV, Marcus F, Krahn AD. Early repolarization: an epidemiologist's and a clinician's view. *J Electrocardiol*. 2013.

20. Antzelevitch C, Yan GX. J wave syndromes. *Heart Rhythm*. 2010;7:549–558.

21. Tikkanen JT, Anttonen O, Junttila MJ, et al. Long-term outcome associated with early repolarization on electrocardiography. *New Engl J Med*. 2009;361:2529–2537.

22. Tikkanen JT, Junttila MJ, Anttonen O, et al. Early repolarization: electrocardiographic phenotypes associated with favorable long-term outcome. *Circulation*. 2011;123:2666–2673.

9

Myocardial Ischemia and Infarction

DAVID G. STRAUSS, PETER M. VAN DAM, TOBIN H. LIM, AND GALEN S. WAGNER

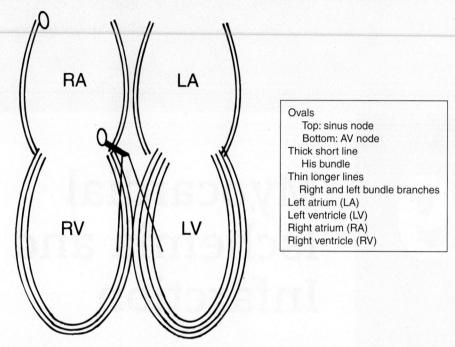

FIGURE 9.1. Schematic comparison of the relative thickness of the myocardium in the four cardiac chambers along with the sinoatrial node, AV node, His bundle, and right and left bundles. (Modified from Wagner GS, Waugh RA, Ramo BW. *Cardiac Arrhythmias.* New York, NY: Churchill Livingstone; 1983:2, with permission.)

The energy required to maintain the cardiac cycle is generated by a process known as *aerobic metabolism*, in which oxygen is required for energy production. Oxygen and essential nutrients are supplied to the cells of the myocardium in the blood via the *coronary arteries (myocardial perfusion)*. If the blood supply to the myocardium becomes insufficient, an energy deficiency occurs. To compensate for this diminished aerobic metabolism, the myocardial cells initiate a different metabolic process, *anaerobic metabolism*, in which oxygen is not required. In this process, the cells use their reserve supply of glucose stored in glycogen molecules to generate energy. Anaerobic metabolism, however, is less efficient than aerobic metabolism, producing enough energy to survive but not function. It is also temporary, operating only until this glycogen is depleted.

In the period during which perfusion is insufficient to meet the myocardial demand required for both survival and function, the myocardial cells are ischemic. To sustain themselves, myocardial cells with an energy deficiency must uncouple their electrical activation from mechanical contraction and remain in their resting state. This has been termed myocardial *stunning* during acute, sudden-onset ischemia and *hibernation* during chronic ischemia.[1] Thus, the area of the myocardium that is ischemic cannot participate in the pumping process of the heart.[2,3]

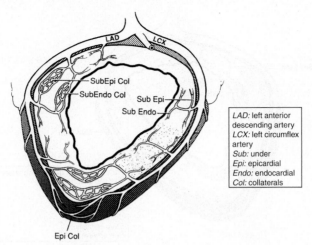

FIGURE 9.2. Cross-section of the left ventricle from the left anterior oblique view. The epicardial courses of the main branches of the main coronary arteries and their intramyocardial branches are shown. (Modified from Califf RM, Mark DB, Wagner GS, eds. *Acute Coronary Care*. 2nd ed. Chicago, IL: Mosby-Year Book; 1994, with permission.)

Various areas of the myocardium are more or less susceptible to ischemia. There are several determining factors:

1. Proximity to the intracavitary blood supply.
2. Distance from the major coronary arteries.
3. Workload as determined by the pressure required to pump blood.

Proximity to the Intracavitary Blood Supply

The internal layers of myocardial cells (endocardium) have a secondary source of nutrients, the intracavitary blood, which provides protection from ischemia.[4,5] The entire myocardium of the right and left atria has so few cell layers that it is almost all endocardium and subendocardium (Fig. 9.1). In the ventricles, however, only the innermost cell layers are similarly protected. The Purkinje system is located in these layers and is therefore well protected against ischemia.[6]

Distance from the Major Coronary Arteries

The ventricles consist of multiple myocardial layers that depend on the coronary arteries for their blood supply. These arteries arise from the aorta and course along the epicardial surfaces before penetrating the thickness of the myocardium. They then pass sequentially through the epicardial, middle, and subendocardial layers (Fig. 9.2). The subendocardial layer is the most distant, innermost layer of the myocardium and is subjected to the highest myocardial wall tension, resulting in greater oxygen needs.[7] Thus, it is the most susceptible to ischemia.[8] The thicker walled left ventricle is much more susceptible to insufficient perfusion than is the thinner walled right ventricle because of both the wall thickness itself and the greater workload of the left ventricle.

Workload as Determined by the Pressure Required to Pump Blood

The greater the pressure required by a cardiac chamber to pump blood, the greater its workload and the greater its metabolic demand for oxygen. The myocardial workload is smallest in the atria, intermediate in the right ventricle, and greatest in the left ventricle. Therefore, the susceptibility to ischemia is also lowest in the atria, intermediate in the right ventricle, and greatest in the left ventricle.

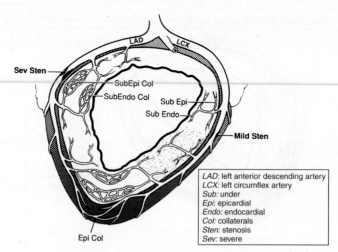

FIGURE 9.3. Stenosis of coronary arteries. (From Califf RM, Mark DB, Wagner GS, eds. *Acute Coronary Care.* 2nd ed. Chicago, IL: Mosby-Year Book; 1994, with permission.)

Ischemia is a relative condition that depends on the balance among the coronary blood supply, the level of oxygenation of the blood, and the myocardial workload. Theoretically, an individual with normal coronary arteries and fully oxygenated blood could develop *myocardial ischemia* if the workload were increased either by an extremely elevated arterial blood pressure or an extremely high heart rate. Alternatively, an individual with normal coronary arteries and a normal myocardial workload could develop ischemia if the oxygenation of the blood became extremely diminished. Conversely, the myocardium of someone with severe narrowing (stenoses) in all coronary arteries might never become ischemic if the cardiac workload remained low and the blood was well oxygenated.

When ischemia is produced by an increased workload, it is normally reversed by returning to the resting state before the myocardial cells' reserve supply of glycogen is entirely depleted. However, a condition that produces myocardial ischemia by decreasing the coronary blood supply may not be reversed so easily.

Coronary arteries may gradually become partly obstructed by plaques in the chronic process of atherosclerosis (Fig. 9.3). This condition produces ischemia when, even though the myocardial blood supply is sufficient at a resting workload, it becomes insufficient when the workload is increased by either emotional or physical stress. The gradual progression of the atherosclerotic process is accompanied by growth of collateral arteries, which supply blood to the myocardium beyond the level of obstruction. Indeed, these collateral arteries may be sufficient to entirely replace the blood-supplying capacity of the native artery if it becomes completely obstructed by the atherosclerotic plaque.[9]

Partially obstructed atherosclerotic coronary arteries may suddenly become completely obstructed by the acute processes of spasm of their smooth-muscle layer or *thrombosis* within the remaining arterial lumen.[10,11] In either of these conditions, ischemia develops immediately unless the resting metabolic demands of the affected myocardial cells can be satisfied by the collateral blood flow. If the spasm is relaxed or the thrombus is resolved (thrombolysis) before the glycogen reserve of the affected cells is severely depleted, the cells promptly resume their contraction. However, if the acute, complete obstruction continues until the myocardial cells' glycogen is severely depleted, they become stunned.[12] Even after blood flow is restored, these cells are unable to resume contraction until they have repleted their glycogen reserves. If the complete obstruction further persists until the myocardial cells' glycogen is entirely depleted, the cells are unable to sustain themselves, are irreversibly damaged, and become necrotic. This clinical process is termed a heart attack or *myocardial infarction* (MI).

ELECTROCARDIOGRAPHIC CHANGES

Electrophysiologic Changes during Ischemia

Knowledge of the action potential changes that occur during ischemia and the location of ischemia allows one to understand what ECG changes will occur during ischemia. This will be illustrated with the use of the interactive ECG simulation program, ECGSIM.[13] With the onset of ischemia, there are three principle changes that occur to the action potential:

1. Action potential duration shortens
2. Action potential amplitude decreases
3. Depolarization of the action potential is delayed (slowed conduction velocity)

Experimental and simulation studies have shown that changes in extracellular potassium and pH, along with opening of ATP-dependent potassium channels (K_{ATP}), can account for the AP changes that occur in acute ischemia.

Electrocardiographic Changes during Supply Ischemia (Insufficient Blood Supply)

Figure 9.4 and its accompanying Video 9.1 demonstrate the individual and the combined effect of these three action potential changes during demand ischemia (insufficient blood supply) due to sudden occlusion of the distal left anterior descending coronary artery. The principal ECG changes that occur are seen in the ECG leads that are directly above the ischemic area. In this case, they are leads V3 and V4.

1. Action potential duration shortening causes increased T-wave amplitude.
2. Decreased action potential amplitude causes increased ST-segment elevation.
3. Delayed depolarization causes the QRS complex to become more positive (increased R wave and decreased S wave).

Figure 9.4 shows the combined effect of all three action potential changes during ischemia. When the location of ischemia occurs in a different part of the left ventricle, the same changes to the ECG occur in the leads that are above the ischemic area. This will be discussed in more detail in Chapter 11.

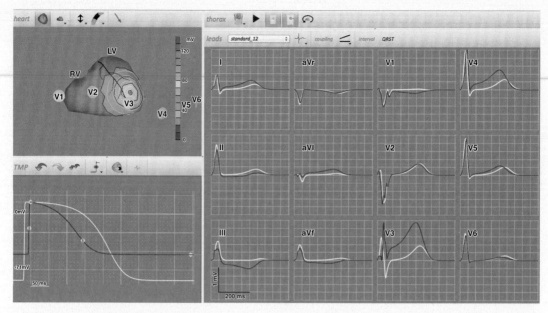

FIGURE 9.4. Simulation of transmural myocardial ischemia from insufficient blood supply with ECGSIM. **A.** Heart – upper left: The right and left ventricles (RV and LV) are shown with the left anterior descending (LAD) coronary artery (red) running down between the two ventricles. An area of ischemic myocardium has been highlighted that appears as a lighter yellow color and correlates to transmural ischemia that could occur from a mid-to-distal LAD occlusion. The spatial location of the 6 precordial electrodes are shown. **B.** TMP– lower left: The action potential (also known as transmembrane potential [TMP]) from a cell at the center of the ischemic region is shown. The baseline normal action potential is shown in white and the ischemic action potential is shown in red. The ischemic action potential has a shortened action potential depolarization (early repolarization), decreased action potential amplitude (depolarized baseline) and delayed initiation of the upstroke (delayed depolarization). **C.** Leads – on right: The normal baseline 12-lead ECG is shown in white and the simulated ECG from transmural ischemia is shown in red. The most significant change arrears in lead V3, which has its positive pole most directly above the ischemic region, as seen in the upper left model of the heart. The ECG changes that occur in V3 are an increase in T wave amplitude, ST-segment elevation and changes to the terminal part of the QRS (disappearance of S wave and increase in R wave). These changes also occur in leads V4, I and aVL, which also have positive poles above the ischemic area. The associated video further demonstrates the relation between the individual action potential changes and the ECG changes. ECGSIM can be downloaded for free from www.ecgsim.org. See Video 9.1.

Video 9.1

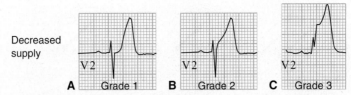

FIGURE 9.5. Lead V2 waveforms in a patient with Sclarovsky–Birnbaum grade 1 ischemia (increase in T-wave amplitude only), grade 2 ischemia (increase in ST segment and T wave) and grade 3 (increase in QRS complex, ST segment, and T wave; "tombstoning").

Based on clinical observations, Sclarovsky and Birnbaum developed a method for classifying the gradation of changes observed in decreased supply and have shown that patient prognosis worsens as the ischemia grade increases:[14]

Grade 1: increase in T-wave amplitude only (Fig. 9.5A),
Grade 2: increase in T waves + ST segments (see Fig. 9.5B),
Grade 3: increase in T waves + ST segments + QRS complexes; "tombstoning"
    (see Fig. 9.5C)

Going back to the lessons learned from ECGSIM (see Fig. 9.4), the least severe grade 1 ischemia (only increase in T-wave amplitude) means that the only ischemic change is a shortening of action potential duration. With grade 2 ischemia, there is also an increase in ST-segment elevation, indicating the presence of decreased action potential amplitude. With grade 3 ischemia, changes to the QRS complex are now present, indicating the presence of delayed depolarization. *Tombstoning* is a descriptive term for this most extreme severity of decreased supply.

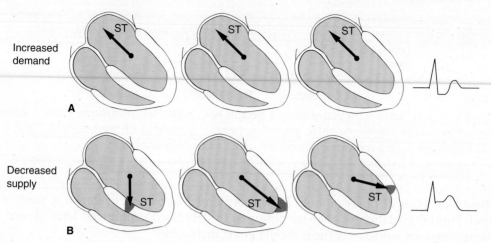

FIGURE 9.6. ECG changes with abnormal perfusion. **A.** Global subendocardial ischemia from increased demand causes the ST-segment vector to point away from the entire left ventricle (appears as ST depression in lead V5). **B.** Transmural ischemia from an occluded coronary artery (i.e., decreased supply) causes the ST-segment vector to point toward the involved region resulting in ST elevation in the ECG leads above the ischemia zone. *Arrows,* ST-segment direction.

Electrocardiographic Changes during Demand Ischemia

An increase in demand is most commonly recognized on the ECG by changes in the ST segments; however, demand ischemia can also result in changes in the QRS complex and T wave.[15] Because increased demand is limited to the subendocardial layer of the left ventricle, it is termed subendocardial ischemia. In addition, demand ischemia usually occurs globally throughout the entire subendocardium of the left ventricle and thus it is not possible to localize demand ischemia to an individual coronary artery territory. Instead of the ST and T waves shifting toward the ischemic area in supply ischemia, with demand ischemia, the ST and T waves shift away from the ischemic area (Fig. 9.6). This results in ST depression and T-wave inversion in most leads on the 12-lead ECG because the positive pole of the lead lies above the epicardium of the left ventricle. However, demand ischemia results in ST elevation and an increase in T-wave amplitude in lead aVR, which has a positive pole that points away from the endocardium of the left ventricle.

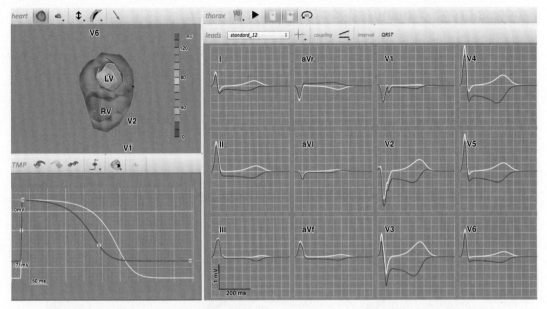

FIGURE 9.7. Simulation of subendocardial ischemia from increased myocardial demand with ECGSIM. **A.** Heart – left upper: The left (top) and right (bottom) ventricles are shown so that the endocardium can be viewed. The entire endocardium of the left ventricle has been highlighted so that it appears as a lighter yellow color. **B.** TMP – left lower: The action potential (also known as transmembrane potential [TMP]) from a cell at the center of the ischemic region is shown. The baseline normal action potential is shown in white and the ischemic action potential is shown in red. The ischemic action potential has a shortened action potential depolarization (early repolarization) and decreased action potential amplitude (depolarized baseline). Depolarization has not been delayed (as was done with transmural ischemia) because this does not normally occur with subendocardial ischemia. **C.** Leads – on right: The normal baseline 12-lead ECG is shown in white and the simulated ECG from global subendocardial ischemia is shown in red. Horizontal or down-sloping ST-segment depression with inverted T-waves occurs in a large number of leads except for aVR, where there is ST segment elevation and a positive T wave. The associated video further demonstrates the relation between the individual action potential changes and the ECG changes. ECGSIM can be downloaded for free from www.ecgsim.org. See Video 9.2.

Figure 9.7 and its accompanying Video 9.2 demonstrate ischemic action potential changes throughout the left ventricular endocardium representative of global subendocardial ischemia.

1. Action potential duration shortening causes T-wave flattening and then inverted T waves in all leads except aVR. In aVR, T waves flip from negative to positive.
2. Decreased action potential amplitude causes ST-segment depression in all leads except aVR, where ST elevation occurs.

Video 9.2

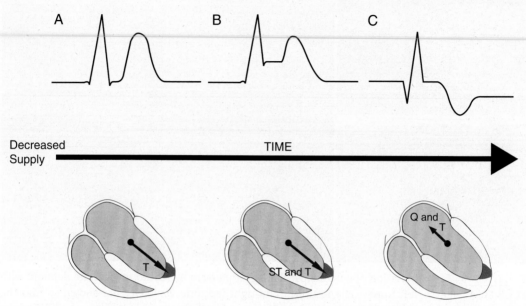

FIGURE 9.8.   Results of myocardial ischemia over time. Early transmural myocardial ischemia produces increased T-wave amplitude **(A)**, which is followed by ST-segment elevation **(B)**. After infarction (cell death occurs), Q waves develop and T waves invert **(C)**.

Insufficient myocardial perfusion of the left ventricle caused by complete coronary arterial occlusion results initially in *hyperacute T-wave* changes (Fig. 9.8A). Unless the occlusion is very brief or the myocardium is very well protected, the epicardial injury current is generated as represented by ST-segment deviation (see Fig. 9.8B). Both the T wave and ST segments deviate toward the involved region. If delayed depolarization occurs, the terminal part of the QRS complex also deviates toward the involved region. If the complete occlusion persists, and myocardial reperfusion is not attained while the cells retain their viability, an MI occurs (see Fig. 9.8C; see Chapter 12). As this infarction process evolves, both the QRS complex and T wave are directed away from the involved region.[16,17]

The abnormal Q wave is the hallmark of an established infarction and the abnormal T wave is termed the *postischemic T wave*.[18] It is inverted in its relationship to the QRS complex in many of the ECG leads (see Fig. 9.8C). The ECG changes associated with each of the three pathologic processes introduced in this chapter are presented in Chapters 10, 11, and 12.

GLOSSARY

Aerobic metabolism: the intracellular method for converting glucose into energy that requires the presence of oxygen and produces enough energy to nourish the myocardial cell and also to cause it to contract.

Anaerobic metabolism: the intracellular method for converting glucose into energy that does not require oxygen but produces only enough energy to nourish the cell.

Coronary arteries: either of the two arteries (right or left) that arise from the aorta immediately above the semilunar valves and supply the tissues of the heart itself.

Hyperacute T waves: T waves directed toward the ischemic area of the left-ventricular epicardium that can be identified in leads involved with the ischemic area by an increased positive amplitude.

Myocardial infarction: death of myocardial cells as a result of failure of the circulation to provide sufficient oxygen to restore metabolism after the intracellular stores of glycogen have been depleted.

Myocardial ischemia: a reduction in the supply of oxygen to less than the amount required by myocardial cells to maintain aerobic metabolism.

Myocardial perfusion: the flow of oxygen and nutrients into the cells of the heart muscle.

Pericarditis: inflammation of the pericardium.

Postischemic T waves: T waves directed away from the ischemic area of the left-ventricular myocardium when the ischemic process is resolving either from infarction or to reperfusion.

Stunned myocardium: a region of myocardium consisting of cardiac cells that are using anaerobic metabolism and are therefore ischemic and incapable of contraction but which are not infarcted.

Thrombosis: the formation or presence of a blood clot within a blood vessel.

Tombstoning: severe demand ischemia that obscures the transition from QRS to ST segment to T wave.

Transmural: involving the full thickness of the myocardial wall.

REFERENCES

1. Kloner RA, Bolli R, Marban E, et al. Medical and cellular implications of stunning, hibernation, and preconditioning: an NHLBI workshop. *Circulation.* 1998;97(18): 1848–1867.

2. Reimer KA, Jennings RB, Tatum AH. Pathobiology of acute myocardial ischemia: metabolic, functional and ultrastructural studies. *Am J Cardiol.* 1983;52(2): 72A–81A.

3. Lanza G, Coli S, Cianflone D. Coronary blood flow and myocardial ischemia. In: Fuster V, Alexander RW, O'Rourke RA, eds. *Hurst's the Heart.* 11th ed. New York, NY: McGraw-Hill; 2004:1153–1172.

4. Reimer KA, Jennings RB. The "wavefront phenomenon" of myocardial ischemic cell death. II. Transmural progression of necrosis within the framework of ischemic bed size (myocardium at risk) and collateral flow. *Lab Invest.* 1979;40(6):633–644.

5. Reimer KA, Lowe JE, Rasmussen MM, et al. The wavefront phenomenon of ischemic cell death. 1. Myocardial infarct size vs duration of coronary occlusion in dogs. *Circulation.* 1977;56(5):786–794.

6. Hackel DB, Wagner G, Ratliff NB, et al. Anatomic studies of the cardiac conducting system in acute myocardial infarction. *Am Heart J.* 1972;83(1):77–81.

7. Reimer KA, Jennings RB. Myocardial ischemia, hypoxia and infarction. In: Fozzard HA, ed. *The Heart and Cardiovascular System.* New York, NY: Raven Press Ltd; 1992: 1875–1973.

8. Bauman R, Rembert J, Greenfield J. The role of the collateral circulation in maintaining cellular viability during coronary occlusion. In: Califf RM, Mark DB, Wagner GS, eds. *Acute Coronary Care.* 2nd ed. Chicago, IL: Mosby-Year Book; 1994.

9. Cohen M, Rentrop KP. Limitation of myocardial ischemia by collateral circulation during sudden controlled coronary artery occlusion in human subjects: a prospective study. *Circulation.* 1986;74(3):469–476.

10. Kolodgie FD, Virmani R, Burke AP, et al. Pathologic assessment of the vulnerable human coronary plaque. *Heart*. 2004;90(12): 1385–1391.

11. Davies MJ, Fulton WF, Robertson WB. The relation of coronary thrombosis to ischemic myocardial necrosis. *J Pathol*. 1979;127(2):99–110.

12. Cooper HA, Braunwald E. Clinical importance of stunned and hibernating myocardium. *Coron Artery Dis*. 2001;12(5):387–392.

13. van Oosterom A, Oostendorp TF. ECGSIM: an interactive tool for studying the genesis of QRST waveforms. *Heart*. 2004; 90(2):165–168.

14. Billgren T, Birnbaum Y, Sgarbossa EB, et al. Refinement and interobserver agreement for the electrocardiographic Sclarovsky-Birnbaum Ischemia Grading System. *J Electrocardiol*. 2004;37(3):149–156.

15. Michaelides AP, Triposkiadis FK, Boudoulas H, et al. New coronary artery disease index based on exercise-induced QRS changes. *Am Heart J*. 1990;120(2):292–302.

16. Wagner N, Wagner G, White R. The twelve-lead ECG and the extent of myocardium at risk of acute infarction: cardiac anatomy and lead locations, and the phases of serial changes during acute occlusion. In: Califf RM, Mark DB, Wagner GS, eds. *Acute Coronary Care in the Thrombolytic Era*. Chicago, IL: Mosby-Year Book; 1988:31–45.

17. Sclarovsky S. Electrocardiography of acute myocardial ischemic syndromes. London, United Kingdom: Martin Duntz; 1999: 99–122.

18. Surawicz B. ST-T abnormalities. In: MacFarlane PW, Lawrie TDV, eds. *Comprehensive Electrocardiology*. New York, NY: Pergamon Press; 1988:511–563.

10

Subendocardial Ischemia from Increased Myocardial Demand

DAVID G. STRAUSS, TOBIN H. LIM, AND GALEN S. WAGNER

CHANGES IN THE ST SEGMENT

Normal Variants

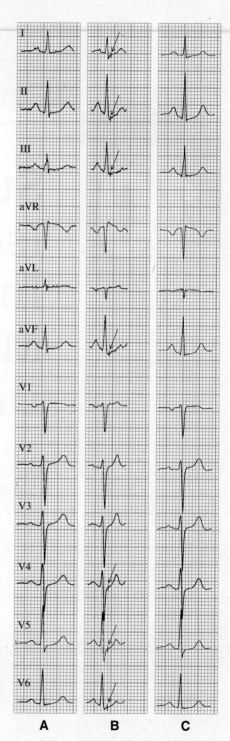

FIGURE 10.1. Twelve-lead ECGs recorded from a 54-year-old man at rest **(A)**, during an exercise stress test **(B)**, and immediately after the test **(C)**. *Arrows* indicate the depression of the ST-J point in many leads in **B**. This minor ST-J point depression with upward sloping ST segments is a benign common normal variation in the ECG during exercise.

Normally, the ST segment on the electrocardiogram (ECG) is at approximately the same baseline level as the PR and TP segments (Fig. 1.12). Observation of the stability of the position of the ST segment on the ECG during a graded exercise stress test provides clinical information about the presence or absence of myocardial ischemia.[1] If coronary blood flow is capable of increasing to a degree sufficient to satisfy the metabolic demands even of the cells in the left-ventricular subendocardium, there is minimal alteration in the appearance of the ST segment. However, there are often some changes in the ST segment that may be falsely considered "positive" for ischemia. A common normal variation in the 12-lead ECG before, during, and after exercise stress testing[2] is shown in Figure 10.1A, B, and C, respectively. Note the minor depression of the J point with the ST segment upsloping toward the upright T wave (arrows). The apparent ST-J point depression with upward sloping ST segment may occur because at faster heart rates, ventricular repolarization occurs sooner (note the shorter length of the ST segment and shorter overall QT interval in B during exercise) and the QRS and T wave almost merge together.

Typical Subendocardial Ischemia

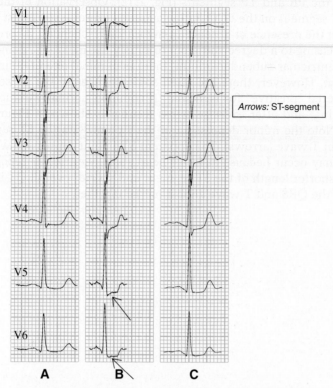

Arrows: ST-segment

A   **B**   **C**

FIGURE 10.2. Serial recordings of the six precordial leads from a 60-year-old man with a history of exertional chest pain made at rest **(A)**, during exercise at a heart rate of 167 beats per minute **(B)**, and 5 minutes after exercise **(C)**. *Arrows* indicate the horizontal ST-segment depression in leads V5 and V6 in **B**.

Partial obstructions within the coronary arteries do not produce insufficient blood supply and therefore cannot be detected on the resting ECG (Fig. 10.2A). However, when such a partial obstruction prevents myocardial blood flow from increasing enough to meet the increased metabolic demand during stress, the resulting ischemia (limited to the subendocardial layer of the left ventricle) is manifested by horizontal (see Fig. 10.2B) or downsloping ST-segment depression.[3] The ST-segment depression typically disappears within several minutes after the demand on the myocardium is returned to baseline levels by stopping the exercise (see Fig. 10.2C) because the myocardial cells have been only reversibly ischemic.

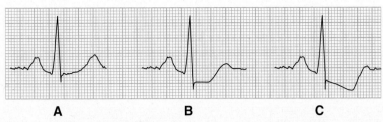

FIGURE 10.3. Single ECG waveforms at rest (A) and two variations of the abnormal condition of exercise-induced subendocardial ischemia (B and C).

A combination of two diagnostic criteria in at least one ECG lead is typically required for diagnosing left-ventricular subendocardial ischemia (Fig. 10.3):

1. ST-segment depression of ≥1 mm (0.10 mV) at the J point.
2. Either a horizontal or a downward slope toward the end of the ST segment at its junction with the T wave.

The terminal part of the T wave typically remains positive (see Fig. 10.3A–C) but with progressively diminished amplitude from Figure 10.3B and C.

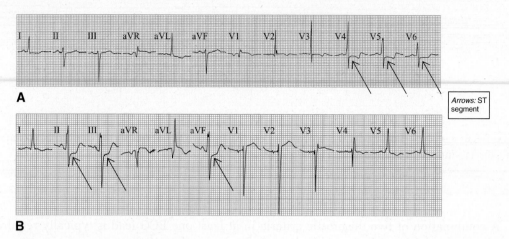

A

Arrows: ST segment

B

FIGURE 10.4. Twelve-lead ECGs from two different patients with left-ventricular subendocardial ischemia. Patient **A** has most prominent ST-segment depression in leads V4 to V6 (*arrows*), with a negative beginning of the T wave in these leads. Patient **A** also has slightly depressed ST segments in I and aVL. Patient **B** has prominent ST-segment depression in leads II, III, and aVF. All of these leads have positive poles pointing away from the epicardium of the left ventricle, thus ST depression occurs with subendocardial ischemia.

As indicated in Chapter 2, the positive poles of most of the standard limb and precordial ECG leads are directed toward the left ventricle. Subendocardial ischemia causes the ST segment to move generally away from the left ventricle (see Fig. 9.6A). The changes in the ST segment appear negative or depressed in the leftward (I, aVL, or V4 to V6) and inferiorly oriented leads (II, III, and aVF), which have their positive poles directed toward the left ventricle (Fig. 10.4A, B). As previously stated in Chapter 9, the location of the ECG leads showing ST-segment depression is not indicative of the involved region of left-ventricular subendocardial ischemia. In leads that have their positive poles directed away from the left ventricle (limb lead aVR and precordial leads V1 and V2), ST elevation is typically present (see Fig. 10.4A, B).

It may be useful to now return to the Video 9.2 (QR code below) which demonstrates how ischemic action potentials in the subendocardium create the ECG pattern of subendocardial ischemia.

Video 9.2

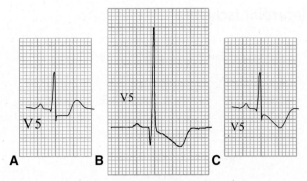

FIGURE 10.5. **A.** Horizontal ST-segment depression with upright T wave consistent with subendocardial ischemia. **B.** Left-ventricular strain causing ST-segment depression; however, it is accompanied by increased QRS voltage and an inverted T wave. **C.** Diagnostic dilemma (subendocardial ischemia versus left-ventricular strain) of depressed ST segment and inverted T wave but normal QRS voltage.

The change in the ST segments that occurs with left-ventricular subendocardial ischemia (Fig. 10.5A) is similar to that described in Chapter 5 for left-ventricular strain. However, left-ventricular strain also causes the T waves to be directed away from the left ventricle and is accompanied by the QRS changes of left-ventricular hypertrophy (LVH; see Fig. 10.5B). Therefore, a diagnostic dilemma exists when a patient with symptoms suggesting an acute coronary syndrome has a resting ECG not suggestive of LVH but with ST depression and inverted T waves (see Fig. 10.5C).

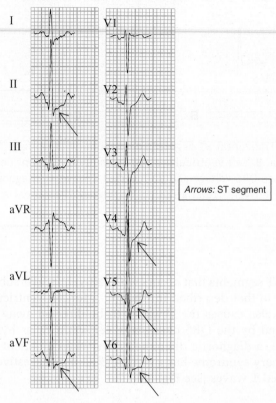

Arrows: ST segment

FIGURE 10.6. ST-J point depression with an upsloping ST segment that may be indicative of subendocardial ischemia. See Table 10.1 for proposed criteria for subendocardial ischemia.

Deviation of the junction of the ST segment with the J point, followed by an upsloping ST segment, may also be indicative of subendocardial ischemia.[2] A 0.1- to 0.2-mV depression of the J point, followed by an upsloping ST segment that remains 0.1 mV depressed for 0.08 seconds[3] or by a 0.2-mV depression of the J point followed by an upsloping ST segment that remains 0.2-mV depressed for 0.08 second, may also be considered "diagnostic" of subendocardial ischemia[4] (Fig. 10.6; Table 10.1).

Table 10.1.		
Varying Electrocardiographic Criteria for Subendocardial Ischemia		
J Point Depression (mV)	Slope	J + 0.08-s Depression
≥0.1	Flat, down	≥ same level
0.1–0.2	Up	≥0.1 mV
≥0.2	Up	≥0.2 mV

Normal Variant or Subendocardial Ischemia

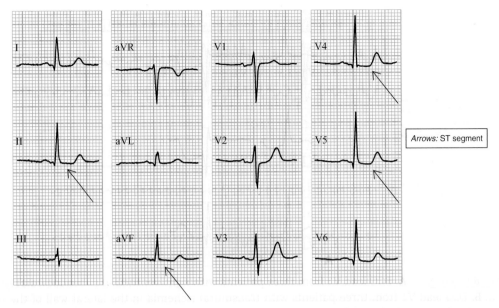

FIGURE 10.7. Twelve-lead ECG from a 69-year-old woman with severe substernal pain at rest and who was transported by ambulance to the emergency department of a hospital. *Arrows* indicate minimal ST-segment depression in many leads. This could be representative of subendocardial ischemia or could be a normal variant.

Lesser deviations of the ST segments (Fig. 10.7) could be caused by subendocardial ischemia or could be a variation of normal. Even the ST-segment changes "diagnostic" of left-ventricular subendocardial ischemia could be an extreme variation of normal. When these lesser ECG changes appear, they should be considered in the context of other manifestations of coronary insufficiency, such as precordial pain, decreased blood pressure, or cardiac arrhythmias.[5,6] Additional stress testing using cardiac imaging end points are typically required for definitive diagnosis or exclusion of insufficient myocardial perfusion.

GLOSSARY

Holter monitoring: continuous ECG recording of one or more leads, either for the detection of abnormalities of morphology suggestive of ischemia or abnormalities of rhythm.

Silent ischemia: evidence of myocardial ischemia appearing on an ECG recording in the absence of any awareness of symptoms of ischemia.

Subendocardial ischemia: a condition marked by deviation of the ST segments of an ECG away from the ventricle (always the left ventricle) and in which only the inner part of the myocardium is ischemic.

Ventricular strain: deviation of the ST segments and T waves of an ECG away from the ventricle in which there is either a severe systolic overload or marked hypertrophy.

REFERENCES

1. Ryik TM, O'Connor FC, Gittings NS, et al. Role of nondiagnostic exercise-induced ST-segment abnormalities in predicting future coronary events in asymptomatic volunteers. *Circulation.* 2002;106: 2787-2792.
2. Sansoy V, Watson DD, Beller GA. Significance of slow upsloping ST-segment depression on exercise stress testing. *Am J Cardiol.* 1997;79:709-712.
3. Rijnek RD, Ascoop CA, Talmon JL. Clinical significance of upsloping ST segments in exercise electrocardiography. *Circulation.* 1980;61:671-678.
4. Kurita A, Chaitman BR, Bourassa MG. Significance of exercise-induced junctional ST depression in evaluation of coronary artery disease. *Am J Cardiol.* 1977;40: 492-497.
5. Ellestad MH, Cooke BM, Greenberg PS. Stress testing; clinical application and predictive capacity. Prog *Cardiovasc Dis.* 1979;21:431-460.
6. Ellestad MH, Savitz S, Bergdall D, et al. The false-positive stress test: multivariate analysis of 215 subjects with hemodynamic, angiographic and clinical data. *Am J Cardiol.* 1977;40:681-685.
7. Shah A, Wagner GS, Green CL, et al. Electrocardiographic differentiation of the ST-segment depression of acute myocardial injury due to left circumflex artery occlusion from that of myocardial ischemia of nonocclusive etiologies. *Am J Cardiol.* 1997;80:512-513.
8. Hurst JW, Logue RB. *The Heart: Arteries and Veins.* New York, NY: McGraw-Hill; 1966:147.
9. Cohn PF, Fox KM. Silent myocardial ischemia. *Circulation.* 2003;108:1263-1277.
10. Krucoff MW, Pope JE, Bottner RK, et al. Dedicated ST-segment monitoring in the CCU after successful coronary angioplasty: incidence and prognosis of silent and symptomatic ischemia. In: van Armin T, Maseri A, eds. *Silent Ischemia: Current Concepts and Management.* Darmstadt, Germany: Steinkopff Verlag; 1987:140-146.

11

Transmural Myocardial Ischemia from Insufficient Blood Supply

DAVID G. STRAUSS, TOBIN H. LIM, AND GALEN S. WAGNER

CHANGES IN THE ST SEGMENT

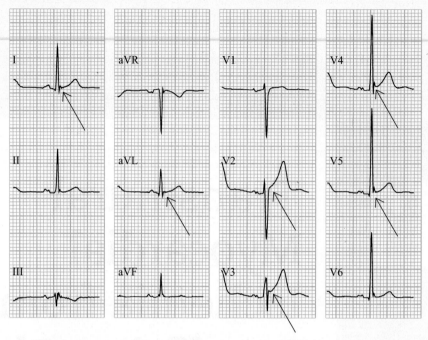

FIGURE 11.1. A 12-lead ECG from a 34-year-old man presenting for the fourth time within a year to an emergency room with severe chest pain. However, the patient had no other signs of ischemia and his ECG did not change from visit-to-visit. Individuals without ischemia can have ST elevation on routine standard ECGs. *Arrows* indicate ST-segment elevation in many leads.

Just as changes in the ST segment of the electrocardiogram (ECG) are reliable indicators of subendocardial ischemia (caused by increased myocardial demand), they are also reliable indicators of transmural myocardial ischemia from insufficient coronary blood flow. Observation of the position of the ST segments (relative to the PR and TP segments) in a patient experiencing acute precordial pain provides clinical evidence of the presence or absence of severe transmural myocardial ischemia that typically progress to myocardial infarction (MI). However, many normal individuals show ST-segment elevation on their routine standard ECGs in the absence of ischemia (Fig. 11.1).[1-3]

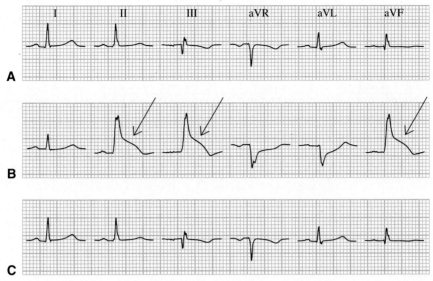

FIGURE 11.2. The six limb leads of the ECG recorded serially from a 58-year-old man with chest pain on exertion caused by a 90% obstruction of the right coronary artery. ECGs before **(A)**, during **(B)**, and after **(C)** 2 minutes of angioplasty balloon occlusion. *Arrows,* ST-segment elevation in leads II, III, and aVF that move toward the involved myocardial region during transmural myocardial ischemia.

When a sudden, complete occlusion of a coronary artery prevents blood flow from reaching an area of myocardium, the resulting transmural myocardial ischemia[4-6] is manifested by deviation of the ST segment toward the involved region. This is shown in the ECG of a patient before, during, and after receiving brief therapeutic balloon occlusion with percutaneous transluminal coronary angioplasty (Fig. 11.2A–C). The ST-segment changes typically disappear abruptly when coronary blood flow is restored by deflating the angioplasty balloon after a brief period. This indicates that the myocardial cells have been reversibly ischemic and have not actually become infarcted.

It may be difficult to differentiate the abnormal changes in the ST segment produced by transmural myocardial ischemia from variations of normal, particularly when the deviation of the ST segment is minimal. Presence of one of the following criteria is typically required for the diagnosis of transmural myocardial ischemia[7]:

1. Elevation of the origin of the ST segment at its junction (J point) with the QRS complex in two or more leads of:

   - 0.1 mV (1 mm) in any lead except for leads V2 and V3
   - in leads V2 and V3 ST-J elevation should be:
     a. 0.25 mV (2.5 mm) in men less than 40 years of age
     b. 0.20 mV (2.0 mm) in men 40 years of age or older
     c. 0.15 mV (1.5 mm) in women of any age.

2. Depression of the origin of the ST segment at the J point of 0.10 mV (1 mm) in two or more of leads V1-V3.

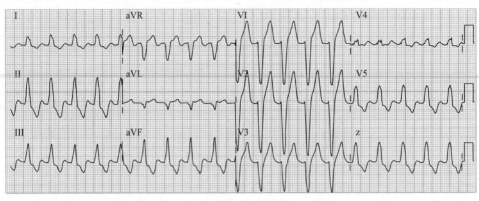

FIGURE 11.3. A 12-lead ECG of a patient with LBBB. ST-segment elevation in leads V1 to V3 is normal in LBBB and should exceed 5 mm (0.5 mV) in order to be diagnostic of acute transmural myocardial ischemia. See Table 11.1 for a complete description of criteria to diagnose acute transmural myocardial ischemia in the presence of LBBB.

A greater threshold is required for ST-segment elevation in leads V2 to V3 because a normal, slight elevation of the ST segment is often present (see Fig. 3.12). In addition, younger men are most likely to have "normal" ST elevation in leads V2 to V3, which is the reason for different thresholds by age and gender.

When the amplitude and duration of the terminal S wave is further increased in leads V1 to V3 as a result of left-ventricular dilation (see Fig. 5.8) or left-bundle-branch block (LBBB) (Fig. 11.3), an even greater "normal" elevation of the ST segment is typically present. A study has shown that elevation of the ST segment to ≥0.5 mV is required in leads V1 to V3 to diagnose acute anterior transmural myocardial ischemia in the presence of LBBB.[8] This and other electrocardiographic criteria are presented in Table 11.1. However, the 0.1-mV threshold remains applicable for diagnosis of acute transmural ischemia when the deviation of the ST segment is in the same direction (concordant with) as that of the terminal QRS waveform.

Table 11.1.

Electrocardiographic Criteria of Actue Myocardial Infarction in the Presence of Left-Bundle-Branch Block

Criteria

- ST-segment elevation ≥1 mm and concordant with a predominantly negative QRS complex.
- ST-segment depression ≥1 mm in leads V1, V2, or V3.
- ST-segment elevation ≥5 mm and discordant with a predominantly negative QRS complex.

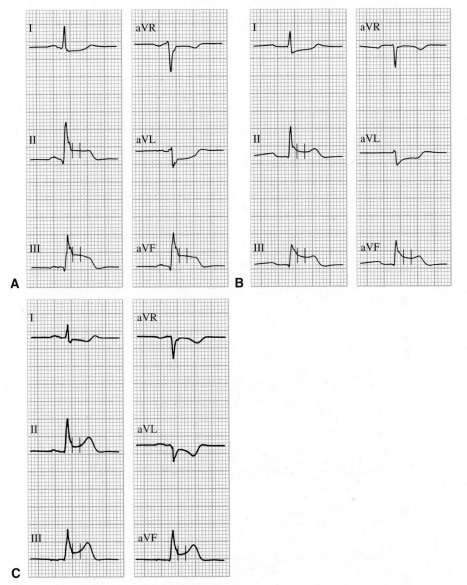

FIGURE 11.4. Variations in the appearances of the ST-segment changes of transmural myocardial ischemia in three patients during occlusion of the RCA. *Vertical lines*, locations of J and J + 0.08-second time points for measuring the amount of ST-segment deviation from the horizontal PR–TP baseline.

Various positions along the ST segment are sometimes selected for measuring the amount of deviation from the horizontal PR-TP baseline. Measurement of ST-segment deviation is either for establishing the diagnosis of transmural myocardial ischemia or for estimating its extent. "J" and "J + 0.08 second" have been used in some clinical situations (Fig. 11.4). The deviated ST segment may be horizontal (see Fig. 11.4A), downsloping (see Fig. 11.4B), or upsloping (see Fig. 11.4C). The sloping produces different amounts of deviation of the ST segment as it moves from the J point toward the T wave. Note that the J point is more elevated than the J + 0.08-second point in Figure 11.4B, equally elevated in Figure 11.4A, and less elevated in Figure 11.4C. The ECG criteria for ST-elevation myocardial infarction (STEMI) may be accompanied by other manifestations of insufficient myocardial perfusion, such as typical or atypical precordial pain, decreased blood pressure, or cardiac arrhythmias.

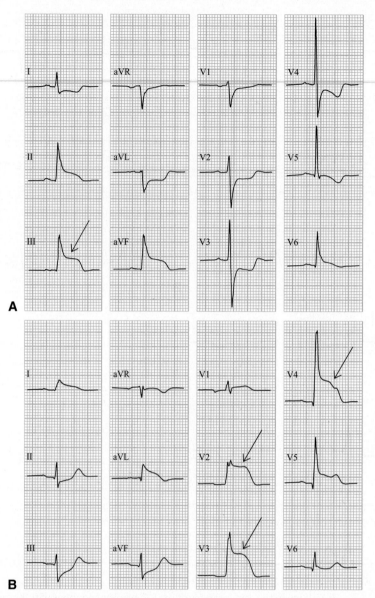

FIGURE 11.5. Twelve-lead ECGs illustrating acute transmural myocardial ischemia after 1 minute of balloon occlusion in the mid-RCA of a 47-year-old man with symptoms of unstable angina **(A)** and the proximal LAD of a 73-year-old woman with a recent acute anterior infarction **(B)**. *Arrows*, maximal ST-segment deviation directed toward the involved regions.

Because the ST-segment axis in transmural myocardial ischemia deviates toward the involved area of myocardium, the changes described appear positive or elevated in leads with their positive poles pointing toward ischemic inferior (Fig. 11.5A) or anterior (see Fig. 11.5B) aspects of the left ventricle (LV). Often, both ST-segment elevation and depression appear in different leads of a standard 12-lead ECG. Usually, the direction of greater deviation should be considered primary and the direction of lesser deviation should be considered secondary or *reciprocal*. When transmural myocardial ischemia involves both inferior and lateral aspects of the LV, the ST-segment depression of lateral involvement in leads V1 to V3 may equal or exceed the elevation produced by inferior involvement in leads II, III, and aVF.

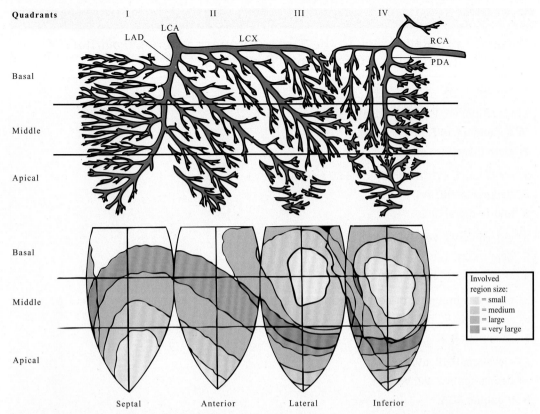

FIGURE 11.6. The 12 sections of the LV myocardium defined by the four quadrants and the three levels. The distributions of the coronary arteries (left coronary artery [LCA], left anterior descending artery [LAD] coronary artery, left circumflex artery [LCX], right coronary artery [RCA], and posterior descending [PDA]) **(top)** are related to the distributions of insufficient blood supply resulting from occlusion of the respective arteries **(bottom)**. The four grades of shading from light to dark indicate the size of the involved region as small, medium, large, and very large, respectively. (Adapted from Califf RM, Mark DB, Wagner GS. *Acute Coronary Care in the Thrombolytic Era.* Chicago, IL: Year Book; 1988:20–21, with permission.)

As when considering a map of the earth, these "Mercator" views provide a planar perspective of the spatial relationships of the anatomy and pathology to the basal, middle, and apical segments of the four quadrants or "walls" of the LV in Figure 11.6.[9] The LV is typically divided into septal, anterior, lateral, and inferior quadrants. Distributions of the major coronary arteries (left coronary artery [LCA], left anterior descending [LAD] coronary artery, left circumflex artery [LCX], right coronary artery [RCA], and the posterior descending artery [PDA]; see Fig. 11.6, top) are related to the distributions of insufficient blood supply resulting from occlusions of the respective arteries (see Fig. 11.6, bottom).

Table 11.2.

Seven Culprit Risk Areas in the Three Coronary Arteries (*Bold/Italics* indicates usual leads with maximal deviation)

1. Proximal LAD

ST elevation: V1, **V2**, **V3**, V4, I, aVL
ST depression: *aVF*, **III**

2. Main diagonal LAD

ST elevation: I, aVL (minimal-to-no ST elevation in V1, V2, V3)
ST depression: **III**, *aVF*

3. Mid-to-distal LAD

ST elevation: V3, **V4**, **V5**, V6, I, **II**, aVF
ST depression: aVR

4. Nondominant LCX

ST elevation: (minimal-to-no ST elevation in II, III, aVF)
ST depression: V1, **V2**, **V3**, V4

5. Dominant LCX

ST elevation: II, **III**, *aVF*
ST depression: V1, **V2**, **V3**, V4

6. Proximal RCA

ST elevation: II, **III**, *aVF*, V4R
ST depression: V1, V2, V3

7. Distal RCA

ST elevation: II, **III**, *aVF*
ST depression: (minimal-to-no ST depression in V1, V2, V3)

Transmural myocardial ischemia most commonly occurs in the distal aspect of the area of the left-ventricular myocardium supplied by one of the three major coronary arteries. Note that involvement of basal and middle segments of the lateral quadrant may be due to occlusion of the proximal LCX or a large (marginal) branch. The relationship between seven culprit areas in the three coronary arteries and the leads commonly with ST elevation or depression are shown in Table 11.2.

In about 90% of individuals, the PDA originates from the RCA, and the LCX supplies only part of a single left-ventricular quadrant. This has been termed *right coronary dominance*. In the other 10% of individuals with *left coronary dominance*, the PDA originates from the LCX, and the RCA supplies only the right ventricle.

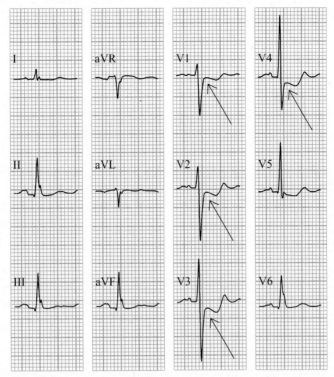

FIGURE 11.7. A 12-lead ECG recorded after 1 minute of balloon occlusion in the mid-LCX of a 54-year-old man with symptoms of acute unstable angina. *Arrows* indicate ST-segment depression in leads V1 to V4 from transmural myocardial ischemia in the lateral wall of the left ventricle.

The basal and middle sectors of the lateral quadrant of the LV typically supplied by the LCX and its branches are located distant from the positive poles of all 12 of the standard ECG leads. Therefore, occlusion of the LCX is typically indicated by ST-segment depression rather than elevation (Fig. 11.7). Note that no ST-segment elevation is present in any standard lead. Consideration of the mirror-lake image obtained by viewing the recording upside down and backward, or placement of additional leads on the posterior–lateral thorax would be required to visualize ST-segment elevation due to transmural myocardial ischemia in this area.[10]

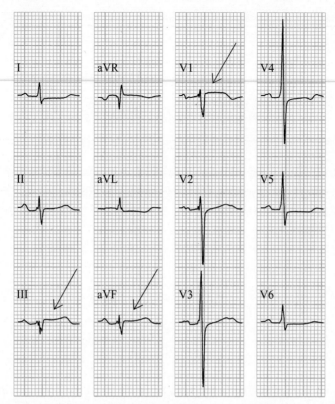

FIGURE 11.8. A 12-lead ECG after 1 minute of balloon occlusion in the proximal RCA in a 65-year-old woman presenting with acute precordial pain of sudden onset. *Arrows* indicate the transmural myocardial ischemia appearing as ST-segment elevation in leads III and aVF and transmural myocardial ischemia in the right ventricle appearing as ST-segment elevation in lead V1.

Transmural myocardial ischemia may also involve the thinner walled right-ventricular myocardium when its blood supply via the RCA becomes insufficient. Right-ventricular transmural myocardial ischemia is represented on the standard ECG as ST-segment elevation in lead V1 greater than V2 (Fig. 11.8). There would be even greater ST elevation present in the more rightward additional leads V3R and V4R than in lead V1, which is also be considered lead V2R.

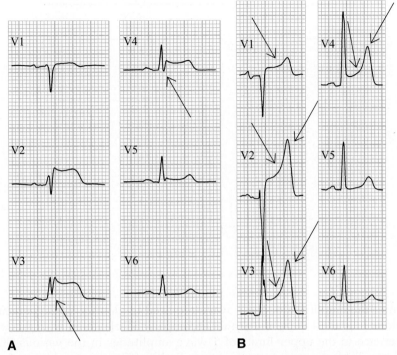

FIGURE 11.9. The six precordial leads of the ECG after 1 minute of balloon occlusion of the LAD in **(A)** a 74-year-old woman with a 5-year history of exertional angina and **(B)** a 51-year-old man with an initial episode of precordial pain. **A.** *Arrows,* disappearance of the S wave from below the TP–PR segment baseline. **B.** *Arrows,* ST-segment elevation and hyperacute T waves.

Although the T waves are not typically recognized as indicators of ischemia caused by increased myocardial demand, they are reliable indicators of ischemia from insufficient coronary blood supply (see Chapter 9). Figure 11.9 presents the changes in ST segments and T waves immediately after acute balloon occlusion of the LAD of two patients. In both examples, the ST segments and T waves deviate toward the involved anterior aspect of the LV. In some patients, the degree of deviation of the T wave is similar to that of the ST segment (see Fig. 11.9A). In other patients, there is the markedly greater deviation of the T-wave axis that is characteristic of "hyperacute" T waves (see Fig. 11.9B). These T-wave elevations typically persist only transiently after acute coronary thrombosis.[11] Hyperacute T waves may therefore be useful in timing the duration of the ischemia/infarction process when a patient presents with acute precordial pain.

Table 11.3.

T-Wave Amplitude Normal Limits (mV)

Lead[a]	Males 40–49	Females 40–49	Males ≥50	Females ≥50
aVL	0.30	0.30	0.30	0.30
I	0.55	0.45	0.45	0.45
−aVR	0.55	0.45	0.45	0.45
II	0.65	0.55	0.55	0.45
aVF	0.50	0.40	0.45	0.35
III	0.35	0.30	0.35	0.30
V1	0.65	0.20	0.50	0.35
V2	1.45	0.85	1.40	0.70
V3	1.35	0.85	1.35	0.85
V4	1.15	0.85	1.10	0.75
V5	0.90	0.70	0.95	0.70
V6	0.65	0.55	0.65	0.50

[a] Cabrera sequence

Definition of the amplitude of the T wave required to identify the hyperacute changes that occur alone in grade 1 ischemia or that accompany ST elevation with grade 2 ischemia requires reference to the upper limits of T-wave amplitudes in the various ECG leads of normal subjects. Table 11.3 presents the upper limits of T-wave amplitudes (in millivolts) in each of the 12 standard ECG leads for women and men in the >40-year-old age group in the normal data base from Glasgow, Scotland.[12] A rough estimate of the normal upper limits of T-wave amplitude would be ≥0.50 mV in the limb leads and ≥1.00 mV in the precordial leads.

CHANGES IN THE QRS COMPLEX

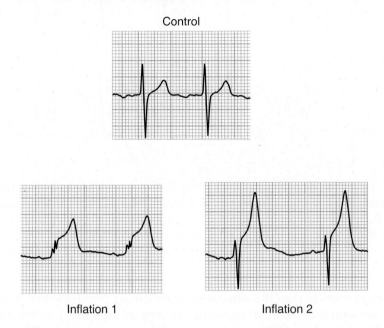

Control

Inflation 1   Inflation 2

FIGURE 11.10.   Recordings of two cardiac cycles in lead V2 from baseline (control) and after 2 minutes each of two different periods of balloon occlusion of the LAD. (From Wagner NB, Sevilla DC, Krucoff MW, et al. Transient alterations of the QRS complex and ST segment during percutaneous transluminal balloon angioplasty of the left anterior descending coronary artery. *Am J Cardiol.* 1988;62:1038–1042, with permission.)

The ECG manifestation of transmural myocardial ischemia, like that of the subendocardial ischemia described in Chapter 10, is most prominently the changes in the ST segment. This may be accompanied by deviation of the adjacent waveforms (QRS complex and T wave) in the same direction of the ST segments, as illustrated in LAD balloon inflation 2 (Fig. 11.10). This deviation affects the amplitudes of the later QRS waveforms to a greater extent than those of the earlier QRS waveforms as can be seen by comparing the inflation 2 and control recordings.[13] During inflation 1, the distortion of the QRS complex is much greater, indicating that there is a delayed depolarization of the ischemic zone. However, during the second inflation, there is minimal change in the QRS complex but significantly greater increase in T-wave amplitude. This may be due to "preconditioning", where an initial sublethal ischemic episode protects the myocardium from future ischemic episodes.[14]

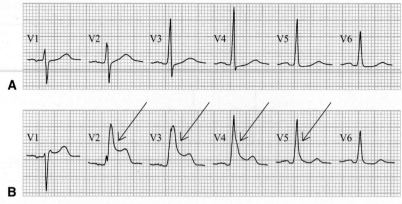

FIGURE 11.11. The six precordial leads of the ECG are presented from serial recordings from a 64-year-old man with acute unstable angina. **A.** Baseline recording prior to angiography after pain had resolved. **B.** After 2 minutes of the initial balloon occlusion of the LAD. *Arrows* indicate the increased QRS complex duration in **B** that is apparent in leads V2 to V5.

The primary changes in the QRS complexes representing "tombstoning" may occur after the onset of transmural myocardial ischemia, as seen in inflation 1 of Figures 11.10 and 11.11B. The deviation of the QRS complex toward the area of transmural ischemia occurs because of slowed conduction (delayed depolarization) in the ischemic zone (lead V2 of Fig. 11.11B). The duration of the QRS complex may also be prolonged, as in the patient whose ECG is shown in the figure above. Typically, acute ischemia of a higher grade of severity (grade 3) occurs during initial balloon occlusion when either collateral arteries or preconditioning provide the least protection. The ischemic zone is activated late, thereby producing an unopposed positive QRS complex waveform. With transmural myocardial ischemia in the lateral wall of the LV (typically from LCX occlusion), the QRS complex would deviate in the negative direction in leads V1 to V3.[15]

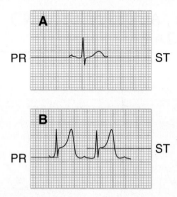

FIGURE 11.12. **A.** An ECG recording made before balloon inflation, in which the PR and ST baselines are at the same level and a 0.03-mV S wave is present. PR and ST baselines. **B.** During balloon occlusion, the ST segment is elevated by 0.03 mV by the epicardial injury current, and the S wave also deviates upward so that it just reaches the PR-segment baseline.

The deviation of the ST segments in transmural myocardial ischemia confounds measurement of the amplitudes of the QRS complex waveforms of the ECG because there are no longer isoelectric PR–ST–TP segments. As illustrated in Figure 11.12, the baseline of the PR segment remains as the reference for the initial waveform of the QRS complex, but with deviation of the QRS complex (see Fig. 11.12B), the terminal waveform maintains its relationship with the ST-segment baseline. The S-wave amplitude of 0.03-mV measured from the ST-segment baseline is the same in Figure 11.12A and B.

Having now learned more about the ST-segment, T-wave and QRS-complex changes during transmural ischemia, it is recommended to return to Video 9.1. Video 9.1 uses the simulation program ECGSIM to make the connection between ischemic action potential changes and the characteristic ECG patterns of transmural ischemia.

Video 9.1

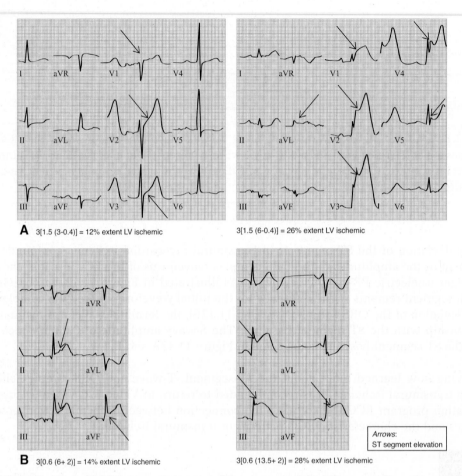

A 3[1.5 (3-0.4)] = 12% extent LV ischemic

3[1.5 (6-0.4)] = 26% extent LV ischemic

B 3[0.6 (6+ 2)] = 14% extent LV ischemic

3[0.6 (13.5+ 2)] = 28% extent LV ischemic

Arrows:
ST segment elevation

FIGURE 11.13. Aldrich score estimates of the percent of the LV myocardium that is ischemic for two anterior infarcts **(A)** and two inferior infarcts **(B)**. *Arrows* show leads with ST elevation that are counted in the Aldrich score.

The ECG evaluation in patients with acute myocardial ischemia/MI includes consideration of indices in three key aspects of this pathologic process: extent, acuteness, and severity. Algorithms for each of these have been developed. Presenting ECGs of patients with anterior or inferior STEMI can be used for calculating the extent (Aldrich score), acuteness (Anderson-Wilkins score), and severity (Sclarovsky–Birnbaum grade).

In the following section, each of these three indices is calculated on the presenting ECGs of two patients with anterior infarcts and two patients with inferior infarcts.

Extent

The Aldrich score has been developed for estimating the extent of myocardium at risk for infarction by quantitating initial ST-segment changes on the presenting ECG.[16] This score is expressed as "% myocardium at risk of infarction" as illustrated above in Figure 11.13.[16] Aldrich scoring formulas for anterior and inferior STEMI are as follows:

% anterior LV infarcted = 3(1.5 [number of leads with ST elevation − 0.4])
% inferior LV infarcted = 3(0.6[ΣST elevation in leads II, III, aVF] + 2.0)

Observation of all of the 11 leads is required for estimating the extent of anterior infarcts (see Fig. 11.13A) because counting the number of leads with ST elevation is required. However, observation of only the limb leads II, III, and aVF is required for estimating the extent of inferior infarcts (see Fig. 11.13B) because only the sum of ST elevation in these is considered.

Table 11.4.

Thresholds for Anderson-Wilkins Acuteness Score

Leads	Tall T Waves (mV)	Abnormal Q Waves (s)
I	0.5	0.02
II	0.5	0.02
III	0.25	Only if abnormal in aVF
aVR	—	—
aVL	0.25	0.02
aVF	0.5	0.02
V1	0.5	0.20
V2	1.0	0.85
V3	1.0	0.85
V4	1.0	Any
V5	0.75	0.02
V6	0.75	0.02

Acuteness

Anderson-Wilkins and colleagues[17,18] developed an ECG acuteness score (Anderson-Wilkins score) to augment the historical timing of acute symptom onset in guiding the clinician about the potential for using reperfusion therapy to achieve myocardial salvage.

The Anderson-Wilkins score is provided as a continuous scale from 4.0 (hyperacute) to 1.0 (subacute) based on the comparative hyperacute T waves versus abnormal Q waves in each of the leads with ST-segment elevation. (See Table 11.4 for T wave amplitude and Q wave duration thresholds) There are two steps in the acuteness scoring process as indicated:

1. Determine the phase of the infarction process (from IA to IIB) in all leads with either ST-segment elevation or abnormally tall T waves (Table 11.5);
2. Calculate the acuteness score for the entire 12-lead ECG.

$$\frac{4(\# \text{ leads IA}) + 3(\# \text{ leads IB}) + 2(\# \text{ leads IIA}) + (\# \text{ leads IIB})}{\text{Total } \# \text{ leads IA, IB, IIA, and IIB}}$$

Table 11.5.

Phase of Infarction Process: To Be Determined in Leads with Either ST-Segment Elevation or Tall T Waves

	Abnormal Q Waves	
Tall T Waves	No	Yes
Yes	I A	II A
No	I B	II B

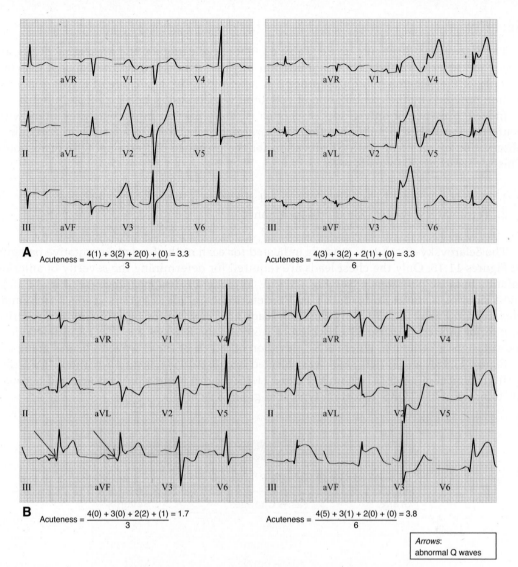

A Acuteness = $\dfrac{4(1) + 3(2) + 2(0) + (0)}{3} = 3.3$

Acuteness = $\dfrac{4(3) + 3(2) + 2(1) + (0)}{6} = 3.3$

B Acuteness = $\dfrac{4(0) + 3(0) + 2(2) + (1)}{3} = 1.7$

Acuteness = $\dfrac{4(5) + 3(1) + 2(0) + (0)}{6} = 3.8$

Arrows:
abnormal Q waves

FIGURE 11.14. Anderson-Wilkins acuteness score estimates of the "acuteness" of ischemia. A score of 4 indicates early (hyperacute) ischemia (tall T waves without Q waves). A score of 1 indicates subacute ischemia (Q waves present, no tall T waves). **A.** Acute anterior infarcts. **B.** Acute inferior infarcts.

Observation of all 12 leads is required for determination of the acuteness scores of both anterior (Fig. 11.14A) and inferior (see Fig. 11.14B) infarcts. The morphologies of Q and T waves in all leads with either ST elevation or tall T waves must be considered. Earliness is indicated by tall T waves without abnormal R waves in both examples of anterior infarcts (see Fig. 11.14A) but only the second example of inferior infarcts (see Fig. 11.14B) due to the already abnormal Q waves in the first example.

Severity

The Sclarovsky–Birnbaum grade (Table 11.6) for application on the presenting ECG estimates the severity of the ischemia/infarction process. It is based on the concept that the severity of the ischemia/infarction process is determined by the degree of myocardial protection provided by the combination of collateral vessels and ischemic preconditioning.

Indeed, presence of only grade 1 ischemia is rarely present in patients presenting with acute myocardial ischemia/infarction. Differentiation between grades 2 and 3 requires observation of each lead with ST elevation for the presence of "terminal QRS distortion." This is characterized in leads with:

1. Terminal R wave by a large ST-segment elevation to R-wave amplitude ratio.
2. Terminal S wave by its total disappearance.

The Sclarovsky–Birnbaum grade is indicated for each of the four representative patients in Figures 11.15. Only the chest leads are required for determining the severity of anterior infarcts because persistence (see Fig. 11.15A, left side) or disappearance (see Fig. 11.15A, right side) of S waves in leads V1 to V3 determines grade 2 versus grade 3 ischemia. However in Figure 11.15B, only the limb leads are required for determining the severity of inferior infarcts because ST elevation of <50% of the R wave (see Fig. 11.15B, left side) indicates grade ischemia, whereas ST elevation of ≥50% of the R wave indicates grade 3.

Figure 11.15A and B (left side) was selected because of ST elevation without "QRS distortion" typical of grade 2 ischemia. Figure 11.15A and B (right side) was selected because of "tombstone-like" QRS distortion typical of grade 3 ischemia.

Table 11.6.		
Sclarovsky–Birnbaum Grade		
Grade	ECG Changes	Severity
1	T wave	Least
2	ST segment	Moderate
3	QRS complex	Most

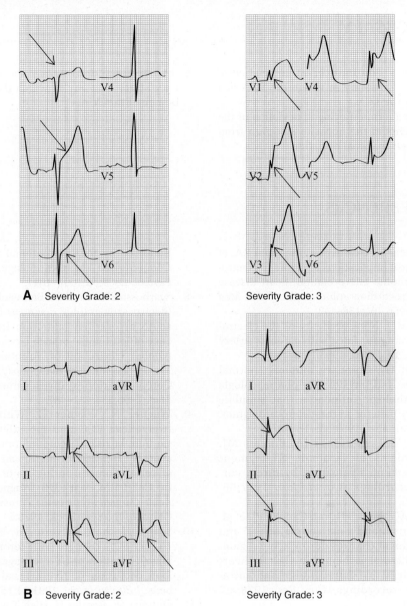

FIGURE 11.15. Sclarovsky–Birnbaum grades of ischemia. **A.** ECGs of patients with anterior infarcts with grade 2 ischemia (ST elevation without QRS distortion) and grade 3 (ST elevation with QRS distortion defined by loss of S waves). **B.** ECGs of patients with inferior infarcts with grade 2 ischemia (ST elevation <50% R-wave amplitude) and grade 3 ischemia (ST elevation ≥50% R-wave amplitude).

Left coronary dominance: an unusual coronary artery anatomy in which the PDA is a branch of the LCX.

Reciprocal: a term referring to deviation of the ST segments in the opposite direction from that of their maximal deviation.

Right coronary dominance: the usual coronary artery anatomy in which the PDA is a branch of the RCA.

REFERENCES

1. Prinzmetal M, Goldman A, Massumi RA, et al. Clinical implications of errors in electrocardiographic interpretation; heart disease of electrocardiographic origin. *J Am Med Assoc*. 1956;161:138–143.

2. Levine HD. Non-specificity of the electrocardiogram associated with coronary artery disease. *Am J Med*. 1953;15:344–355.

3. Marriott HJ. Coronary mimicry: normal variants, and physiologic, pharmacologic and pathologic influences that simulate coronary patterns in the electrocardiogram. *Ann Intern Med*. 1960;52:413–427.

4. Vincent GM, Abildskov JA, Burgess MJ. Mechanisms of ischemic ST-segment displacement. Evaluation by direct current recordings. *Circulation*. 1977;56:559–566.

5. Kleber AG, Janse MJ, van Capelle FJ, et al. Mechanism and time course of S-T and T-Q segment changes during acute regional myocardial ischemia in the pig heart determined by extracellular and intracellular recordings. *Circ Res*. 1978;42:603–613.

6. Janse MJ, Cinca J, Morena H, et al. The "border zone" in myocardial ischemia. An electrophysiological, metabolic, and histochemical correlation in the pig heart. *Circ Res*. 1979;44:576–588.

7. Wagner GS, Macfarlane P, Wellens H, et al. AHA/ACCF/HRS recommendations for the standardization and interpretation of the electrocardiogram: part VI: acute ischemia/infarction: a scientific statement from the American Heart Association Electrocardiography and Arrhythmias Committee, Council on Clinical Cardiology; the American College of Cardiology Foundation; and the Heart Rhythm Society. Endorsed by the International Society for Computerized Electrocardiology. *J Am Coll Cardiol*. 2009;53:1003–1011.

8. Sgarbossa EB, Pinski SL, Barbagelata A, et al. Electrocardiographic diagnosis of evolving acute myocardial infarction in the presence of left bundle-branch block. GUSTO-1 (Global Utilization of Streptokinase and Tissue Plasminogen Activator for Occluded Coronary Arteries) Investigators. *N Engl J Med*. 1996;334:481–487.

9. Wagner N, Wagner G, White R. The twelve-lead ECG and the extent of myocardium at risk of acute infarction: cardiac anatomy and lead locations, and the phases of serial changes during acute occlusion. In: Califf RM, Mark DB, Wagner GS, eds. *Acute Coronary Care in the Thrombolytic Era*. Chicago, IL: Year Book; 1988:31–45.

10. Seatre H, Startt-Selvester R, Solomon J. 16-lead ECG changes with coronary angioplasty: location of ST-T changes with balloon occlusion of five arterial perfusion beds. *J Electrocardiol*. 1991;24:153–162.

11. Dressler W, Roesler H. High T waves in the earliest stage of myocardial infarction. *Am Heart J*. 1947;34:627–645.

12. Macfarlane P, Lawrie T, eds. *Comprehensive Electrocardiography*. New York, NY: Pergamon Press; 1989:1446–1457.

13. Wagner NB, Sevilla DC, Krucoff MW, et al. Transient alterations of the QRS complex and ST segment during percutaneous transluminal balloon angioplasty of the left anterior descending coronary artery. *Am J Cardiol*. 1988;62:1038–1042.

14. Murry CE, Jennings RB, Reimer KA. Preconditioning with ischemia: a delay of lethal cell injury in ischemic myocardium. *Circulation*. 1986;74:1124–1136.

15. Selvester RH, Wagner NB, Wagner GS. Ventricular excitation during percutaneous transluminal angioplasty of the left anterior descending coronary artery. *Am J Cardiol.* 1988;62:1116–1121.

16. Aldrich HR, Wagner NB, Boswick J, et al. Use of initial ST-segment deviation for prediction of final electrocardiographic size of acute myocardial infarcts. *Am J Cardiol.* 1988;61:749–753.

17. Anderson ST, Wilkins M, Weaver WD, et al. Electrocardiographic phasing of acute myocardial infarction. *J Electrocardiol.* 1992;25(Supp l):3–5.

18. Corey KE, Maynard C, Pahlm O, et al. Combined historical and electrocardiographic timing of acute anterior and inferior myocardial infarcts for prediction of reperfusion achievable size limitation. *Am J Cardiol.* 1999;83:826–831.

12

Myocardial Infarction

DAVID G. STRAUSS, TOBIN H. LIM, AND
GALEN S. WAGNER

INFARCTING PHASE

Transition from Ischemia to Infarction

When insufficient coronary blood supply persists after myocardial energy reserves have been depleted, the myocardial cells become irreversibly ischemic and the process of necrosis termed "myocardial infarction" occurs. The QRS complex is the most useful aspect of the electrocardiogram (ECG) for evaluating the presence, location, and extent of myocardial infarction (MI), which will be discussed in detail in this chapter.

The end of Chapter 11 discusses the transition from acute myocardial ischemia to cellular necrosis (infarction) and how ECG scores can be used to estimate the extent,[1] severity,[2] and acuteness[3] of ischemia. The Anderson-Wilkins acuteness score can estimate where in the process from acute ischemia to completed infarction a particular patient is. A key message is that during acute transmural ischemia, the electrical vector (axis) of the QRS complex, ST segment, and T wave all point toward the ischemic region. In other words, in ECG leads above the ischemic region, S waves disappear and/or R waves increase; ST-segment elevation develops; and T waves increase in amplitude. However, as the process of ischemia transitions to infarction, T waves decrease in amplitude (later becoming negative); Q waves develop; and ST segments decrease in amplitude.

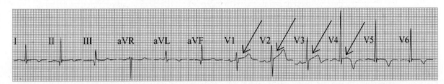

FIGURE 12.1. A 12-lead ECG from a 68-year-old man 4 days after thrombolytic therapy for an acute infarction. Acute chest pain has returned and new ST-segment elevation is apparent. *Arrows,* ST-segment elevation in multiple leads.

The changes in the ST segment that are prominent during transmural myocardial ischemia typically disappear when the jeopardized myocardium either infarcts or is salvaged. The time course of resolution of the injury current is accelerated by therapeutic reperfusion via the culprit artery[4] (see Chapter 11). Schroder and coworkers[5] identified the threshold of ≥70% reduction in ST-segment elevation in the maximally involved lead as indicative of successful reperfusion.

When re-elevation of the ST segments is observed, further myocardial ischemia is suggested (Fig. 12.1). The reperfusing phase may be complicated by infarction of the myocardium in the periphery of the initially ischemic area. The initially occluding thrombus may embolize downstream to interfere with salvage that would have been attained via collateral channels.

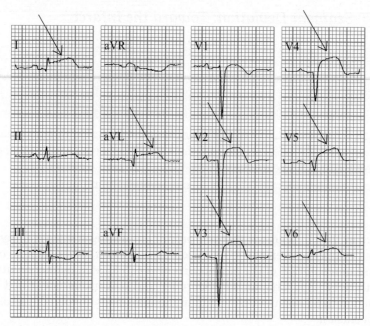

FIGURE 12.2. A 12-lead ECG obtained 2 weeks after an acute LAD occlusion leading to an extensive anteroseptal infarction. *Arrows*, indicate persistent ST-segment elevation without evolution of T-wave inversion.

In some patients, the ST-segment elevation does not completely resolve and T-wave inversion fails to occur during the reperfusing phase of an MI (Fig. 12.2). This condition more commonly occurs with anterior infarcts than with those in the other locations in the left ventricle (LV).[6] The lack of ST-segment resolution has been associated acutely with failure to reperfuse and chronically with thinning of the left-ventricular wall caused by *infarct expansion*.[7,8] The most extreme manifestation of infarct expansion is the development of a *ventricular aneurysm*, but this is almost always prevented by successful reperfusion therapy.

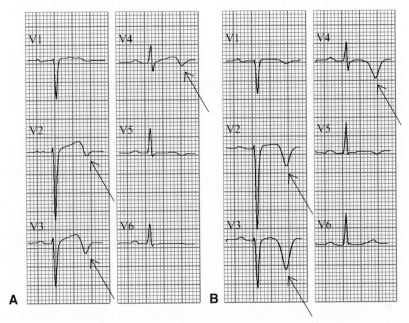

FIGURE 12.3. Serial 12-lead ECGs from a 64-year-old woman at 3 days **(A)** and 7 days **(B)** after an uncomplicated acute anteroseptal infarction. *Arrows,* indicate the terminal T-wave negativity **(A)** and total T-wave negativity **(B)**.

The movement of the T waves toward the involved region of the LV also resolves as the jeopardized myocardium either recovers or infarcts. Unlike the ST segment, however, T waves do not typically return only to their original positions. The T waves typically migrate past the isoelectric baseline until they are directed away from the involved region.[9] They assume an appearance identical to that described in Chapter 9 as "postischemic T waves," indicating that there is no ongoing myocardial ischemia. This evolution of the T wave is illustrated in serial ECGs at 3 and 7 days post *anterior infarction* (Fig. 12.3A, B). Typically, the terminal portion of the T wave is the first to become inverted, followed by the middle and initial portions.

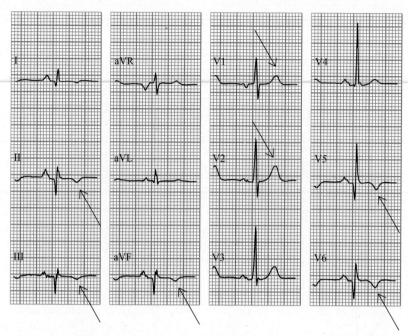

FIGURE 12.4. A 12-lead ECG from a 53-year-old man 5 days after an infarction involving the inferior and lateral walls extending to the apex. *Arrows* indicate negative T waves in leads with abnormal Q waves but positive T waves in leads with abnormal R waves.

Similarly, when the lateral wall of the LV is involved, the T waves eventually become markedly positive in the leads in which the injury current was represented by ST depression. Figure 12.4 illustrates the prominent positive T waves (arrows) with abnormal R waves in leads V1 and V2 that accompany the negative T waves (arrows) with abnormal Q waves in other leads (II, III, aVF, V5, and V6) during the healing phase of an extensive inferior infarction.

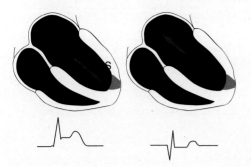

FIGURE 12.5.   Schematic cross-sections.

The QRS complex is the key waveform for evaluating the presence, location, and extent of a healing or chronic MI. As indicated in Chapter 11, almost immediately after a complete coronary artery occlusion, the QRS complex deviates toward the involved myocardial region, primarily because of delay in myocardial activation and secondarily because of the ischemia current of injury. Because the process of infarction begins in the most poorly perfused subendocardial layer of the myocardium, the deviation of the terminal QRS waveforms toward the ischemic region is replaced by deviation of the initial QRS waveforms away from the infarcted region (Fig. 12.5).[10] Absence of any electrical activation of the infarcted myocardium has replaced the delayed activation of the severely ischemic myocardium, as illustrated in Figure 12.5.

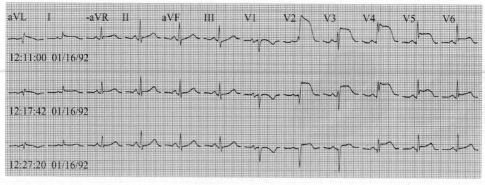

FIGURE 12.6. Continuous ECG monitoring during the first 27 minutes of intravenous thrombolytic therapy (begun at 12:00:00) in a 69-year-old man with acute thrombotic occlusion of the LAD. The 12 standard leads of the ECG are presented in panoramic format after 11, 17, and 27 minutes of therapy.

The evolving appearance of the abnormalities of the QRS complex produced by an anterior infarction during the first few minutes of intravenous thrombolytic therapy with continuous monitoring for ischemia is shown in Figure 12.6. Secondary changes in the morphology of the QRS complex during transmural myocardial ischemia have shifted the axis of the complex toward the anterior left-ventricular wall. Myocardial reperfusion is accompanied by rapid resolution of the transmural myocardial ischemia and a shift of the QRS complex away from the anterior left-ventricular wall. Although it may appear that the reperfusion itself has caused the infarction, it is much more likely that the infarction occurred before initiation of the therapy that led to reperfusion and that its detection on the ECG was obscured by the secondary changes of the QRS complex caused by the ischemic injury currents.

Transmural myocardial ischemia involving the thin right-ventricular free wall may be manifested on the ECG by deviation of the ST segment (see Chapter 11), but right-ventricular infarction is not manifested by significant alteration of the QRS complex. This is because activation of the right-ventricular free wall is insignificant in comparison with activation of the thicker interventricular septum and left-ventricular free wall. MI evolves from transmural myocardial ischemia in the distal aspects of the left-ventricular myocardium supplied by one of the three major coronary arteries (see Fig. 11.6).[11]

QRS Complex for Diagnosing

Table 12.1.			
Abnormal Q Waves Suggesting MI			
Limb Leads		Precordial Leads	
Lead	Criteria for Abnormal	Lead	Criteria for Abnormal
I	≥0.03 s	V1	Any Q
II	≥0.03 s	V2	Any Q
III	None	V3	Any Q
aVR	None	V4	≥0.02 s
aVL	≥0.03 s	V5	≥0.03 s
aVF	≥0.03 s	V6	≥0.03 s

Modified from Wagner GS, Freye CJ, Palmeri ST, et al. Evaluation of a QRS scoring system for estimating myocardial infarct size. I. Specificity and observer agreement. *Circulation.* 1982;65:345, with permission.

The initial portion of the axis of the QRS complex deviates most prominently away from the area of infarction and is represented on the ECG by a prolonged Q-wave duration. As presented in Figure 3.6, the initial QRS waveform may normally be negative in all leads except V1 to V3. The presence of any Q wave is considered abnormal only in these 3 of the 12 standard ECG leads. Table 12.1 indicates the upper limits of normal Q-wave duration in the various ECG leads.[12] The duration of the Q wave should be the primary measurement used in the definition of abnormality, because the amplitudes of the individual QRS waveforms vary with the overall amplitude of the QRS complex. As discussed in the next section, Q-wave amplitude should be considered abnormal only in relation to the amplitude of the following R wave.

Many cardiac conditions other than MI are capable of producing abnormal initial QRS waveforms. As indicated in Chapters 5 through 7, abnormalities that commonly prolong the duration of the Q wave are:

1. ventricular hypertrophy;
2. intraventricular conduction abnormalities; and
3. ventricular preexcitation.

The term "Q wave" as used here also refers to the Q-wave equivalent of abnormal R waves in leads V1 and V2. Therefore, the following steps should be considered in the evaluation of Q waves for the presence of MI:

1. Are abnormal Q waves present in any lead?
2. Are criteria present for other cardiac conditions that can produce abnormal Q waves?
3. Does the extent of Q-wave abnormality exceed that which could have been produced by some other cardiac condition?

Table 12.2.

Abnormally Small R Waves Suggesting MI

Limb Leads		Precordial Leads	
Lead	Criteria for Abnormal	Lead	Criteria for Abnormal
I	R amp ≤0.20 mV	V1	None
II	None	V2	R dur ≤0.01 s or amp ≤0.10 mV
III	None	V3	R dur ≤0.02 s or amp ≤0.20 mV
aVR	None	V4	R amp ≤0.70 mV or ≤Q amp
aVL	R amp ≤Q amp	V5	R amp ≤0.70 mV or ≤2 × Q amp
aVF	R amp ≤2 × Q amp	V6	R amp ≤0.60 mV or ≤3 × Q amp

amp, amplitude; dur, duration.

The deviation of the QRS axis away from the area of an MI may, in the absence of abnormal Q waves, be represented by diminished R waves. Table 12.2 indicates the leads in which R waves of less than a certain amplitude or duration may be indicative of MI.[2]

Infarction in the lateral wall of the LV is represented by a positive rather than a negative deviation of the QRS complex. This results in an increased rather than a decreased R-wave duration and amplitude in precordial leads VI and V2[13] (Table 12.3).

Table 12.3.

Abnormally Large R Waves Suggesting MI

Lead	Criteria for Abnormal
V1	R dur ≥0.04 s, R amp ≥0.60 mV, R amp ≥S amp
V2	R dur ≥0.05 s, R amp ≥1.50 mV, R amp ≥1.5 × S amp

amp, amplitude; dur, duration.

Table 12.4.
Infarction Terminology Relationships
Septal Wall - LAD occlusion **Q waves or diminished R waves: V1-V3** (V4-V5 if extends toward apex)
Anterior Wall - LAD occlusion **Q waves or diminished R waves: I, aVL** (V3-V5 if extends toward septum and apex)
Inferior Wall Infarct - RCA occlusion **Q waves or diminished R waves: II, III, aVF** (V6 if extends toward apex)
Lateral Wall Infarct - LCX occlusion **Large R Waves: V1, V2** (Q Waves or diminished R waves in V6 if extends toward apex)

LAD, left anterior descending; LCX, left circumflex artery; LV, left ventricle; RCA, right coronary artery; RV, right ventricle.

Table 12.4 indicates the relationships among the coronary arteries, left-ventricular walls, and ECG leads that provide a basis for localizing MIs.[14] It may also be helpful to refer to Figure 11.6 as this learning unit is read.

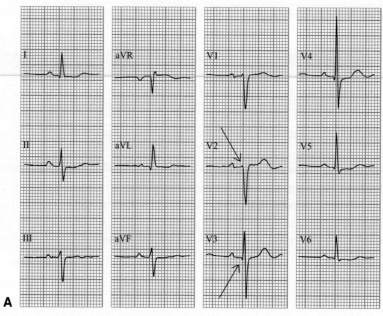

A

FIGURE 12.7. Twelve-lead ECGs from a 75-year-old man with a previous infarct limited to the septum **(A)**, a 61-year-old man with a previous infarct involving the anterior wall **(B)**, and a 55-year-old man with a previous anterior infarct involving multiple apical sectors **(C)**. *Arrows,* Q waves or diminished R waves.

An infarct produced by insufficient blood flow via the left anterior descending (LAD) coronary artery and limited to the septal quadrant (Fig. 12.7A) is termed an "anteroseptal infarct." When the infarct extends into the anterior quadrant (see Fig. 12.7B) and/or into the apical segments of other quadrants (see Fig. 12.7C), it is commonly referred to as an "extensive anterior" infarct. Although these two additional myocardial regions that may be infarcted by occlusion of the LAD are anatomically separate, they commonly share the same "apical" designation.

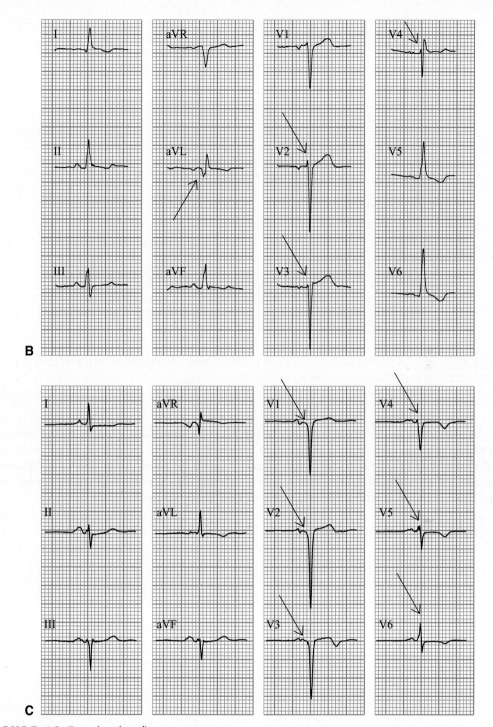

FIGURE 12.7.   (continued)

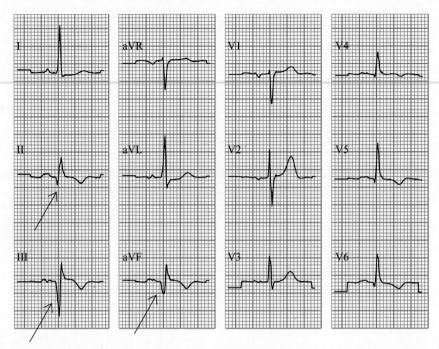

FIGURE 12.8. A 12-lead ECG from a 72-year-old woman 3 days after an acute inferior myocardial infarction from occlusion of the RCA. *Arrows*, abnormal Q.

In most individuals, the right coronary artery (RCA) is "dominant" (supplying the posterior descending artery). Its complete obstruction typically produces an *inferior infarction* involving the basal and middle segments of the inferior quadrant resulting in abnormal Q waves. Figure 12.8 was recorded 3 days after an acute inferior MI. Abnormal Q waves appear only in the three limb leads with inferiorly oriented positive poles (leads II, III, and aVF).

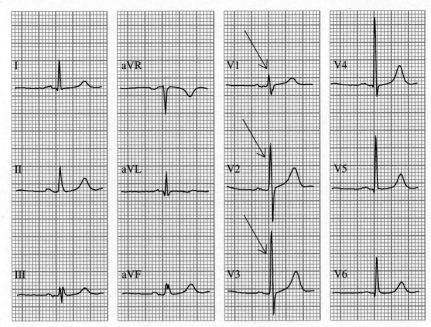

FIGURE 12.9. A 12-lead ECG from a 70-year-old man 1 year after an acute lateral-wall myocardial infarction. Coronary angiography showed complete occlusion of a nondominant LCX (the RCA supplied the posterior descending artery). *Arrows*, abnormally prominent R waves.

Also, when the RCA is dominant, the typical distribution of the left circumflex artery (LCX) supplies only the left-ventricular free wall between the distributions of the LAD and posterior descending artery. The basal and middle segments of the lateral wall of the LV are located away from the positive poles of all 12 of the standard ECG leads. Therefore, complete occlusion of a nondominant LCX is indicated by a positive (in leads V1 and V2) rather than a negative deviation of the QRS complex (Fig. 12.9) and termed *lateral infarction* (formerly termed *posterior* or "posterolateral"). Additional leads on the posterior thorax are required to record the elevation of the ST segment caused by transmural myocardial ischemia and the negative deviation of the QRS complex caused by MI in this region.[13]

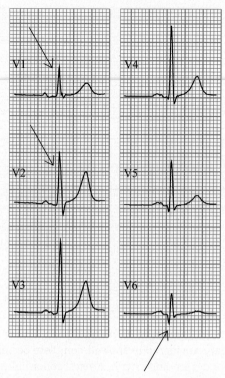

FIGURE 12.10. The six precordial leads of the ECG from a 63-year-old man 1 week after an acute infarction of the lateral wall of the left ventricle from an LCX occlusion. *Arrows,* abnormally large R waves in V1 and V2 and presence of a Q wave in aVF.

Figure 12.10 presents an example of the almost complete QRS-axis deviation away from the left-ventricular free wall expected from a more extensive infarction of the LV lateral wall. Note the almost completely positive QRS forces in leads V1 to V3 and the abnormal Q wave in lead V6.

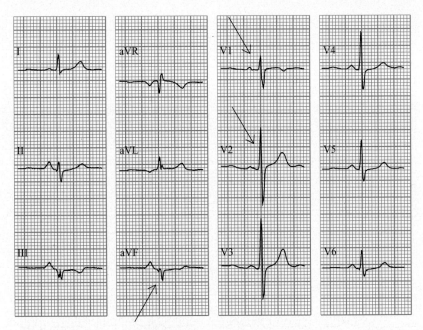

FIGURE 12.11. A 12-lead ECG from a 70-year-old woman with a healed interolateral infarction. *Arrows,* abnormal Q wave in aVF and abnormally prominent R waves in V1 to V2.

When the left coronary artery is dominant (supplying the posterior descending artery), a sudden complete obstruction of the RCA can produce infarction only in the right ventricle, which is not likely to produce changes in the QRS complex. The LCX supplies the middle and basal segments of both the lateral and inferior LV walls, and its obstruction can produce an inferolateral infarction (Fig. 12.11). This same combination of left-ventricular locations can be involved when there is dominance of the RCA and one of its branches extends into the typical distribution of the LCX. The ECG in this instance indicates the region infarcted, but not whether the RCA or the LCX is the "culprit artery."

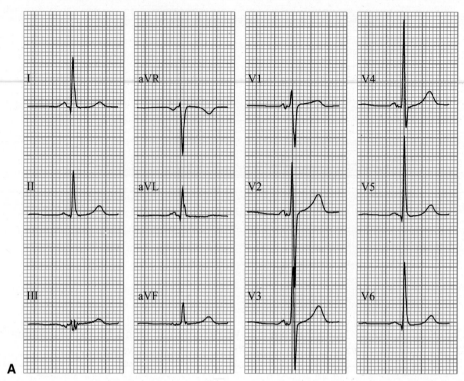

A

FIGURE 12.12. Serial 12-lead ECGs from a previous routine examination **(A)**, the time of hospital admission **(B)**, and the time of hospital discharge **(C)** of an 81-year-old man.

The lateral wall of the apex of the heart may be involved when either a dominant RCA or LCX is acutely obstructed and inferior, lateral, and *apical* locations of infarctions are apparent on the serial 12-lead ECGs (Fig. 12.12). A patient's baseline ECG is shown in Figure 12.12A without abnormal QRS forces. The ECG at the time of hospital admission (see Fig. 12.12B) already shows abnormal Q waves, and the recording at hospital discharge (see Fig. 12.12C) shows that an abnormally prominent R wave has appeared in leads V1 and V2.

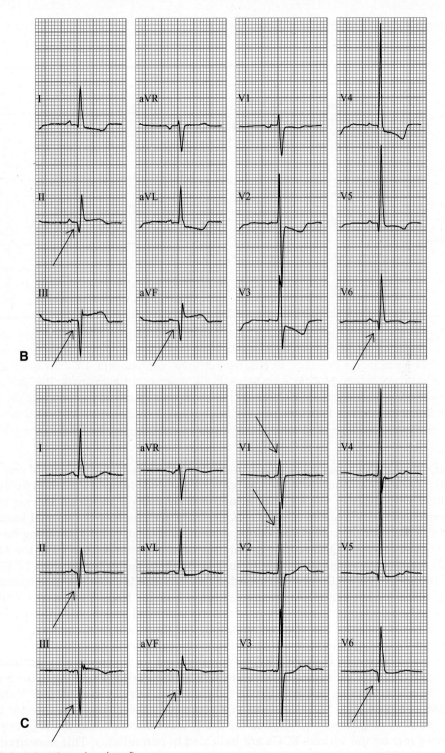

FIGURE 12.12. *(continued)*

Complete 50-Criteria, 31-Point QRS Scoring System*

Lead	Maximum Lead Points	Criteria	Points
I	(2)	Q≥30 ms	(1)
		{ R/Q ≤1	(1)
		{ R≤0.2 mV	(1)
II	(2)	{ Q≥40 ms	(2)
		{ Q≥30 ms	(1)
aVL	(2)	Q≥30 ms	(1)
		R/Q ≤1	(1)
aVF	(5)	{ Q≥50 ms	(3)
		{ Q≥40 ms	(2)
		{ Q≥30 ms	(1)
		{ R/Q ≤1	(2)
		{ R/Q ≤2	(1)

V_1
- Anterior (1) — Any Q (1)
- Lateral (4) — R/S ≥1 (1)
  - { R≥50 ms (2)
  - { R≥1.0 mV (2)
  - { R≥40 ms (1)
  - { R≥0.6 mV (1)
- Q and S ≤0.3 mV (1)

V_2
- Anterior (1) — Any Q (1)
  - { R≤10 ms (1)
  - { R≤0.1 mV (1)
  - { R≤R V, mV (1)
- Lateral (4) — R/S ≥1.5 (1)
  - { R≥60 ms (2)
  - { R≥2.0 mV (2)
  - { R≥50 ms (1)
  - { R≥1.5 mV (1)
- Q and S ≤0.4 mV (1)

V_3 (1)
- { Any Q (1)
- { R≤20 ms (1)
- { R≤0.2 mV (1)

V_4 (3) — Q≥20 ms (1)
- { R/S ≤0.5 (2)
- { R/Q ≤0.5 (2)
- { R/S ≤1 (1)
- { R/Q ≤1 (1)
- { R≤0.7 mV (1)

V_5 (3) — Q≥30 ms (1)
- { R/S ≤1 (2)
- { R/Q ≤1 (2)
- { R/S ≤2 (1)
- { R/Q ≤2 (1)
- { R≤0.7 mV (1)

V_6 (3) — Q≥30 ms (1)
- { R/S ≤1 (2)
- { R/Q ≤1 (2)
- { R/S ≤3 (1)
- { R/Q ≤3 (1)
- { R≤0.6 mV (1)

FIGURE 12.13. Selvester QRS score for estimating myocardial infarct size. See Loring Z, Chelliah S, Selvester RH, et al. A detailed guide for quantification of myocardial scar with the Selvester QRS score in the presence of electrocardiogram confounders. *J Electrocardiol.* 2011;44: 544–554 for additional details. (Modified from Selvester RH, Wagner GS, Hindman NB. The Selvester QRS scoring system for estimating myocardial infarct size. The development and application of the system. *Arch Intern Med.* 1985;145:1877–1881, with permission. Copyright 1985, American Medical Association.)

An individual patient may have single or multiple infarcts in the regions of any of the three major coronary arteries. Selvester and coworkers[15-17] developed a method for estimating the total percentage of the LV that is infarcted by using a weighted scoring system. Computerized simulation of the sequence of electrical activation of the normal human LV provided the basis for their 30-point scoring system, with each point accounting for 3% of the LV.[15-17] The Selvester QRS scoring system includes 50 criteria from 10 of the 12 standard ECG leads, with weights ranging from 1 to 3 points per criterion (Fig. 12.13). The maximal number of points that can be awarded for each lead is shown in parentheses after each lead name (or left-ventricular region within a lead for leads V1 and V2). Only one criterion can be selected from each group of criteria within a bracket. All criteria involving R/Q or R/S ratios consider the relative amplitudes of these waves. Criteria in precordial leads V1 and V2 for both anterior and lateral infarct locations are described. In addition to the Q-wave and decreased R-wave criteria typically used for diagnosis and localization of infarcts, this system for estimating infarct size also contains criteria relating to the S wave.[2]

In the Selvester scoring system, Q-wave duration is heavily considered. Variations of the QRS complex (Fig. 12.14) in lead aVF represents the changes of inferior infarction. The number of QRS points assigned for the Q-wave duration and the R/Q amplitude ratio criteria met by the various ECGs are indicated in parentheses. This measurement is easy when the QRS complex has discrete Q and R waves (see Fig. 12.14A–C, E, and G).[6]

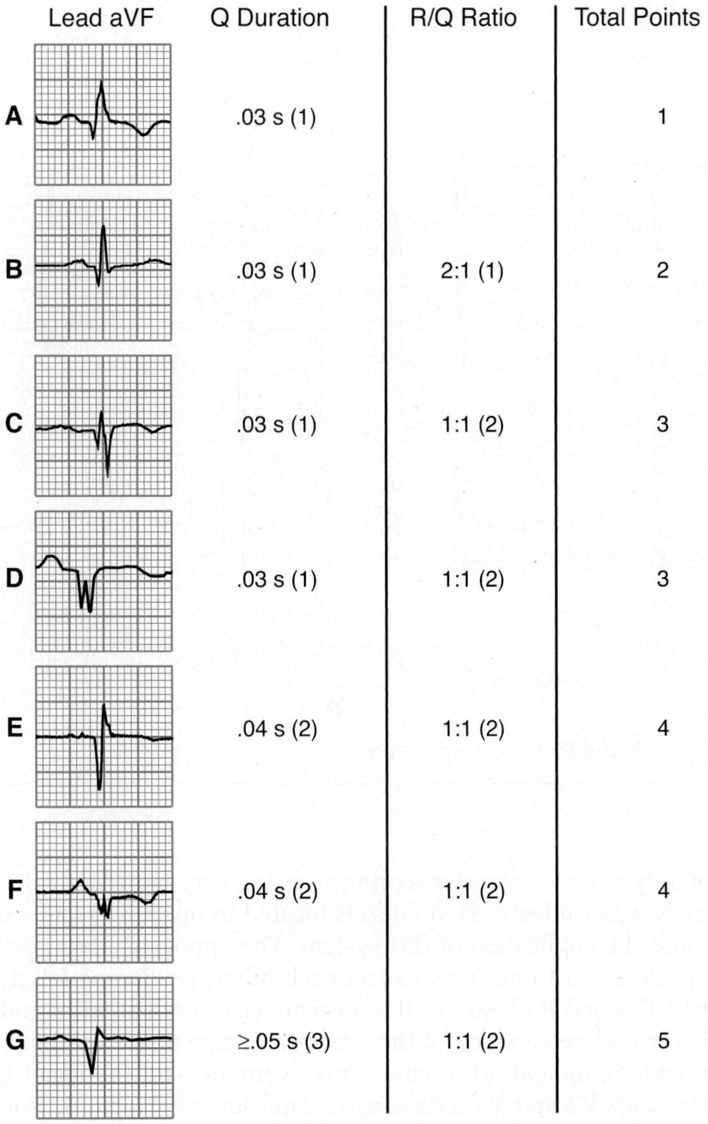

Lead aVF	Q Duration	R/Q Ratio	Total Points
A	.03 s (1)		1
B	.03 s (1)	2:1 (1)	2
C	.03 s (1)	1:1 (2)	3
D	.03 s (1)	1:1 (2)	3
E	.04 s (2)	1:1 (2)	4
F	.04 s (2)	1:1 (2)	4
G	≥.05 s (3)	1:1 (2)	5

FIGURE 12.14. **A–G.** Variations in the appearance of the QRS complex in lead aVF representing the changes of inferior infarction. The numbers of QRS points awarded for the Q-wave duration and the R/Q amplitude ratio criteria met in the various ECGs given as examples are indicated in parentheses. The total number of QRS points awarded for lead aVF is indicated for each example in the final column. (Modified from Wagner GS, Freye CJ, Palmeri ST, et al. Evaluation of a QRS scoring system for estimating myocardial infarct size. I. Specificity and observer agreement. *Circulation.* 1982;65:342–347, with permission.)

The other panels in the figure (see Fig. 12.14D, F) present small upward deflections in a generally negative QRS complex that cannot be termed R waves because they never reach the positive side of the baseline. This type of QRS complex variation should be termed QS. The true Q-wave duration should be measured along the ECG baseline from the onset of the initial negative deflection to the point directly at or above the peak of the notch in the negative deflection. The total number of points awarded for lead aVF is indicated for each example in the final column.

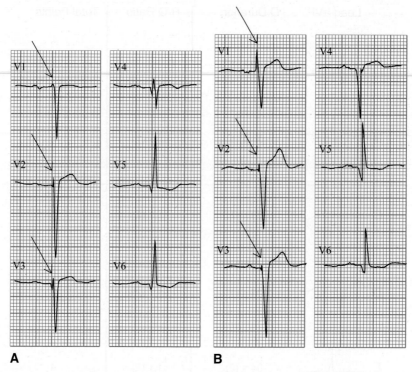

FIGURE 12.15.   **A and B.** *Arrows,* abnormal initial QRS waveforms.

Satisfaction of only a single Selvester scoring criterion may represent either a normal variant or an extremely small infarct. Two infarcts located in opposite sectors of the LV, however, may confound the application of this system. The opposing effects on the summation of the ventricular electrical forces may cancel each other, producing falsely negative ECG changes. Figure 12.15A and B illustrates the coexistence of both anterior and lateral infarcts and the potential for underestimation of the total percentage of the LV that is infarcted. The 0.04 R wave in lead V1 indicates the lateral involvement, and the small Q wave preceding the R wave in leads V2 and V3 indicates the anterior involvement. Note there are also abnormal initial negative QRS waveforms in leads V4 to V6 in Figure 12.15A and B.

MYOCARDIAL INFARCTION AND SCAR IN THE PRESENCE OF CONDUCTION ABNORMALITIES

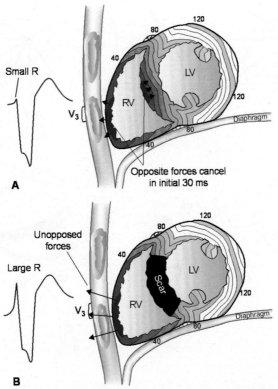

FIGURE 12.16. Electrical activation sequence in left-bundle-branch block (LBBB) and the effect of septal scar. **(A)** LBBB conduction begins in the endocardium of the right ventricle (RV), and electrical forces from the septum and RV free wall go in opposite directions and cancel each other out, producing an isoelectric segment or small R wave in leads V1 to V3. However, in the presence of septal scar **(B)**, the RV free wall forces are unopposed, producing large R waves in leads V1 to V3. LV, left ventricle. (Modified from Strauss DG, Selvester RH, Lima JA, et al. ECG quantification of myocardial scar in cardiomyopathy patients with or without conduction defects: correlation with cardiac magnetic resonance and arrhythmogenesis. *Circ Arrhythm Electrophysiol.* 2008;1:327–336, with permission.)

Bundle-branch and fascicular blocks have traditionally been thought to conceal the typical ECG signs of MI. However, computer simulations suggested that once the correct underlying activation sequence is taken into account, modified ECG criteria can be developed to detect and quantify MI in the presence of conduction abnormalities.[17,18]

Figure 12.16A illustrates the electrical activation through the ventricles in LBBB and a representative ECG waveform representative of leads V1 to V3 without infarction/scar, whereas Figure 12.16B shows activation and the ECG waveform in the presence of septal scar. As opposed to normal conduction where septal infarction causes Q waves in V1 to V3, in the presence of LBBB, septal scar has the opposite effect: it causes large R waves. This is apparent from understanding the activation in LBBB. In LBBB, activation begins in the endocardium of the RV, going in opposite directions (see arrows in 12.16A), resulting in cancellation of electrical forces and producing an isoelectric segment or small R wave at the beginning of the QRS. However, septal scar causes unopposed electrical forces from the RV free wall that causes a large R wave in V1 to V3 in LBBB.

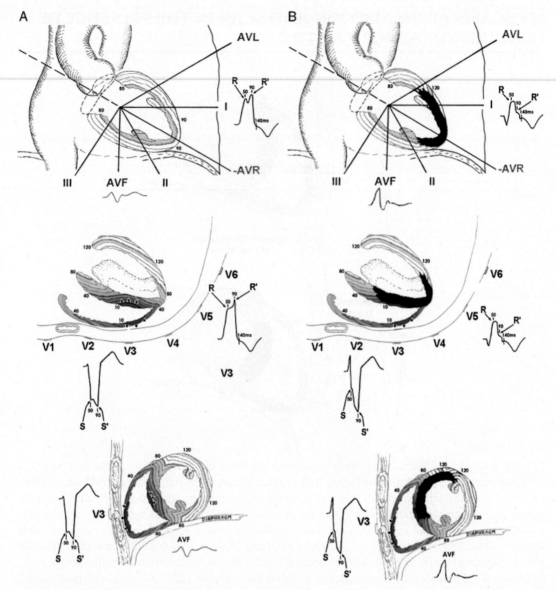

FIGURE 12.17. Left-bundle-branch block activation patterns. All panels demonstrate the ventricular activation pattern in LBBB and ECG waveforms seen from the frontal plane **(top)**, horizontal plane **(middle)**, and sagittal plane **(bottom)** in LBBB without infarction **(A)**, LBBB with extensive anterior infarction **(B)**, LBBB with lateral infarction **(C)**, and LBBB with inferior infarction **(D)**. *(continued)*

Selvester and colleagues developed a complete QRS scoring system for quantifying infarction/scar in the presence of LBBB (along with separate scores for other "ECG confounders" of diagnosing chronic infarction, including right-bundle-branch block, left anterior fascicular block, and left-ventricular hypertrophy). The reader is referred to prior publications for details on the QRS score in the presence of conduction abnormalities.[17-19] Figure 12.17 highlights the main ECG changes that occur in LBBB with infarcts in the three major coronary artery territories (Fig. 12.17B, chronic LAD infarct; Fig. 12.17C, chronic LCX infarct; and Fig. 12.17D, chronic inferior infarct).

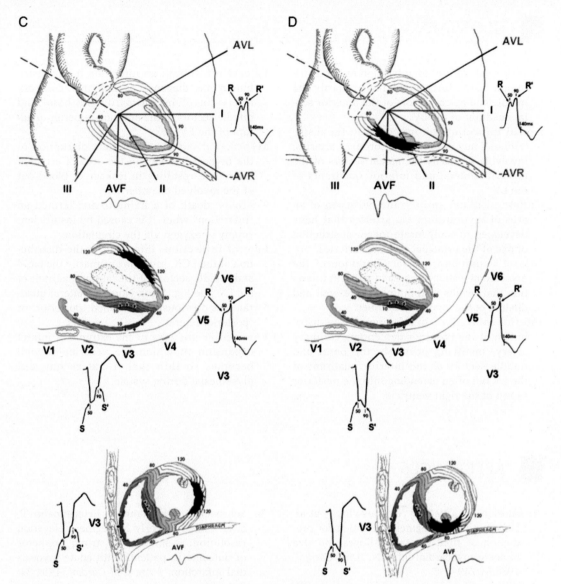

FIGURE 12.17. *(continued)* *Colored lines* represent areas of myocardium activated within the same 10-millisecond period *(isochrones)*. *Numbers* represent milliseconds since beginning of activation. Key ECG changes include the development of large R waves in V1 and V2 with anteroseptal infarction **(B)**, increased R/R' amplitude ratios in V5 and V6 with apical infarction **(B)**, increased S/S' amplitude ratios in V1 and V2 with lateral wall infarction **(C)**, and Q waves and decreased R/Q or R/S in aVF amplitude ratios with inferior wall infarction **(D)**. (Modified from Loring Z, Chelliah S, Selvester RH, et al. A detailed guide for quantification of myocardial scar with the Selvester QRS score in the presence of electrocardiogram confounders. *J Electrocardiol*. 2011;44:544–554, with permission.)

GLOSSARY

Anterior infarction: an infarction in the distribution of the LAD, involving primarily the middle and apical sectors of the anterior septal quadrant of the LV.

Apical infarction: an infarction in the distribution of any of the major coronary arteries, involving primarily the apical sectors of the posterior–lateral and inferior quadrants of the LV.

Collateral blood supply: the perfusion of an area of myocardium via arteries that have developed to compensate for an obstruction of one of the principal coronary arteries.

Infarct expansion: partial disruption of the myocardial wall in the area of a recent infarction that results in thinning of the wall and dilation of the involved chamber.

Inferior infarction: an infarction in the distribution of the posterior descending coronary artery, involving primarily the basal and middle sectors of the inferior quadrant of the LV but often extending into the posterior aspect of the right ventricle.

Lateral infarction: an infarction in the distribution of a "diagonal" or "marginal" coronary artery, involving primarily the basal and middle sectors of the anterior–superior quadrant of the LV.

Myocardial rupture: complete disruption of the myocardial wall in the area of a recent infarction, resulting in leakage of blood out of the involved chamber.

Necrosis: death of a living tissue; termed an "infarction" when it is caused by insufficient supply of oxygen via the circulation.

Lateral infarction: infarction in the distribution of the LCX, involving primarily the basal and middle sectors of the lateral quadrant of the LV (see Fig. 11.6). Note this lateral quadrant has previously been called "posterior" or "posterior-lateral".

Ventricular aneurysm: the extreme of infarct expansion in which the ventricular wall becomes so thin that it bulges outward (dyskinesia) during systole.

REFERENCES

1. Aldrich HR, Wagner NB, Boswick J, et al. Use of initial ST-segment deviation for prediction of final electrocardiographic size of acute myocardial infarcts. *Am J Cardiol.* 1988;61:749–753.
2. Billgren T, Birnbaum Y, Sgarbossa EB. Refinement and interobserver agreement for the electrocardiographic Sclarovsky-Birnbaum Ischemia Grading System. *J Electrocardiol.* 2004;37:149–156.
3. Corey KE, Maynard C, Pahlm O, et al. Combined historical and electrocardiographic timing of acute anterior and inferior myocardial infarcts for prediction of reperfusion achievable size limitation. *Am J Cardiol.* 1999;83:826–831.
4. de Lemos JA, Antman EM, Giugliano RP, et al. ST-segment resolution and infarct-related artery patency and flow after thrombolytic therapy. Thrombolysis in Myocardial Infarction (TIMI) 14 investigators. *Am J Cardiol.* 2000;85:299–304.
5. Schroder R, Dissmann R, Bruggemann T, et al. Extent of early ST segment elevation resolution: a simple but strong predictor of outcome in patients with acute myocardial infarction. *J Am Coll Cardiol.* 1994;24:384–391.
6. Arvan S, Varat MA. Persistent ST-segment elevation and left ventricular wall abnormalities: 2-dimensional echocardiographic study. *Am J Cardiol.* 1984;53:1542–1546.
7. Lindsay J Jr, Dewey RC, Talesnick BS, et al. Relation of ST segment elevation after healing of acute myocardial infarction to the presence of left ventricular aneurysm. *Am J Cardiol.* 1984;54:84–86.
8. Oliva PB, Hammill SC, Edwards WD. Electrocardiographic diagnosis of post infarction regional pericarditis: ancillary observations regarding the effect of reperfusion on the rapidity and amplitude of T wave inversion after acute myocardial infarction. *Circulation.* 1993;88:896–904.

9. Mandel WJ, Burgess MJ, Neville J Jr, et al. Analysis of T wave abnormalities associated with myocardial infarction using a theoretic model. *Circulation.* 1968;38:178–188.

10. Wagner NB, White RD, Wagner GS. The 12-lead ECG and the extent of myocardium at risk of acute infarction: cardiac anatomy and lead locations, and the phases of serial changes during acute occlusion. In: Califf RM, Mark DB, Wagner GS, eds. *Acute Coronary Care in the Thrombolytic Era.* Chicago, IL: Year Book; 1988:36–41.

11. Wagner GS, Wagner NB. The 12-lead ECG and the extent of myocardium at risk of acute infarction: anatomic relationships among coronary, Purkinje, and myocardial anatomy. In: Califf RM, Mark DB, Wagner GS, eds. *Acute Coronary Care in the Thrombolytic Era.* Chicago, IL: Year Book; 1988:16–30.

12. Wagner GS, Freye CJ, Palmeri ST, et al. Evaluation of a QRS scoring system for estimating myocardial infarct size. I. Specificity and observer agreement. *Circulation.* 1982;65:342–347.

13. Flowers NC, Horan LG, Sohi GS, et al. New evidence for inferior-posterior myocardial infarction on surface potential maps. *Am J Cardiol.* 1976;38:576–581.

14. Bayés de Luna A, Wagner G, Birnbaum Y, et al. A new terminology for the left ventricular walls and for the locations of Q wave and Q wave equivalent myocardial infarcts based on the standard of cardiac magnetic resonance imaging. A statement for healthcare professionals from a committee appointed by the international society for holter and non invasive electrocardiography. *Circulation.* 2006;114:1755–1760.

15. Selvester RH, Wagner JO, Rubin HB. Quantitation of myocardial infarct size and location by electrocardiogram and vectorcardiogram. In: *Boerhave Course in Quantitation in Cardiology.* Leyden, The Netherlands: Leyden University Press; 1972:31.

16. Selvester RH, Soloman J, Sapoznikov D. Computer simulation of the electrocardiogram. In: *Computer Techniques in Cardiology.* New York, NY: Marcel Dekker; 1979:417.

17. Strauss DG, Selvester RH. The QRS complex—a biomarker that "images" the heart: QRS scores to quantify myocardial scar in the presence of normal and abnormal ventricular conduction. *J Electrocardiol.* 2009;42:85–96.

18. Strauss DG, Selvester RH, Lima JA, et al. ECG quantification of myocardial scar in cardiomyopathy patients with or without conduction defects: correlation with cardiac magnetic resonance and arrhythmogenesis. *Circ Arrhythm Electrophysiol.* 2008;1:327–336.

19. Loring Z, Chelliah S, Selvester RH, et al. A detailed guide for quantification of myocardial scar with the Selvester QRS score in the presence of electrocardiogram confounders. *J Electrocardiol.* 2011;44:544–554.

13

Miscellaneous Conditions

GALEN S. WAGNER AND
DAVID G. STRAUSS

Chapters 9 through 12 present the electrocardiographic waveform changes caused by myocardial ischemia and infarction. This chapter concludes the section on abnormal wave morphology by presenting the various miscellaneous cardiac and noncardiac conditions that can be diagnosed by interpretation of the electrocardiogram (ECG). This chapter begins with the nonischemic cardiomyopathies. The following learning units consider the ECG waveform changes representing abnormalities of the pericardial linings of the heart and the other major intrathoracic organ, the lungs. Conditions affecting more remote parts of the body, including the brain and endocrine glands, and abnormal amounts of either internally produced or ingested substances in the circulating blood that may also be suspected or even diagnosed by ECG waveform changes are considered in the final section.

CARDIOMYOPATHIES

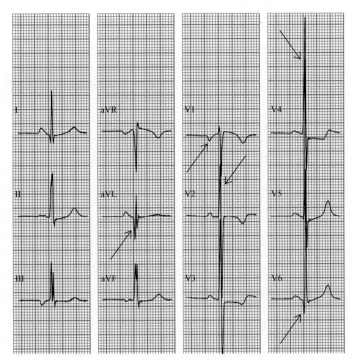

FIGURE 13.1. *Arrows,* waveforms most characteristic of hypertrophic obstructive cardiomyopathy.

"Cardiomyopathy" is a general term applied to all conditions in which the myocardium does not function normally. The primary diagnostic classifications of cardiomyopathy are "ischemic" and "nonischemic." Ischemic cardiomyopathy may either be potentially reversible (hibernation) or irreversible (infarction), resulting in the ECG changes of ischemia, injury, and infarction discussed in Chapters 9 through 12. *Hypertrophic cardiomyopathy* is a common nonischemic cardiomyopathy that occurs when a hypertrophied ventricle either fails to maintain or interferes with normal function. The hypertrophy may either be secondary to pressure overload (see Chapter 5) or may be a primary cardiac condition. Primary hypertrophic cardiomyopathy may involve both ventricles, one entire ventricle, or only a portion of one ventricle.

A common localized variety of this condition is hypertrophic obstructive cardiomyopathy (HOCM), in which the hypertrophied interventricular septum obstructs the aortic outflow tract during systole, resulting in *subaortic stenosis.* HOCM is associated with the many different ECG manifestations, none of which are typical.

A spectrum of ECG changes may occur in hypertrophic cardiomyopathy regardless of whether or not the problem is localized to the septum, as illustrated in Figure 13.1.[1,2]

1. Typical left-ventricular hypertrophy (tall precordial R waves in leads V2 to V5; see Chapter 5).
2. Deep, narrow Q waves in the leftward-oriented leads (aVL and V6).
3. Left atrial enlargement (increased terminal P-wave negativity in lead V1; see Chapter 5).

Amyloidosis

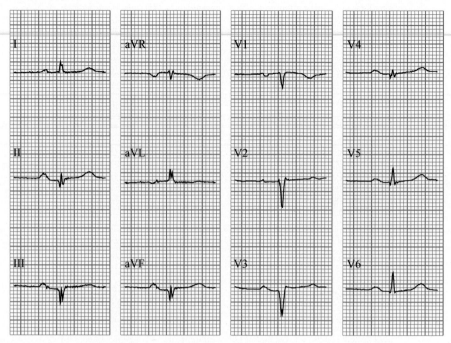

FIGURE 13.2.

An abnormal protein called amyloid is deposited in the heart during various disease processes. Its accumulation causes cardiac amyloidosis, which eventually may produce sufficient cardiomyopathy to cause heart failure. Amyloidosis may be suspected when the following combination of ECG changes appear[1]:

1. Low voltage of all waveforms in the limb leads.
2. Marked left-axis deviation typical of left-anterior fascicular block.
3. Pseudo infarct changes.
4. A prolonged atrioventricular (AV) conduction time.

Characteristics 1 and 3 are apparent in an elderly patient with severe heart failure but no history of ischemic heart disease (Fig. 13.2). Note the extremely low voltage in both limb and precordial leads and pseudo infarct changes; Q waves are typically seen with both inferior and anterior infarcts.

PERICARDIAL ABNORMALITIES

A small, fluid-filled space called the *pericardial sac* separates the heart from the other structures in the thorax. The sac is lined by two layers of connective tissue referred to as the *pericardium*. The innermost of these two layers (visceral pericardium) adheres to the myocardium, and the outer layer (parietal pericardium) encloses the pericardial fluid. These two layers of tissue can become inflamed for many reasons (*pericarditis*). The inflammation usually resolves after an acute phase but may progress to a chronic phase. The acute phase may be complicated by the collection of excess pericardial fluid, a condition termed *pericardial effusion*. Chronic persistence of the inflammatory process may result in thickening of the pericardial tissues and is called *constrictive pericarditis*.

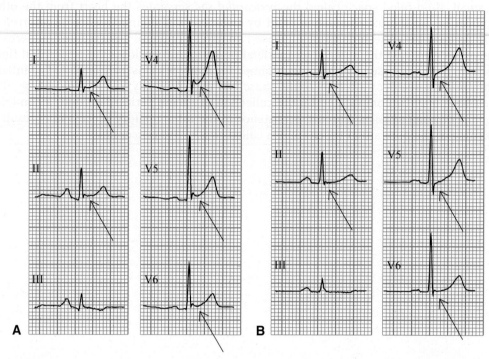

FIGURE 13.3. **A.** *Arrows*, ST-segment elevation. **B.** *Arrows*, ST-segment resolution.

Typically, acute pericarditis persists for 3 or 4 weeks, and the ECG changes it produces evolve through two stages. The recordings in Figure 13.3 are from a patient presenting with the chest pain of acute pericarditis (see Fig. 13.3A) and returning to the clinic 1 month later (see Fig. 13.3B). The characteristic ECG abnormality during the earliest stage of acute pericarditis is elevation of the ST segments in many leads, accompanied by upright T waves (see Fig. 13.3A).[2] Depression of the PR segment was also present in half of a series of consecutive patients with acute pericarditis.[3] When the ST segments return to the isoelectric level, the ECG may appear normal (see Fig. 13.3B).

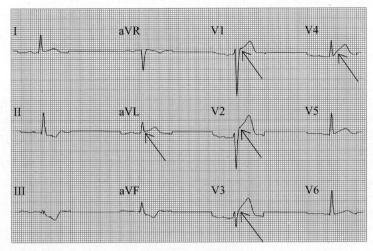

FIGURE 13.4. *Arrows*, leads with ST-segment elevation.

The ST-segment elevation in the first stage of acute pericarditis occurs because the inflammation also involves the immediately adjacent epicardial layer of myocardium, producing an epicardial "injury current" similar to transmural myocardial ischemia discussed in Chapter 11. When the epicardial injury is caused by insufficient myocardial perfusion (i.e. ischemia), the ST-segment elevation is restricted to the ECG leads that overlie the myocardial region supplied by the obstructed coronary artery. Because pericarditis usually involves the entire epicardium, there is ST-segment elevation in all of the standard leads that are positive leftward and anteriorly and with ST depression in lead aVR. However, differentiation between acute pericarditis and acute myocardial ischemia becomes difficult when the pericarditis is localized, creating ST-segment elevation in only a few leads.

Figure 13.4 illustrates such an example with a 12-lead ECG from a woman with breast carcinoma and acute chest pain. In both acute pericarditis and acute myocardial infarction, the patient may present with precordial pain, and additional clinical evaluation is necessary to reach the appropriate diagnosis. Serial ECG recordings are useful because the acute epicardial injury current of decreased coronary flow is transient and resolves when the region is either infarcted or reperfused, but the changes of pericarditis persist until the inflammation resolves.

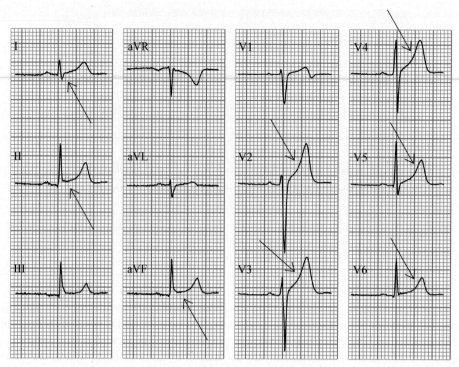

FIGURE 13.5. *Arrows,* multiple leads with ST-segment elevation.

Acute pericarditis also often resembles the normal variant termed "early repolarization" discussed in Chapter 3. Figure 13.5 presents a typical example of a routine 12-lead ECG recorded from a healthy young man that could represent either the early repolarization or the first stage of acute pericarditis.

A factor on this example that favors a diagnosis of acute pericarditis is the widespread ST elevation, but another factor that favors early repolarization is the increased T-wave amplitude in several leads (see Table 12.1). This emphasizes the point that it is often not possible to distinguish on the ECG between these very different conditions.

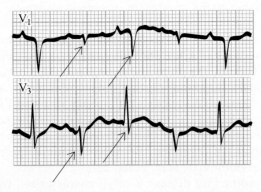

FIGURE 13.6. *Arrows*, markedly different P-wave and QRS-complex waveforms alternating on consecutive cycles.

Small and even moderate amounts of pericardial effusion or constriction may have little or no effect on the ECG. However, a generalized decrease in all of the ECG waveform amplitudes (*low voltage*) occurs if significant pericardial effusion or thickening develops. This probably occurs because the cardiac impulses are dampened by the pericardial fluid or fibrotic thickening. Because both of these pathologic conditions have similar effects on the cardiac electrical activity and its transmission to the body surface, they are considered together. A triad of ECG changes that is virtually diagnostic of pericardial effusion or constriction is presented below:

1. Low voltage.
2. Widespread ST-segment elevation.
3. Total electrical alternans.

These changes are observed in ECG leads V1 and V3 recorded from a patient with carcinoma of the lung and malignant pericardial effusion (Fig. 13.6). *Total electrical alternans* refers to the alternating high and low voltages of all ECG waveforms between cardiac cycles within a given lead.[4,5]

In addition to these ECG effects, chronic constrictive pericarditis may be accompanied by the T-wave inversion that defines the second stage of acute pericarditis.[6] The depth of inversion of the T waves has been reported to correlate with the degree of pericardial adherence to the myocardium. This may be clinically important because surgical "stripping" of the thickened pericardium is more difficult when it is adhered tightly to the myocardium.

PULMONARY ABNORMALITIES

When a pulmonary abnormality creates an increased resistance to blood flow from the right side of the heart, a condition of systolic or pressure overload develops (see Chapter 5). This condition has been termed *cor pulmonale*, and it can occur either acutely or chronically. The most common cause of acute cor pulmonale is *pulmonary embolism*. Chronic cor pulmonale may be produced by the pulmonary congestion that occurs with left-ventricular failure or by the pulmonary hypertension that develops either as a primary disease or as a secondary disease to chronic obstructive pulmonary disease. Right-atrial enlargement commonly occurs with acute and chronic cor pulmonale. In the acute condition, there is right-ventricular dilation, whereas in the chronic condition there is right-ventricular hypertrophy (RVH) at first, then RV dilatation. Because chronic RVH is discussed in detail in Chapter 5, only acute cor pulmonale is included here.

Chronic obstructive pulmonary disease is often characterized by *emphysema*, in which the lungs become overinflated. This produces anatomic changes that affect the ECG in unique ways. The ECG changes of pulmonary emphysema may occur alone or in combination with the changes of RVH because emphysema may or may not be accompanied by the obstruction of the airways. When CO_2 is unable to escape through the tracheal–bronchial system, the condition of hyperventilation occurs. The resultant hypercapnia (elevated blood CO_2 levels) and respiratory acidosis cause the pulmonary arterial constriction leading to the compensatory RVH that is termed chronic cor pulmonale.

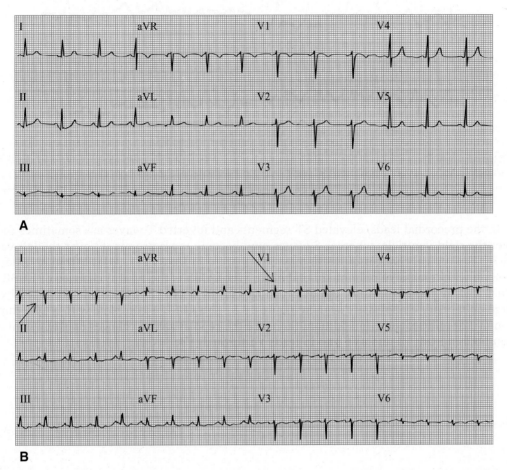

FIGURE 13.7. **A and B.** *Arrows,* terminal rightward (*I*) and anterior (*V1*) shift in QRS waveforms.

Acute cor pulmonale in the absence of evidence of the changes of RVH owing to chronic cor pulmonale is most commonly seen in pulmonary embolism. Acute cor pulmonale can occur in the presence or absence of chronic changes of RVH. The ECG changes considered herein are those in the absence of RVH. The RV distortion produced by an acute outflow obstruction such as pulmonary embolism causes delayed conduction through the right bundle and/or the RV myocardium, resulting in the ECG pattern of incomplete or even complete right-bundle-branch block (RBBB; see Chapter 6). The subtraction of the RV contribution from the initial portion of the QRS complex shifts the waveforms away from both the inferior (limb leads) and anterior (chest leads), mimicking both inferior and anterior infarcts. This shift to the QRS beyond the completion of LV activation produces unopposed terminal rightward and anterior forces.[7] The rightward direction is represented primarily by an S wave in lead I and the anterior direction by an R′ wave in V1. Figure 13.7 presents recordings from before (A) and after (B) sudden dyspnea in an elderly man who had received prostate surgery.

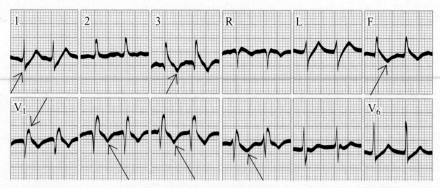

FIGURE 13.8. Lead I: *arrow*, rightward axis shift. Leads II, aVF, and V2–V4: *arrows*, inverted T waves. Lead V1: *arrow*, prominent R' wave.

In the precordial leads, elevated ST segments and inverted T waves are sometimes seen over the right ventricle, whereas S waves may become more prominent over the left ventricle. The typical changes of RBBB may be apparent in lead V1 (a 12-lead from an elderly woman with a massive pulmonary embolism who exhibits the typical changes of RBBB is illustrated in Fig. 13.8). All of the ECG changes of the acute cor pulmonale produced by a large pulmonary embolus are seen in Figure 13.8. The RBBB is complete with a QRS duration of 120 milliseconds. In addition, there are the repolarization changes of T-wave inversion both in leads III and aVF and in leads V1 through V4.

Pulmonary Emphysema

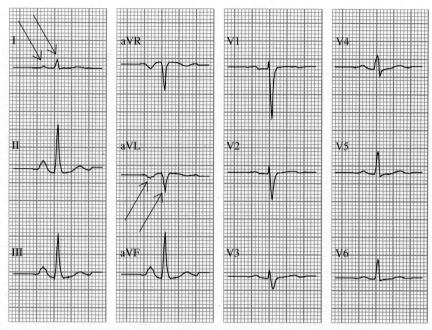

<u>FIGURE 13.9.</u>   *Arrows*, rightward axis shift of the P and QRS waveforms.

The five most typical findings in emphysema have been grouped together as follows[8]:

1. Tall P waves in leads II, III, and aVF.
2. Exaggerated atrial repolarization waves producing ≥0.10-mV PR and ST-segment depression in leads II, III, and aVF.
3. Rightward shift of the axis of the QRS complex in the frontal plane.
4. Decreased progression of the R-wave amplitudes in the precordial leads.
5. Low voltage of the QRS complexes, especially in the left precordial leads.

Figure 13.9 presents a typical example of pulmonary emphysema with all five of these characteristics. Rightward shifts of both the P waves and QRS complexes (negative in lead aVL and only slightly positive in lead I) and a low voltage in the leftward (V4 to V6) precordial leads are illustrated (Fig. 13.9). Note the prominent P waves in II, III, and aVF followed by PR- and ST-segment depression below the TP baseline.

These ECG changes are produced because the hyperexpanded emphysematous lungs compress the heart, lower the diaphragms, and increase the space between the heart and the recording electrodes.

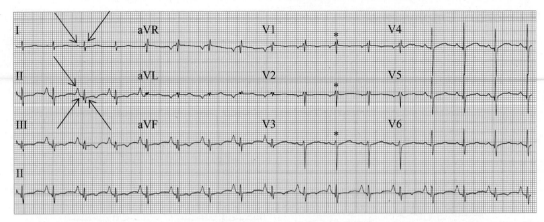

FIGURE 13.10. A 12-lead ECG recording from a patient with pulmonary emphysema. The *arrows* in lead I indicate the isoelectric P wave and low-voltage QRS complex, and the *arrows* in lead II indicate the prominent P wave and PR and ST segments depressed below the TP-segment baseline. *Asterisks* indicate the absence of decreased R-wave progression from leads V1 to V3.

The QRS axis in the frontal plane is occasionally indeterminate (Fig. 13.10).[9] This occurs because pulmonary emphysema directs the QRS complex posteriorly so that minimal upward or downward deviation swings the frontal plane axis of the complex from +90 degrees to −90 degrees. Figure 13.10 also illustrates criteria 1, 2, 3, and 4 in the list given above.

Selvester and Rubin[10] have developed quantitative ECG criteria for both definite and possible emphysema (Table 13.1).

These criteria achieve approximately 65% sensitivity for the diagnosis of emphysema and 95% specificity for the exclusion of emphysema in normal control subjects and in patients with congenital heart disease or myocardial infarction.[9] This good performance relative to that of other systems is most likely the result of combining quantitative criteria for the frontal plane P-wave axis with criteria for both the frontal and transverse plane amplitudes of the QRS complex.

Table 13.1.

Electrocardiographic Criteria for Emphysema

Definite Emphysema	Possible Emphysema
A. P axis >+60 degrees in limb leads and either	P axis >+60 degrees in limb leads and either
B. 1. R and S amp ≤0.70 mV in limb leads and 2. R amp ≤0.70 mV in V6 or	1. R and S amp ≤0.70 mV in limb leads or 2. R amp ≤0.70 mV in V6
C. SV4 ≥ RV4	

From Rubin LJ, ed. *Pulmonary Heart Disease.* Boston, MA: Martinus Nijhoff; 1984:122, with permission.

INTRACRANIAL HEMORRHAGE

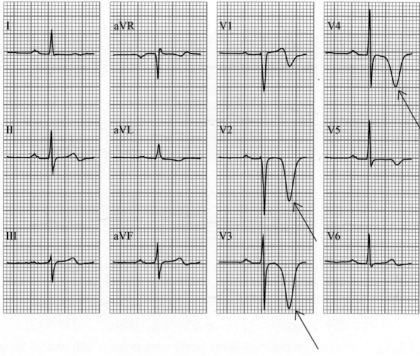

FIGURE 13.11. *Arrows*, unusually prominent inverted T waves.

Hemorrhage into either the intracerebral or subarachnoid spaces can produce dramatic changes in the ECG, presumably because of increased intracranial pressure.[11-14] Less severe ECG changes occur with nonhemorrhagic cerebrovascular accidents.[15] The three most common ECG changes in intracranial hemorrhage are:

1. Widening and inversion of T waves in the precordial leads.
2. Prolongation of the QTc interval.
3. Bradyarrhythmias.

Figure 13.11 presents a 12-lead ECG recording that is a typical example of characteristic 1. ST elevation or depression can occasionally occur, mimicking cardiac ischemia. In some cases, regional wall motion abnormalities are observed in subarachnoid hemorrhage (SAH) associated with ST elevation, or "neurogenic stunned myocardium."[16]

Thyroid Abnormalities

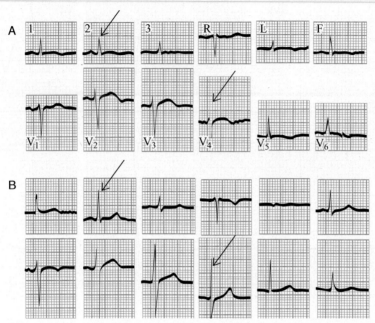

FIGURE 13.12. *Arrows*, contrasting R-wave amplitudes in leads 2(II) and V4 before **(A)** and after treatment **(B)**.

The extreme hypothyroid condition is termed *myxedema* and the extreme hyperthyroid condition is termed *thyrotoxicosis*. Both are often accompanied by typical changes in ECG waveform morphology. Because the thyroid hormone thyroxin mediates sympathetic nervous activity, a hypothyroid state is accompanied by a slowing of the sinus rate (sinus bradycardia). Conversely, a hyperthyroid state is accompanied by an acceleration of the sinus rate (*sinus tachycardia*).[17] Similarly, AV conduction may be impaired in hypothyroidism and accelerated in hyperthyroidism.[18]

Hypothyroidism

The diagnosis of hypothyroidism should be suspected when the following combination of ECG changes is present (Fig. 13.12):

1. Low voltage of all waveforms.
2. Inverted T waves without ST-segment deviation in many or all leads.
3. Sinus bradycardia.

QT prolongation and AV or intraventricular conduction delay may also occur. These changes may be related to cardiac deposits of the gelatinous connective tissue typical of myxedema, diminished sympathetic nervous activity, and/or the effect on the myocardium of reduced levels of thyroxin.[19]

Hyperthyroidism

The diagnosis of hyperthyroidism should be suspected when the amplitudes of all of the ECG waveforms are increased.[20] This simulates right-atrial and left-ventricular enlargement (see Chapter 5). The heart rate is rapid because of the increased levels of thyroxin. The cardiac rhythm may reflect an acceleration of normal sinus impulse formation (*sinus tachycardia*), or the abnormal atrial tachyarrhythmia known as *atrial fibrillation* (see Chapter 17). Although the QT interval decreases as the heart rate increases, the corrected QT interval (QTc) may be prolonged.[21]

Hypothermia

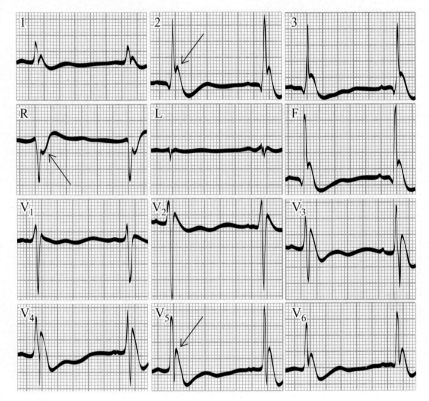

FIGURE 13.13. *Arrows,* Osborn waves.

Hypothermia has been defined as a rectal temperature <36° C or <97° F. At these lower temperatures, characteristic ECG changes develop. All intervals of the ECG (including the RR, PR, QRS, and QT intervals) may lengthen. Characteristic *Osborn waves* appear as deflections at the J point in the same direction as that of the QRS complex.[22] Figure 13.13 illustrates these changes in an elderly man exposed to the cold with a body temperature of 32.8° C or 91° F. The height of the Osborn waves is roughly proportional to the degree of hypothermia.

Obesity

Obesity has the potential to affect the ECG as follows:

1. Displacing the heart by elevating the diaphragm.
2. Increasing cardiac workload.
3. Increasing the distance between the heart and the recording electrodes.

In a study of >1,000 obese individuals, the heart rate, PR interval, QRS interval, QRS voltage, and QTc interval all showed an increase with increasing obesity.[23] The QRS axis also tended to shift leftward. Interestingly, only 4% of this population had low QRS voltage. One study has reported an increased incidence of false-positive criteria for inferior myocardial infarction in both obese individuals and in women in the final trimester of pregnancy (presumably because of diaphragmatic elevation).[24]

ELECTROLYTE ABNORMALITIES

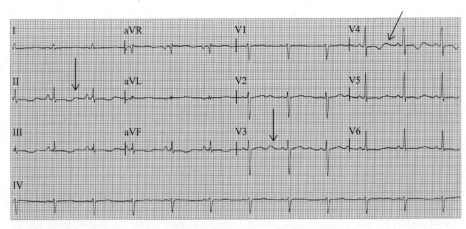

FIGURE 13.14. *Arrows,* prominent U waves.

Either abnormally low (hypo-) or high (hyper-) serum levels of the electrolytes potassium or calcium may produce marked abnormalities of the ECG waveforms. Indeed, typical ECG changes may provide the first clinical evidence of the presence of these conditions.

Potassium

The terms *hypokalemia* and *hyperkalemia* are commonly used for alterations in serum levels of potassium. Because abnormalities in either of these conditions may be life threatening, an understanding of the ECG changes they produce is important.

Hypokalemia

Hypokalemia may have many causes,[25] often occurs with other electrolyte disturbances (e.g., reduced serum magnesium levels), and is particularly dangerous in the presence of *digitalis* therapy. The typical ECG signs of hypokalemia may appear when the serum potassium concentration is within normal limits, and conversely, the ECG may be normal when serum levels of potassium are elevated. The ECG changes in hypokalemia are[26]:

1. Flattening or inversion of the T wave.
2. Increased prominence of the U wave.
3. Slight depression of the ST segment.
4. Increased amplitude and width of the P wave.
5. Prolongation of the PR interval.
6. Premature beats and sustained tachyarrhythmias.
7. Prolongation of the QTc interval.

Figure 13.14 illustrates characteristics 1, 2, and 4 from a patient receiving diuretic therapy for chronic heart failure. The serum potassium level was 1.7 mEq/L (normal range, 4 to 5 mEq/L).

The characteristic reversal in the relative amplitudes of the T and U waves is the most characteristic change in waveform morphology in hypokalemia. The U-wave prominence is caused by prolongation of the recovery phase of the cardiac action potential. This can lead to the life-threatening *torsades de pointes* type of ventricular tachyarrhythmia (see Chapter 19).[27] Hypokalemia also potentiates the tachyarrhythmias produced by digitalis toxicity (see Chapter 16).

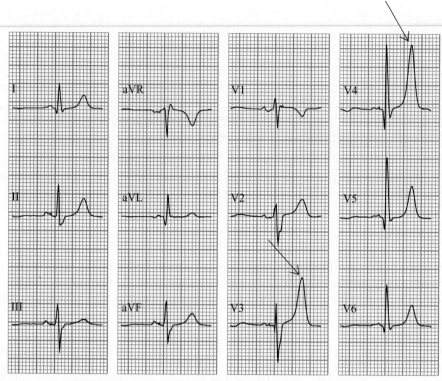

FIGURE 13.15. *Arrows*, unusually prominent and peaked positive T waves.

As in hypokalemia, there may be a poor correlation between serum potassium levels and the typical ECG changes of hyperkalemia.[28] The earliest ECG evidence of hyperkalemia usually appears in the T waves (Fig. 13.15). With increasing severity of hyperkalemia, the following ECG changes occur:

1. Increased amplitude and peaking of the T wave.
2. Prolongation of the QRS interval.
3. Prolongation of the PR interval.
4. Flattening of the P wave.
5. Loss of P wave.
6. Sine wave appearance.

The AV conduction in hyperkalemia may become so delayed that advanced AV block appears[29] (see Chapter 22). Prolongation of the QRS complex and flattening of the P waves occur because the high potassium levels in hyperkalemia delay the spread of the cardiac activating impulse through the myocardium. This abnormally slow conduction can lead to cardiac arrest from ventricular fibrillation (see Chapter 19).[30]

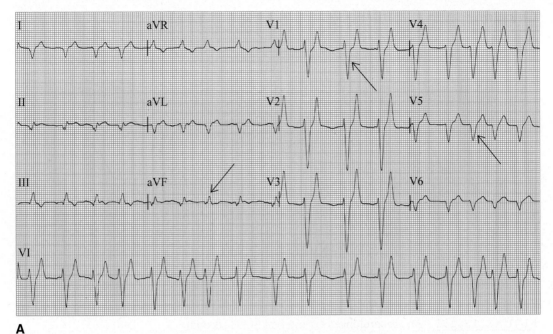

A

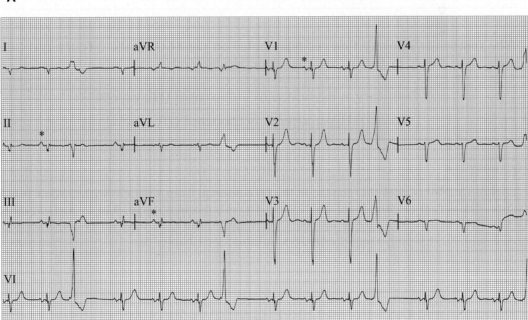

B

FIGURE 13.16. **A.** *Arrows*, markedly prolonged QRS complexes. **B.** *Asterisks*, reappearing P waves.

Figure 13.16A is from a patient with end-stage renal disease and an initial serum potassium level of 7.8 mEq per L. It demonstrates peaked T waves, QRS prolongation, and an absence of P waves. In Figure 13.16B, the T waves and the QRS complexes return to their normal duration and the P waves reappear when the serum potassium concentration returns to normal (corrected with dialysis to 4.5 mEq/L). Hyperkalemia may also reduce the myocardial response to artificial pacemaker stimulation.[31]

Calcium

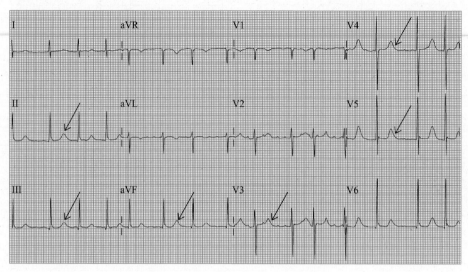

FIGURE 13.17. *Arrows*, prolonged QT interval (0.434 second).

The ventricular recovery time, as represented on the ECG by the QTc interval (see Chapter 3), is altered by the extremes of serum calcium levels:

> Deficiency = Hypocalcemia → Prolonged QTc interval
>
> Excess = Hypercalcemia → Shortened QTc interval

Hypocalcemia

Figure 13.17 illustrates this change in the QTc interval from a patient with chronic renal failure. The serum calcium level was 7.2 mg/100 mL (normal range, 9 to 11 mg/100 mL). Because the ventricular rate is 88 beats per minute, the QTc interval is 0.483 second (0.434 + [0.00175 × 28]; using the Hodges formula; see Chapter 3).

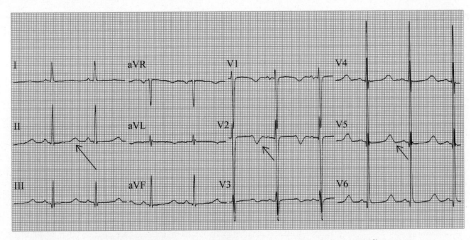

FIGURE 13.18. *Arrows,* markedly prolonged QT interval (0.500 second).

In *hypocalcemia,* the prolonged QT interval may be accompanied by terminal T-wave inversion in some leads. Figure 13.18 illustrates the prolonged QT interval with some terminal T-wave changes in a patient with chronic renal failure. The serum calcium level was 4.7 mEq/L. The ventricular rate is 100 beats per minute, therefore the QTc = 0.570 second (0.500 + [0.00175 × 40]; using the Hodges formula).

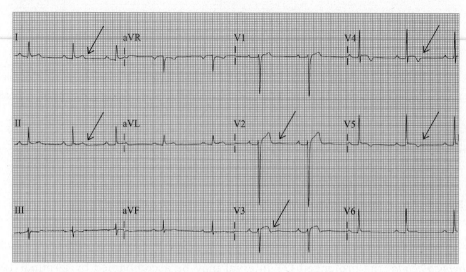

FIGURE 13.19. *Arrows,* short QT interval (0.307 second).

In *hypercalcemia,* the proximal limb of the T wave acutely slopes to its peak, and the ST segment may not be apparent, as illustrated in leads V2 and V3 in Figure 13.19.[32] In extreme hypercalcemia, an increase in amplitude of the QRS complex, biphasic T waves, and Osborn waves has been described.[33,34] Because the heart rate is 56 beats per minute, the QTc is 0.300 second (0.307+[0.00175 × 4]).

DRUG EFFECTS

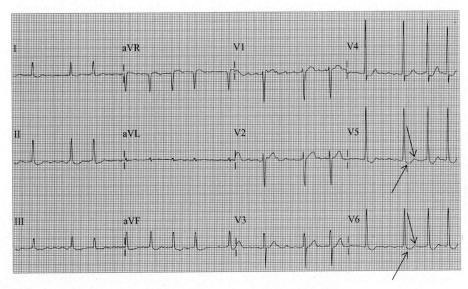

FIGURE 13.20. *Arrows,* coved St segments and flattened T waves.

Either therapeutic or toxic cardiac effects of various medications can sometimes be detected on the ECG. The term *drug effect* refers to the therapeutic cardiac manifestations of a drug on the ECG, and the term *drug toxicity* refers to the cardiac *arrhythmias* caused by various medications (see Chapters 19 and 22). The level of a drug in blood and tissue at which toxicity occurs can vary widely depending on the underlying pathology for which the drug is being used, the patient's premedication ECG status, the variations in electrolytes such as potassium, and the presence of other drugs.

Digitalis

Digitalis is commonly used to treat cardiac failure and slow the ventricular rate in atrial tachyarrhythmias. It causes characteristic ECG changes termed *digitalis effect* because the recovery or repolarization of the myocardial cells occurs earlier than it normally does (Fig. 13.20). This is manifested on the ECG by:

1. "Coved" ST-segment depression.
2. A flattened T wave.
3. A decreased QTc interval.

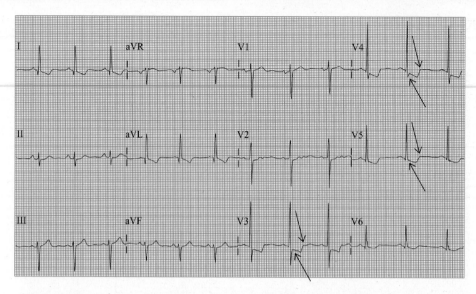

FIGURE 13.21. *Arrows*, marked ST-segment depression with decreased T-wave amplitude.

Occasionally, the ST-J point is depressed, mimicking myocardial injury. Figure 13.21 illustrates this mimicry of myocardial injury from a patient with congestive heart failure. The ECG changes, including ST-segment depression, developed at the time of administering digitalis loading doses. This extreme example of digitalis effect usually occurs only in those leads with tall R waves. Another manifestation of digitalis effect is the vagally mediated slowing of AV nodal conduction (see Chapter 22). In sinus rhythm, there is a slight increase in the PR interval; in atrial fibrillation, there is a decrease in the ventricular rate (see Chapter 17).

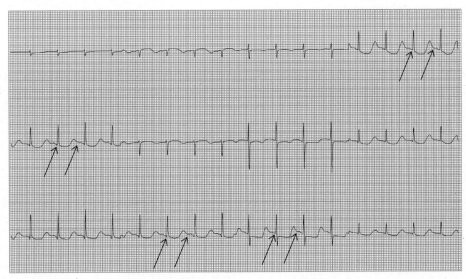

FIGURE 13.22. *Arrows*, markedly prolonged QT interval from the QRS complex onset to the end of the T wave.

The effect of an antiarrhythmic drug may be modified by the underlying cardiac disorder for which it is being used, by coexisting electrolyte imbalance, and by interaction of the drug with other drugs. An example of a drug interaction is the marked increase in blood levels of drug A (e.g., digitalis) that occurs with the introduction of drug B (e.g., quinidine and amiodarone). The commonly used antiarrhythmic drugs are classified as follows according to Vaughan Williams and associates.[35,36]

Class 1 Drugs

Drugs in class 1 of the Vaughan Williams classification have direct action on the sodium channels of the myocardial cell membrane and have been subdivided according to their effect on the different phases of the action potential. The more common drugs and their effects on the action potential are as follows:

CLASS IA (INCLUDING QUINIDINE, PROCAINAMIDE, AND DISOPYRAMIDE). In contrast to digitalis, the effect of *quinidine* is produced by a delay in the recovery or repolarization of myocardial cells. This results in prolongation of the QTc interval,[37] a decreased T-wave amplitude, and an increased U-wave amplitude. These changes are illustrated in Figure 13.22 from a patient with recent acute anterior infarction complicated by ventricular tachycardia. The arrhythmia was controlled by quinidine, and a quinidine effect appeared on the ECG. In this example, the QT interval is 0.39 second, and because the ventricular rate is 100 beats per minute, the QTc interval is prolonged to 0.49 second. Minimal prolongation of the QRS complex occurs rarely with quinidine effect; an increase in duration of the QRS complex of 25% to 50% is evidence of quinidine toxicity. Quinidine effect is also exaggerated by the presence of digitalis. The phenothiazine group of drugs, which are commonly used in treating psychiatric disorders, produce ECG changes similar to quinidine effect.

CLASS IB (LIDOCAINE AND MEXILETINE). Usually, the surface ECG is unaltered by lidocaine and mexiletine.

CLASS IC (FLECAINIDE). Flecainide produces broadening of the QRS complex, with the interval between the J point and the end of the T wave remaining unaltered, thus slightly prolonging the QT interval.

Class 2 Drugs

The drugs in class 2 of the Vaughan Williams classification system are the β-adrenergic blocking agents. By decreasing sympathetic effect on the heart, there is a slowing of rate due to the decreased sinoatrial (SA) node impulse formation. Conduction through the AV node is also delayed, prolonging the PR interval of the ECG. If there is underlying SA or AV nodal dysfunction, these changes may be increased.

Class 3 Drugs

The drugs in class 3 of the Vaughan Williams system prolong myocardial repolarization and may therefore markedly prolong the QTc interval on the ECG. Among the class 3 drugs are the following:

SOTALOL. Sotalol has both class 2 and 3 drug effects and may therefore produce SA and AV nodal suppression and also prolongation of the QTc interval.

AMIODARONE. Amiodarone has class 1, 2, and 3 effects.

Class 4 Drugs

Drugs in class 4 of the Vaughan Williams classification system block calcium channels and as a result slow both SA and AV nodal functions. Their effects are therefore similar to those of drugs in class 2.

Arrhythmia: any cardiac rhythm other than regular sinus rhythm.

Atrial fibrillation: the tachyarrhythmia at the rapid end of the flutter/fibrillation spectrum produced by macro–re-entry within multiple circuits in the atria and characterized by irregular multiform F waves.

Constrictive pericarditis: thickening of the pericardium caused by chronic inflammation and resulting in interference with myocardial function.

Cor pulmonale: an acute or chronic pressure overload of the right side of the heart caused by increased resistance to blood flow through the lungs.

Digitalis: a drug that occurs naturally in the foxglove plant and is used both to increase contraction of the cardiac muscle and decrease conduction through the AV node.

Emphysema: a pulmonary disease in which the alveoli are destroyed and the lungs become overinflated.

Hypercalcemia: an abnormally increased level of serum calcium (Ca^{++}), with a serum Ca^{++} concentration >11 mg/100 mL.

Hyperkalemia: an abnormally increased level of serum potassium (K^+), with a serum K^+ concentration >5 mEq/L.

Hypertrophic cardiomyopathy: a condition in which cardiac performance is decreased because of decreased contraction capability of the thickened myocardium.

Hypocalcemia: an abnormally decreased level of serum calcium (Ca^{++}), with a serum Ca^{++} concentration <9 mg/100 mL.

Hypokalemia: an abnormally decreased level of serum potassium (K^+), with a serum K^+ concentration <4 mEq/L.

Hypothermia: subnormal temperature of the body defined as temperature <36° C or <97° F.

Low voltage: a total amplitude of the QRS complex that is <0.70 mV in all limb leads and <1.0 mV in all precordial leads.

Myxedema: severe hypothyroidism characterized by a decreased metabolic state and firm, inelastic edema; dry skin and hair; and loss of mental and physical vigor.

Osborn waves: abnormal ECG waveforms caused by hypothermia.

Pericardial effusion: an increase in the amount of fluid in the pericardial sac.

Pericardial sac: the fluid-filled space between the two layers of the pericardium.

Pericarditis: acute or chronic inflammation of the pericardium.

Pericardium: the two-layered membrane that encloses the heart and the roots of the great blood vessels.

Procainamide: a compound related to the local anesthetic procaine that is used in the treatment of reentrant tachyarrhythmias.

Pulmonary embolism: the sudden obstruction of a pulmonary artery by a dislodged clot or fat originating from the legs or the pelvic region.

Quinidine: a drug that occurs naturally in the bark of the cinchona tree and prolongs myocardial recovery time and protects against some tachyarrhythmias. However, quinidine and other related drugs may also produce tachyarrhythmias by overprolongation of recovery time.

Sinus tachycardia: an acceleration of the normal sinus rhythm beyond the upper limit of 100 beats per minute.

Subaortic stenosis: narrowing of the outflow passage from the left ventricle proximal to the aortic valve to a degree sufficient to obstruct the flow of blood.

Thyrotoxicosis: severe hyperthyroidism characterized by an increased metabolic condition, sweating, and protruding eyes.

Torsades de pointes: a variety of ventricular tachycardia resulting from prolongation of the ventricular recovery time. The term is French for "turning of the points" or turning of the directions of the QRS complex alternately between positive and negative.

Total electrical alternans: alternation in the amplitudes of all of the ECG waveforms in the presence of a regular cardiac cycle lengths.

REFERENCES

1. Cheng Z, Zhu K, Tian Z, et al. The findings of electrocardiography in patients with cardiac amyloidosis. *Ann Noninvasive Electrocardiol.* 2013;18(2):157–162.

2. Bhardwaj R, Berzingi C, Miller C, et al. Differential diagnosis of acute pericarditis from normal variant early repolarization and left ventricular hypertrophy with early repolarization: an electrocardiographic study. *Am J Med Sci.* 2013;345(1):28–32.

3. Bruce MA, Spodick DH. Atypical electrocardiogram in acute pericarditis: characteristics and prevalence. *J Electrocardiol.* 1980;13:61–66.

4. Bashour FA, Cochran PA. The association of electrical alternans with pericardial effusion. *Dis Chest.* 1963;44:146.

5. Nizet PM, Marriott HJL. The electrocardiogram and pericardial effusion. *JAMA.* 1966;198:169.

6. Dalton JC, Pearson RJ, White PD. Constrictive pericarditis: a review and long term follow-up of 78 cases. *Ann Intern Med.* 1956;45:445.

7. Ferrari E, Imbert A, Chevalier T, et al. The ECG in pulmonary embolism. Predictive value of negative T waves in precordial leads—80 case reports. *Chest.* 1997;111(3):537–543.

8. Wasserburger RH, Kelly JR, Rasmussen HK, et al. The electrocardiographic pentalogy of pulmonary emphysema: a correlation of roentgenographic findings and pulmonary function studies. *Circulation.* 1959;20:831–841.

9. Thomas AJ, Apiyasawat S, Spodick DH. Electrocardiographic detection of emphysema. *Am J Cardiol.* 2011;107(7):1090–1092.

10. Selvester RH, Rubin HB. New criteria for the electrocardiographic diagnosis of emphysema and cor pulmonale. *Am Heart J.* 1965;69:437–447.

11. Burch GE, Meyers R, Abildskov JA. A new electrocardiographic pattern observed in cerebrovascular accidents. *Circulation.* 1954;9:719.

12. Hersch C. Electrocardiographic changes in subarachnoid haemorrhage, meningitis, and intracranial spaceoccupying lesion. *Br Heart J.* 1964;26:785.

13. Surawicz B. Electrocardiographic pattern of cerebrovascular accident. *JAMA.* 1966;197:913.

14. Shuster S. The electrocardiogram in subarachnoid haemorrhage. *Br Heart J.* 1960;22:316–320.

15. Fentz V, Gormsen J. Electrocardiographic patterns in patients with cerebrovascular accidents. *Circulation.* 1962;25:22–28.

16. Kono T, Morita H, Kuroiwa T. Left ventricular wall motion abnormalities in patients with subarachnoid hemorrhage: neurogenic stunned myocardium. *J Am Coll Cardiol.* 1994;24:636.

17. Wald DA. ECG manifestations of selected metabolic and endocrine disorders. *Emerg Med Clin North Am.* 2006;24(1):145–157, vii.

18. Vanhaelst L, Neve P, Chailly P, et al. Coronary disease in hypothyroidism: observations in clinical myxoedema. *Lancet.* 1967;2:800–802.

19. Surawicz B, Mangiardi ML. Electrocardiogram in endocrine and metabolic disorders. *Cardiovasc Clin.* 1977;8:243–266.

20. Surawicz B, Mangiardi ML. Electrocardiogram in endocrine and metabolic disorders. In: *Electrocardiographic Correlations.* Philadelphia, PA: FA Davis; 1977:243–266.

21. Harumi K, Ouichi T. Q-T prolongation syndrome (in Japanese). In: *Naika mook.* Tokyo: Kinbara; 1981:210.

22. Okada M, Nishimura F, Yoshino H, et al. The J wave in accidental hypothermia. *J Electrocardiol.* 1983;16:23–28.

23. Frank S, Colliver JA, Frank A. The electrocardiogram in obesity: statistical analysis of 1,029 patients. *J Am Coll Cardiol.* 1986;7:295–299.

24. Starr JW, Wagner GW, Behar VS, et al. Vectorcardiographic criteria for the diagnosis of inferior myocardial infarction. *Circulation.* 1974;49:829–836.

25. Salerno DM, Asinger RW, Elsperger J, et al. Frequency of hypokalemia after successfully resuscitated out-of-hospital cardiac arrest compared with that in transmural acute myocardial infarction. *Am J Cardiol.* 1987;59:84–88.

26. Surawicz B. The interrelationship of electrolyte abnormalities and arrhythmias. In: *Cardiac Arrhythmias: Their Mechanisms, Diagnosis, and Management.* Philadelphia, PA: JB Lippincott; 1980:83.

27. Krikler DM, Curry PVL. Torsades de pointes, an atypical ventricular tachycardia. *Br Heart J.* 1976;38:117–120.

28. Surawicz B. Relationship between electrocardiogram and electrolytes. *Am Heart J.* 1967;73:814–834.

29. Ettinger PO, Regan TJ, Oldewurtel HA. Hyperkalemia, cardiac conduction, and the electrocardiogram. A review. *Am Heart J.* 1974;88:360–371.

30. Sekiya S, Ichikawa S, Tsutsumi T, et al. Nonuniform action potential durations at different sites in canine left ventricle. *Jpn Heart J.* 1983;24:935–945.

31. Bashour TT. Spectrum of ventricular pacemaker exit block owing to hyperkalemia. *Am J Cardiol.* 1986;57:337–338.

32. Nirenburg DW, Ransil BJ. Q-aTc interval as a clinical indicator of hypercalcemia. *Am J Cardiol.* 1979;44:243–248.

33. Douglas PS, Carmichael KA, Palevsky PM. Extreme hypercalcemia and electrocardiographic changes. *Am J Cardiol.* 1984;54: 674–679.

34. Sridharan MR, Horan LG. Electrocardiographic J wave in hypercalcemia. *Am J Cardiol.* 1984;54:672–673.

35. Vaughan Williams EM. Classification of antiarrhythmic drugs. In: Sandoe E, Flensted-Jensen E, Olsen KH, eds. *Cardiac Arrhythmias.* Sodertalje, Sweden: Astra; 1970:449–472.

36. Roden DM. Drug-induced prolongation of the QT interval. *N Engl J Med.* 2004;350:1013–1022.

37. Watanabe Y, Dreifus LS. Interactions of quinidine and potassium on atrioventricular transmission. *Circ Res.* 1967;20:434–446.

14 Introduction to Arrhythmias

GALEN S. WAGNER AND
DAVID G. STRAUSS

APPROACH TO ARRHYTHMIA DIAGNOSIS

The nine features that should be examined in every analysis of the electrocardiogram (ECG) are presented in Chapter 3. The two of these features that are of primary importance in the evaluation of cardiac rhythm are:

1. rate and regularity; and
2. identification of the rhythm.

The method for determining the rates of both regular and irregular rhythms should be reviewed before proceeding with this chapter. Normal sinus rhythm, with its rate limits of 60 to 100 beats per minute, and its slight irregularity due to respiratory variation, is also presented in Chapter 3. Of the original nine features presented in Chapter 3, the additional ECG features that are important aspects of many of the abnormalities of cardiac rhythm include:

1. P-wave morphology;
2. PR interval;
3. QRS complex morphology; and
4. QTc interval.

The term "arrhythmia" is very general, referring to all rhythms other than regular sinus rhythm. Even the slight variation in sinus rate caused by altered autonomic balance during the respiratory cycle is termed "sinus arrhythmia." The term *dysrhythmia* has been proposed by some as an alternative, but "arrhythmia," meaning "imperfection in a regularly recurring motion," is the commonly accepted term for rhythms other than regular sinus rhythm. The presence of an arrhythmia does not necessarily reflect cardiac disease, as indicated by the broad array of abnormal rhythms that commonly occur in healthy individuals of all ages. Arrhythmias are primarily classified according to their rate, and usually, the atria and ventricles have the same rates. However, there are many different atrial/ventricular relationships among the cardiac arrhythmias:

1. The atrial and ventricular rhythms are associated and have the same rate, but (a) the rhythm originates in the atria or (b) the rhythm originates in the ventricles.
2. The atrial and ventricular rhythms are associated, but the atrial rate is faster than the ventricular rate (the rhythm must originate in the atria).
3. The atrial and ventricular rhythms are associated, but the ventricular rate is faster than the atrial rate (the rhythm must originate in the ventricles).
4. The atrial and ventricular rhythms are independent (*atrioventricular [AV] dissociation*) and (a) the atrial and ventricular rates are the same (isorhythmic dissociation), (b) the atrial rate is faster than the ventricular rate, or (c) the ventricular rate is faster than the atrial rate.

When the atrial and ventricular rhythms are associated but have differing rates, the rhythm is named according to the rate of the chamber (atrial or ventricular) from which it originates (e.g., when a rapid atrial rhythm is associated with a slower ventricular rate, the name "atrial tachyarrhythmia" is used). When the atrial and ventricular rhythms are dissociated, names should be given to both of the rhythms (e.g., atrial tachyarrhythmia with ventricular tachyarrhythmia).

The term *bradyarrhythmia* is used to identify any rhythm with a rate <60 beats per minute, and "tachyarrhythmia" is used to identify any rhythm with a rate >100 beats per minute. There are also many arrhythmias that do not alter the rate beyond these normal limits. In contrast to the general terms "bradyarrhythmia" and "tachyarrhythmia," the terms "bradycardia" and "tachycardia" refer to specific arrhythmias such as sinus bradycardia and sinus tachycardia. The two important aspects of arrhythmias that are basic to their understanding are:

1. their mechanism; and
2. their site of origin.

The mechanisms that produce arrhythmias are either:

1. problems of impulse formation (*automaticity*); or
2. problems of impulse conduction (block or reentry).

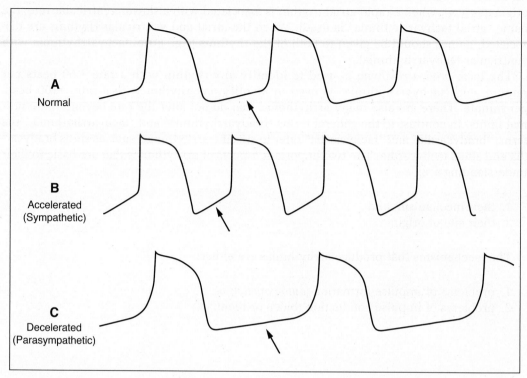

FIGURE 14.1. Schematic action potentials of a pacemaking cell. **A.** Normal sinus rhythm. **B.** Excess sympathetic activity increases the slope of the slow spontaneous depolarization, creating an accelerated rhythm, as in sinus tachycardia. **C.** Excess parasympathetic activity decreases the slope of the slow spontaneous depolarization, creating a decelerated rhythm, as in sinus brachycardia. *Arrows* indicate the slow spontaneous depolarization in all three conditions. See Animation 14.1.

Arrhythmias caused by problems of automaticity can originate in any cell in the pacemaking and conduction system that is capable of *spontaneous depolarization*. Such cells, termed *pacemaker cells*, are present in the:

1. Sinus node.
2. Purkinje cells scattered through the atria.
3. Common (His) bundle.
4. Right and left bundle branches.
5. Purkinje cells in the fascicles and peripheral ventricular endocardial network.

See Chapter 1, Figure 1.7.

Animation 14.1

Normally, the automaticity of the sinus node exceeds that of all other parts of the pacemaking and conduction systems, allowing it to control the cardiac rate and rhythm. This is important because of both the location of the sinus node and its relationship to the parasympathetic and sympathetic components of the autonomic nervous system (see Chapter 3). A site below the sinus node can initiate the cardiac rhythm either because it usurps control from the sinus node by accelerating its own automaticity or because the sinus node abdicates its role by decreasing its automaticity. The term "ectopic" is often applied to rhythms that originate from any site other than the sinus node. Cardiac cells function as pacemakers by forming electrical impulses called action potentials via the process of spontaneous depolarization (Fig. 14.1). When the automaticity of cardiac cells is severely impaired, the therapeutic use of an artificial pacemaker may be required (see Chapter 23). The acceleration of automaticity is limited by the maximal rate of impulse formation in pacemaker cells and therefore rarely causes a clinically important tachyarrhythmia.

The mechanism by which a tachyarrhythmia is perpetuated determines the treatment required for its management. Accelerated automaticity can best be treated by eliminating the cause of the acceleration rather than by treating the acceleration itself. When the accelerated automaticity originates from the sinus node, the cause is increased sympathetic nervous activity resulting from systemic conditions such as exertion, anxiety, fever, decreased cardiac output, or thyrotoxicosis. When the accelerated automaticity originates from another location, the most common causes are ischemia and digitalis toxicity. Therefore, accelerated sinus automaticity is treated by removing the responsible systemic condition, and accelerated nonsinus automaticity, termed "ectopic," is treated by removing the responsible condition.

Table 14.1.

Impulse Conduction Block

Site of Block	Site Primarily Affected
1. Sinus node	1. Atrial myocardium
2. AV node	2. His bundle
3. His bundle	3. Bundle branches
4. Bundle branches	4. Ventricular myocardium

The term *block* is used to refer to the situation in which conduction is slowed or fails to occur at all (e.g., AV block; see Chapter 22) or bundle-branch block (see Chapter 6). Cardiac impulses can be either partly blocked, causing conduction delay (e.g., a prolonged PR interval), or totally blocked, causing conduction failure (e.g., complete AV block). With a partial block of impulses, there is no change in the rate of the affected site, but with a total block of impulses, a bradyarrhythmia is produced in the affected site. Either partial or total block can occur at any site within the pacemaking and conduction system (Table 14.1).

PROBLEMS OF IMPULSE CONDUCTION: REENTRY

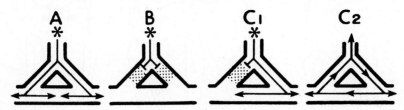

FIGURE 14.2. *Asterisks* indicate sites of impulse formation, *arrows* indicate the directions of impulse conduction, *perpendicular lines* indicate block of impulse conduction, and *shaded areas* indicate areas that have not yet completed the repolarization process. See Animation 14.2.

Although conduction abnormalities sufficient to produce block can occur only within the pacemaking and conduction systems, uneven or *inhomogeneous conduction* can occur in any part of the heart. This inhomogeneous spread of electrical impulses can result in reentry of an impulse into an area that has just previously been depolarized and repolarized.[1] Reentry produces a circular movement of the impulse, which continues as long as the impulse encounters receptive cells, resulting in a single *premature beat*, multiple premature beats, a nonsustained tachyarrhythmia, or even a sustained tachyarrhythmia. There are three prerequisites to the development of reentry:

1. An available circuit.
2. A difference in the refractory periods of the two pathways (limbs) in the circuit.
3. Conduction that is sufficiently slow somewhere in the circuit to allow the remainder of the circuit to recover its responsiveness by the time the impulse returns.

In Figure 14.2, the diagrams represent three different situations regarding the homogeneity of pathway receptiveness to impulse conduction: (A) Both limbs of the pathway are receptive—the left and right limbs have completed the recovery process and are receptive to the entering impulse; (B) both limbs of the pathway are refractory—the left and right limbs are still refractory (because of the persisting depolarized state) to being reactivated by the entering impulse; (C1) one limb of the pathway is receptive and the other is refractory; (C2) the left limb of the pathway is refractory and the right limb is receptive. By the time the impulse reaches the distal end of the left limb (by traveling down the right limb), it is able to reenter because repolarization has been completed. The impulse continues to cycle within the *re-entry circuit* as long as it encounters receptive cells, thus producing a reentrant tachyarrhythmia.

Animation 14.2

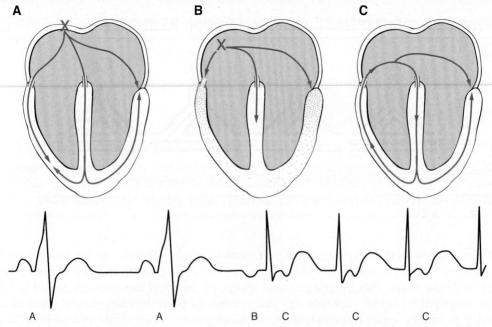

FIGURE 14.3. **Top.** The presence of a Kent bundle is indicated by the open space between the right atrium and ventricle and the AV node by the open space at the summit of the interventricular septum. X, site of the pacemaker in the sinus node **(A)** and in the right atrium **(B)**. No pacemaking is required in **C**. The *arrows* indicate the directions of impulse conduction. **Bottom.** the corresponding ECG, indicating sinus rhythm with a normal P wave immediately followed by the QRS complex, indicating ventricular preexcitation **(A)**; an inverted P wave preceding the QRS complex, indicating an APB without preexcitation **(B)**; and inverted P waves following the QRS complexes, indicating a reentrant junctional tachycardia **(C)**. (Modified from Wagner GS, Waugh RA, Ramo BW. *Cardiac Arrhythmias.* New York, NY: Churchill Livingstone; 1983:13, with permission.) See Animation 14.3.

An example of the development of a "re-entry circuit" in the presence of an accessory AV conduction pathway is presented in Figure 14.3. During sinus rhythm (see Fig. 14.3A), both the AV node and the bundle of Kent have had time to recover from their previous activation. The premature atrial beat in Figure 14.3B encounters persisting refractoriness in the nearby bundle of Kent but encounters receptiveness in the more distant AV node, a situation analogous to that shown in Figure 14.2C1. This leads to the development of a re-entry circuit (see Fig. 14.3C) analogous to that in Figure 14.2C2. Re-entry circuits vary in size from a local area of myocardial fibers (see Fig. 14.2C2) to atrial and ventricular chambers (see Fig. 14.3C).

The term *micro–re-entry* describes the mechanism that occurs when a re-entry circuit is too small for its activation to be represented by a waveform on the surface ECG. The impulses formed within the re-entry circuit spread through the surrounding myocardium just as they would spread from an automatic or pacemaking site. The P waves and QRS complexes on the ECG are produced by this passive spread of activation through the atria and ventricles. Micro–re-entry commonly occurs in the AV node (see Chapter 18) and in the ventricles (see Chapter 19).

The term *macro–re-entry* describes the mechanism that occurs when a re-entry circuit is large enough for its own activation to be represented on the surface ECG (see Fig. 14.3). Cycling of the activating impulse through the right atrium (see Fig. 14.3C) is represented by a portion of the P wave, with the remainder of the P wave produced by spread of the impulse through the uninvolved left atrium. Cycling of the impulse through the right ventricle (see Fig. 14.3C) is represented by a portion of the QRS complex, with the remainder of the QRS complex produced by spread of

Animation 14.3 the impulse through the uninvolved left ventricle.

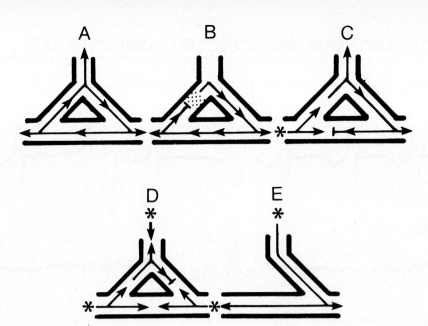

FIGURE 14.4. The diagram in Figure 14.2 is used to illustrate reentry **(A)** and the four mechanisms of termination **(B–E)**. *Asterisks, arrows, perpendiculars,* and *shaded areas* have the same meanings as in Figure 14.3. The *asterisk* in **C** indicates an ectopic site of impulse formation, the *three asterisks* in **D** indicate impulse reception from all sides initiated by the precordial electric shock, and the *single asterisk* in **E** indicates sinus node impulse formation. See Animation 14.4.

There are also forms of macro–re-entry in which the re-entry circuit is entirely within either the atrial or ventricular myocardium. When this occurs, sawtooth-like or undulating ECG waveforms replace discrete P waves (see Chapter 17) or QRS complexes (see Chapter 19).

In attempting to treat reentry, it is important to understand its mechanism. For any re-entry circuit to perpetuate itself, the advancing head of the recycling impulse must not catch up with the refractory tail (Fig. 14.4A). Thus, there must always be a gap of nonrefractory cells between the head and the tail of the recycling impulse. A sustained reentrant tachyarrhythmia can be terminated by:

1. Administering drugs that accelerate conduction of the impulse in the re-entry circuit so that it encounters an area that has not yet recovered (see Fig. 14.4B). Termination also results if a drug prolongs the recovery time.
2. Introducing an impulse from an artificial pacemaker that depolarizes (captures) part of the re-entry circuit, thereby rendering it nonreceptive to the returning impulse (see Fig. 14.4C).
3. Introducing a precordial electrical shock, termed *cardioversion*, that captures all receptive parts of the heart, including those in the re-entry circuit, rendering the circuit nonreceptive to the returning impulse (see Fig. 14.4D).
4. Performing surgical or catheter ablation of one limb of the tissue required for the re-entry circuit. For example, ablation of the accessory AV pathway in a patient with ventricular preexcitation (see Fig. 14.4E).

Animation 14.4

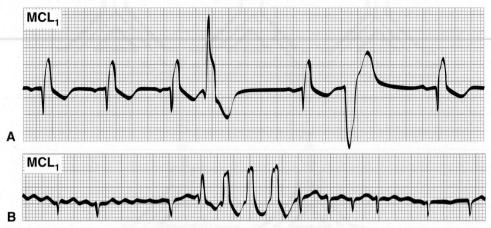

FIGURE 14.5. **A.** Right-bundle-branch block during sinus rhythm, and both lead V1-positive (fourth beat) and lead V1-negative (sixth beat) VPBs (see Chapter 19). **B.** The basic rhythm is atrial fibrillation, with most beats conducted normally; however, beats four through seven are not conducted through the right bundle. Note the typical triphasic appearance of the initial wide QRS complex.

The introduction of coronary care units (CCUs) in the early 1960s stimulated rapid advances in the diagnosis and treatment of cardiac arrhythmias. In the CCU, patients who have either arrhythmias, or a high risk of developing arrhythmias because of conditions such as acute myocardial infarction, are continuously monitored (see Chapter 2). A modified chest lead V1 (MCL$_1$) is commonly used as the display lead because it provides both a good view of atrial activity and of differentiation between right and left ventricular activity (Fig. 14.5).[2] Often, however, multiple leads are displayed on both bedside and central surveillance monitors to provide multiple views of the cardiac electrical activity to facilitate rapid and accurate rhythm interpretation.

DYNAMIC (HOLTER) MONITORING

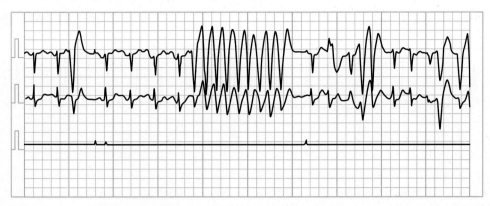

FIGURE 14.6. Holter recording of leads MCL$_1$ and MCL$_5$ revealing VPBs and ventricular tachycardia in a 57-year-old man with dyspnea and palpitations following hospital discharge for an acute myocardial infarction.

A method for continuous ECG monitoring of ambulatory patients in their own environment was developed in the 1960s by Holter[3] and has since been further enhanced.[3] The patient is attached via chest electrodes to a portable recorder that records one to three ECG leads for 24 hours. The patient keeps a diary of activities so that symptoms, activity, and cardiac rhythm can be correlated. Thus, the patient is monitored during situations that actually occur in real-life situations. Holter monitoring is used to identify any correlation between an arrhythmia and symptoms such as *palpitations*, dizziness, syncope, or chest pain (Fig. 14.6).

In a study of 371 patients who received a 24-hour Holter monitoring for detection of cardiac arrhythmias, 174 (47%) had symptoms. However, symptoms coincided with a disturbance of cardiac rhythm in only 48 (27%) of the patients; the remaining 126 patients (73%) experienced their symptoms when their rhythm was entirely normal. Thus, of the original 371 patients who received monitoring, the Holter method revealed whether symptoms were or were not due to the arrhythmias in approximately half. However, the 48 patients in whom arrhythmia was the probable cause of the symptoms represented only about 1 of 8 of the original 371 patients.[4]

Holter monitoring is also of value in specific cardiac diseases or in conditions in which information about the heart's rhythm is important for prognosis and management. These conditions include ischemic heart disease, mitral valve prolapse, cardiomyopathy, conduction disturbances, evaluation of pacemaker function, or Wolff–Parkinson–White syndrome. Holter monitoring may also be helpful in the asymptomatic patient in whom an arrhythmia has been detected on routine examination. In addition, Holter monitoring may be of value in assessing the therapeutic effect of antiarrhythmic drugs and adjusting drug dosages. In this context, however, it is important to realize that the frequency of an arrhythmia may have day-to-day variation of up to 90%[5] and that a marked and consistent reduction in the incidence of the arrhythmia must occur before its successful treatment can be assumed. The limited span of (usually) 24 hours of Holter monitoring makes it unsuitable for detecting infrequent disturbances in cardiac rhythm.

HEART RATE 151   **HEART RATE 154**

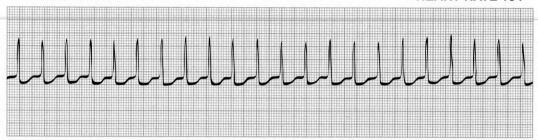

FIGURE 14.7. A single-lead ECG recording from a 17-year-old woman with a history of palpitations, who transmits this rhythm strip by telephone immediately after the recurrence of her symptoms.

The problem of detecting infrequent arrhythmias by Holter monitoring has been largely overcome by *transtelephonic monitoring*.[6,7] When using this method, the patient carries a pocket-sized transmitter and transmits his or her cardiac rhythm via telephone when symptoms occur. This permits more efficient and economical monitoring than with Holter monitoring and facilitates extended periods of monitoring (days to weeks; Fig. 14.7).

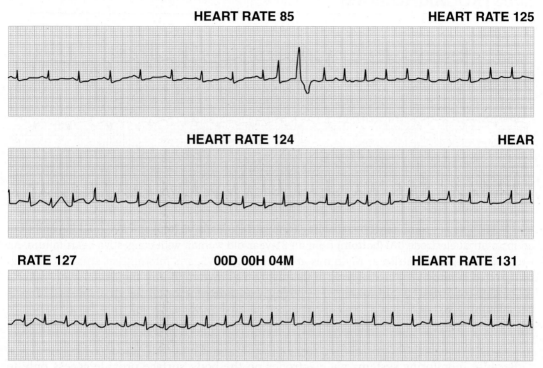

HEART RATE 85 **HEART RATE 125**

HEART RATE 124 **HEAR**

RATE 127 **00D 00H 04M** **HEART RATE 131**

FIGURE 14.8. A continuous recording of the 30 seconds of rhythm stored by the memory loop monitor preceding manual activation (indicated by the *mark in the middle of the bottom strip*). This 72-year-old man had a history of recurrent shortness of breath and activated his recorder as soon as his symptoms began 20 seconds after the onset of his irregularly irregular supraventricular tachycardia that is almost certainly atrial flutter-fibrillation.

It is often clinically important to observe the initiation of an intermittently occurring symptomatic cardiac arrhythmia. This requires a "memory loop" that continually stores the patient's cardiac rhythm for a set period of time.[8] The patient manually activates the permanent recording function of the arrhythmia monitor as soon as symptoms begin. The prior period of rhythm, which has been stored on the memory loop, is captured to reveal the onset of an arrhythmia accompanying the patient's symptoms. This system may reveal the transition from normal rhythm to abnormal brady- or tachyarrhythmias (Fig. 14.8).

INVASIVE METHODS OF RECORDING THE ELECTROCARDIOGRAM

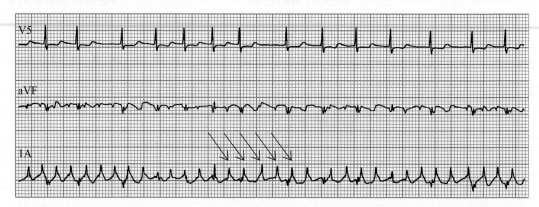

FIGURE 14.9. Simultaneous recording from surface leads V5 **(top)** and aVF **(middle)** and from an intra-atrial electrode (IA) **(bottom)** from an 81-year-old woman with congestive heart failure. An irregularly irregular ventricular rhythm is apparent in lead V5, and intermittent atrial activity can be detected in lead aVF. The diagnosis of the rapid atrial rhythm (flutter-fibrillation) with variable AV block is confirmed by the intra-atrial recording, with *arrows* indicating the atrial rate of 330 beats per minute.

Because monitoring systems via electrodes on the body surface provide access only to electrical activity from the atrial and ventricular myocardia, a definitive rhythm diagnosis is often not possible. The atrial activity may be obscured during a tachyarrhythmia because of superimposed QRS complexes and T waves. When the use of alternate body surface sites for electrodes fails to reveal atrial activity, either transesophageal or intra-atrial recording may be necessary. Figure 14.9 illustrates the ability of intra-atrial recording to reveal diagnostic atrial activity when none is clearly visible on the body surface. The atrial flutter-fibrillation is confirmed in this patient.

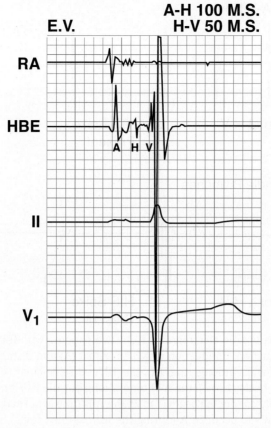

FIGURE 14.10. Electrograms from the right atrium (*RA*) and His bundle (*HBE*) are presented, along with recordings from standard leads II and V1. The atrium-to-His (*A-H*) interval of 100 milliseconds and His-to-ventricle (*H-V*) interval of 50 milliseconds combine to form the 150 milliseconds PR interval. M.S., milliseconds. (From Wagner GS, Waugh RA, Ramo BW. *Cardiac Arrhythmias.* New York, NY: Churchill Livingstone; 1983:117, with permission.)

An even more definitive rhythm diagnosis can be obtained by positioning a multipolar catheter across the tricuspid valve, providing direct access to recording from the common or His bundle.[9-11] With a more proximal electrode in the right atrium, simultaneous recording from multiple intracardiac locations is possible (Fig. 14.10). This diagnostic information is clinically important when AV block is present, and differentiation between AV nodal versus His–Purkinje location cannot be inferred from the surface ECG.

A. Proximal Block—A-V Node

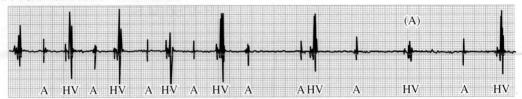

| A | HV | A | HV | A | HV | A | HV | A | | A·HV | A | | HV | | A | | HV |

1° : Long A-H, Normal H-V   2° : HIS Spike
                                          Present

B. Distal Block—Bundle Branches

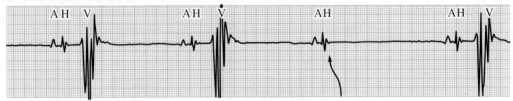

| A·H | V | | A·H | V | | A·H | | | | A·H | V |

1° : Normal A-H, Long H-V   2° : HIS Spike
                                          Present

FIGURE 14.11. His-bundle electrograms from two patients with initial delay and then complete failure of AV conduction. Conduction delays proximal **(A)** and distal **(B)** to the His bundle are indicated by the relationships among atrial (A), His (H), and ventricular (V) spikes. In **A**, during the initial slowly conducted beats (1 to 4), the A-H time is long but the H-V time is normal; however, in **B**, during the initial slowly conducted beats (1 to 2), the A-H time is normal and the H-V time is long. When AV conduction fails to occur in **A** (during the fifth cardiac cycle), no His activation occurs; however, when AV conduction fails to occur in **B** (during the third cardiac cycle), the His activation is present (*arrow*). Slow AV conduction resumes at the end of both **A** and **B**. (From Wagner GS, Waugh RA, Ramo BW. *Cardiac Arrhythmias.* New York, NY: Churchill Livingstone; 1983:119, with permission.)

Recording from the His bundle provides division of the PR interval into its two components: from the atria through the AV node to the His bundle (atrium-to-His interval), and from the His bundle to the ventricles (His-to-ventricle interval). This method provides direct identification of the site of an AV block (Fig. 14.11).[12] His-bundle recordings have provided proof for many of the originally assumed electrocardiographic principles discussed in later chapters.

Many studies have documented high incidences of various arrhythmias in healthy individuals of all ages. In a study of 134 infants during the first 10 days of life,[13] the maximal heart rate reached 220 beats per minute, and the minimal rate was 42 beats per minute. Atrial premature beats (APBs) were found in 19 (14%) of the infants, and sinus pauses occurred in 72%, with the longest pause reaching 1.8 seconds.

In a study of 92 healthy children ages 7 to 11 years,[14] the highest rate attained was 195 beats per minute and the lowest rate was 37 beats per minute. First-degree AV block was found in nine children and second-degree AV block in three. APBs and ventricular premature beats (VPBs) were found in 21% and sinus pauses in 66%.

In a third study, of 131 healthy boys ages 10 to 13 years,[15] waking maximal heart rates ranged between 100 and 200 beats per minute, with minimal rates between 45 and 80 beats per minute. Maximal heart rates during sleep were between 60 and 100 beats per minute, with minimal rates between 30 and 70 beats per minute. First-degree AV block was found in 8% and second-degree AV block in 11%. Single APBs and VPBs were found in 13% and 26%, respectively.

In a study of 50 healthy women ages 22 to 28 years,[16] the waking maximal heart rate ranged from 122 to 189 beats per minute, with minimal rates between 40 and 73 beats per minute. Maximal heart rates during sleep ranged from 71 to 128 beats per minute, with minimal rates between 37 and 59 beats per minute. APBs occurred in 64% and VPBs in 54%. One had one three-beat run of ventricular tachycardia and two (4%) had periods of second-degree AV block.

In a study of 50 healthy male medical students,[17] the waking maximal heart rate ranged from 107 to 180 beats per minute, with minimal rates between 37 and 65 beats per minute. Maximal heart rates during sleep were between 70 and 115 beats per minute, with minimal rates of 33 to 55 beats per minute. Half of the students had sinus arrhythmia sufficient to cause a 100% change in consecutive cycles, and 28% had sinus pauses of >1.75 seconds. APBs were found in 56% of the students, and VPBs were found in 50%. Three (6%) had periods of second-degree AV block.

An investigation of 98 healthy elderly subjects ranging from 60 to 85 years with normal maximal treadmill tests[18] revealed sinus bradycardia in 91%, supraventricular premature beats in 88%, supraventricular tachycardia in 13%, and *atrial flutter* in 1%. Ventricular arrhythmias included premature beats in 78% (many with pairs or multiform beats) and ventricular tachycardia in 4%.

A study of 20 male long-distance runners ranging in age from 19 to 29 years[19] found that all had APBs, 70% had VPBs, and 40% had periods of second-degree AV block. Another study, of 101 healthy women,[20] disclosed VPBs in 34% and complex forms in 10%. Supraventricular premature beats were recorded in 28%, and VPBs were more frequent in women taking contraceptive pills or thyroid medication.

In a study of 50 healthy 80- to 89-year-old men and women,[21] supraventricular premature beats were found in 100%, with 65% having >20 such beats per hour. Supraventricular tachycardia was found in 28%. More than 10 VPBs per hour were found in 32% of the subjects, with multifocal beats in 18%.

Among 147 healthy Swedish workers ranging in age from 15 to 65 years,[22] 95% of those <40 years old had <3 VPBs per hour, whereas in those >40 years old, 95% had >36 VPBs per hour.

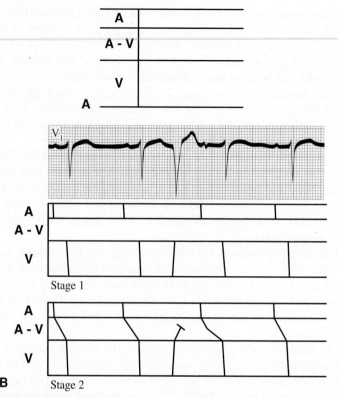

FIGURE 14.12. **A.** The format by which ladder diagrams are constructed: Spaces are provided for representing atrial (A), junctional (AV), and ventricular (V) activation. The two stages of construction of a ladder diagram: *Stage 1* involves the use of *slanted lines* to include the duration of the obvious waveforms representing both atrial and ventricular activation. The forward or backward slope of the *slanted lines* indicates the presumed direction of spread of activation. **B.** *Stage 2* involves constructing lines in the AV junctional space to connect the atrial and ventricular lines to represent the presumed direction of the spread of junctional activation. These lines are terminated and capped with *short perpendicular lines* to indicate the presumed failure of impulse conduction.

Ladder diagrams are often helpful for understanding difficult arrhythmias. These diagrams have rows for indicating atrial (A), atrial-to-ventricular (AV) junction, and ventricular activation (Fig. 14.12A). Additional rows can be added as needed to diagram more complex arrhythmias. The ladder diagram should be constructed directly under or on a photocopy of the ECG recording in two sequential stages as follows:

1. Include what you can see (e.g., draw lines to represent the visible P waves and QRS complexes).
2. Add what you cannot see (e.g., connect the atrial and ventricular lines to represent AV or ventriculoatrial [VA] conduction, and draw lines to represent any missing P waves at regular PP intervals between visible P waves).

Figure 14.12B provides an illustration of the use of ladder diagrams to understand a cardiac arrhythmia with varying PR intervals and varying QRS complex morphologies. In the

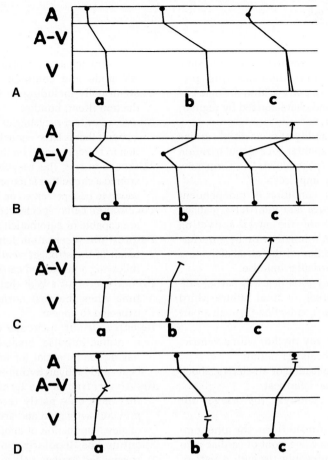

FIGURE 14.13. **A.** A normal sinus beat (*a*) encounters prolonged AV conduction (*b*) and is then replaced by an atrial beat that encounters both prolonged AV conduction and aberrant ventricular conduction (indicated by the *split line*) (*c*). *Solid circles* indicate the site of impulse formation. **B.** AV-junctional beats with progressively longer retrograde conduction times to the atria: in *a*, the P wave precedes the QRS complex, but in *b*, it follows the QRS complex. In *c*, the retrograde conduction time is so long that a second QRS complex is generated. *Arrowheads* have been added to indicate the direction of impulse conduction (*c*), but the direction of the impulse is also indicated by the slopes of the lines. **C.** Ventricular beats with progressively greater penetration into the AV junction: no conduction (*a*), partial conduction (*b*), and complete retrograde VA conduction (*c*). **D.** In *a*, there is complete AV dissociation; in *b*, AV conduction results in "fusion" during the QRS complex; and in *c*, VA conduction results in fusion during the P wave.

first stage of the diagram, all visible P waves and QRS complexes have been represented. Note the reversed slope representing the premature wide QRS complex, indicating the likelihood that it originated from the ventricles. When the lines representing AV conduction are added in the second stage, the prolonged PR interval following the third P wave is indicated by a slant to represent a conduction delay. The VPB must have traveled retrogradely into the AV junction so that the next sinus impulse found the junction *relatively refractory*.

In subsequent chapters, ladder diagrams are used as visual aids to understand mechanisms of arrhythmias. Figure 14.13A–D presents four examples to indicate how various symbols may be used to represent aberrant ventricular conduction (see Fig. 14.13A), *junctional* rhythm (see Fig. 14.13B), ventricular rhythm (see Fig. 14.13C), and dissociation between atrial and ventricular rhythms (see Fig. 14.13D).

GLOSSARY

Atrial flutter: the tachyarrhythmia at the slow end of the flutter/fibrillation spectrum, produced by macro–re-entry within a single circuit in the atria and characterized by regular, uniform F waves.

Automaticity: the ability of specialized cardiac cells to achieve spontaneous depolarization and function as "pacemakers" to form new cardiac-activating impulses.

AV dissociation: a condition of independent beating of the atria and ventricles, caused either by block of the atrial-activating impulse in the AV junction or by interference with conduction of the atrial-activating impulse by a ventricular impulse.

Block: either a delay (first degree), partial failure (second degree), or total failure (third degree) of impulse conduction through a part of the heart.

Bradyarrhythmia: any rhythm with a ventricular rate of <60 beats per minute.

Cardioversion: application of an electric shock to restore a normal heartbeat.

Dysrhythmia: a synonym (by usage) for arrhythmia.

Inhomogeneous conduction: the phenomenon in which the wave front of cardiac activation spreads unevenly through a part of the heart because of varying refractoriness from previous activation, creating the potential for impulse reentry.

Isorhythmic dissociation: AV dissociation, with the atria and ventricles beating at the same or almost the same rate.

Junctional: a term referring to the cardiac structures that electrically connect the atria and ventricles and normally including the AV node and common (His) bundle and abnormally including an accessory AV conduction (Kent) bundle.

Macro–re-entry: recycling of an impulse around a circuit that is large enough for its own activation to be represented on the surface ECG.

Micro–re-entry: the recycling of an impulse around a circuit that is too small for its own activation to be represented on the surface ECG.

Pacemaker cells: specialized cardiac cells that are capable of automaticity.

Palpitation: a sensation felt in the chest as a result of the stronger ventricular contraction following a prolonged cardiac cycle.

Premature beat: a beat that occurs before the time when the next normal beat would be expected to appear.

Re-entry circuit: a circular course traveled by a cardiac impulse, created by reentry, and having the potential for initiating premature beats and tachyarrhythmias.

Relative refractory: a term referring to cells that have only partly recovered from their previous activation and are therefore capable of slow conduction of another impulse.

Spontaneous depolarization: the ability of a specialized cardiac cell to activate by altering the permeability of its membrane to a sufficient degree to attain threshold potential without any external stimulation.

Transtelephonic monitoring: cardiac monitoring in which the patient uses a pocket-sized transmitter to send a cardiac rhythm strip over the telephone when cardiac symptoms occur.

REFERENCES

1. Hoffman BF, Cranefield PF, Wallace AG. Physiological basis of cardiac arrhythmias. *Mod Concepts Cardiovasc Dis*. 1966;35:103.

2. Marriott HJL, Fogg E. Constant monitoring for cardiac dysrhythmias and blocks. *Mod Concepts Cardiovasc Dis*. 1970;39:103.

3. Holter NJ. New method for heart studies: continuous electrocardiography of active subjects over long periods is now practical. *Science*. 1961;134:1214.

4. Zeldis SM, Levine BJ, Michelson EL, et al. Cardiovascular complaints: correlation with cardiac arrhythmias on 24-hour electrocardiographic monitoring. *Chest*. 1982;78:456.

5. Michelson EL, Morganroth J. Spontaneous variability of complex ventricular arrhythmias detected by long-term electrocardiographic recording. *Circulation*. 1980;61:690–695.

6. Grodman PS. Arrhythmia surveillance by transtelephonic monitoring: comparison with

Holter monitoring in symptomatic ambulatory patients. *Am Heart J.* 1979;98:459.

7. Judson P, Holmes DR, Baker WP. Evaluation of outpatient arrhythmias utilizing transtelephonic monitoring. *Am Heart J.* 1979;97:759–761.

8. Cumbee SR, Pryor RE, Linzer M. Cardiac loop ECG recording: a new noninvasive diagnostic test in recurrent syncope. *South Med J.* 1990;83:39–43.

9. Damato AN, Lau SH. Clinical value of the electrogram of the conduction system. *Prog Cardiovasc Dis.* 1970;13:119–140.

10. Goldreyer BN. Intracardiac electrocardiography in the analysis and understanding of cardiac arrhythmias. *Ann Intern Med.* 1972;77:117–136.

11. Vadde PS, Caracta AR, Damato AN. Indications of His bundle recordings. *Cardiovasc Clin.* 1980;11:1–6.

12. Pick A. Mechanisms of cardiac arrhythmias; from hypothesis to physiologic fact. *Am Heart J.* 1973;86:249–269.

13. Southall DP, Richards J, Mitchell P, et al. Study of cardiac rhythm in healthy newborn infants. *Br Heart J.* 1980;43:14–20.

14. Southall DP, Johnston F, Shinebourne EA, et al. A 24-hour electrocardiographic study of heart rate and rhythm patterns in population of healthy children. *Br Heart J.* 1981;45:281–291.

15. Scott O, Williams GJ, Fiddler GI. Results of 24-hour ambulatory monitoring of electrocardiogram in 131 healthy boys aged 10 to 13 years. *Br Heart J.* 1980;44:304–308.

16. Sobotka PA, Mayer JH, Bauernfeind RA, et al. Arrhythmias documented by 24-hour continuous ambulatory electrocardiographic monitoring in young women without apparent heart disease. *Am Heart J.* 1981;101:753–759.

17. Brodsky M, Wu D, Denes P, et al. Arrhythmias documented by 24 hour continuous electrocardiographic monitoring in 50 male medical students without apparent heart disease. *Am J Cardiol.* 1977;39:390–395.

18. Fleg JL, Kennedy HL. Cardiac arrhythmias in a healthy elderly population: detection by 24-hour ambulatory electrocardiography. *Chest.* 1982;81:302–307.

19. Talan DA, Bauernfeind RA, Ashley WW, et al. Twenty-four hour continuous ECG recordings in long-distance runners. *Chest.* 1982;82:19–24.

20. Romhilt DW, Choi SC, Irby EC. Arrhythmias on ambulatory monitoring in women without apparent heart disease. *Am J Cardiol.* 1984;54:582–586.

21. Kantelip JP, Sage E, Duchene-Marullaz P. Findings on ambulatory monitoring in subjects older than 80 years. *Am J Cardiol.* 1986;57:398–401.

22. Orth-Gomer K, Hogstedt C, Bodin L, et al. Frequency of extrasystoles in healthy male employees. *Br Heart J.* 1986;55:259–264.

15

Premature Beats

GALEN S. WAGNER

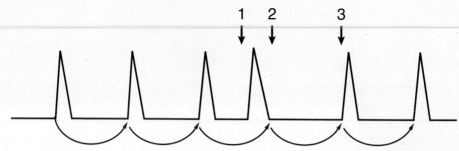

FIGURE 15.1. The timing of a regular underlying rhythm is indicated by the *curved lines* with *arrows*. A PB interrupts this rhythm (1), preventing the occurrence of the next normal beat (2); however, the following normal beat occurs at the expected time (3).

Normal sinus rhythm is commonly interrupted by a premature beat (PB). An alternate term for "beat" is "contraction," with both terms referring to the mechanical event initiated by the early QRS complex on the electrocardiogram (ECG) recording. A PB is recognized by the early appearance of a QRS complex, either normal or abnormal in configuration and either preceded or not preceded by a P wave. Other terms are often substituted for the term "premature beat," including "premature contraction," "early beat," "extrasystole," "premature systole," and *ectopic beat*.

The individual who has a PB may or may not experience a *palpitation*. This palpitation is felt during the next on-time beat because of the increased ventricular contraction strength caused by the higher volume of blood that enters the ventricles during the delay following the PB. Figure 15.1 illustrates the following sequence of events that occur as a result of a single PB:

1. The PB occurs early in the cardiac cycle.
2. The presence of the PB prevents the occurrence of the next normal beat.
3. There is a pause following the PB until the next normal beat occurs.

A single PB is potentially the first beat of a sustained tachyarrhythmia ("tach"). It may be followed by any number of similarly appearing beats to which the terms in the following two paragraphs are applied (Table 15.1).

Table 15.1.	
Terminology of Quantities of Premature Beats	
Number of Consecutive Beats	Term
1	A premature beat
2	A pair or a *couplet*
3—30-s continuation	Nonsustained tach
>30-s continuation	Sustained tach

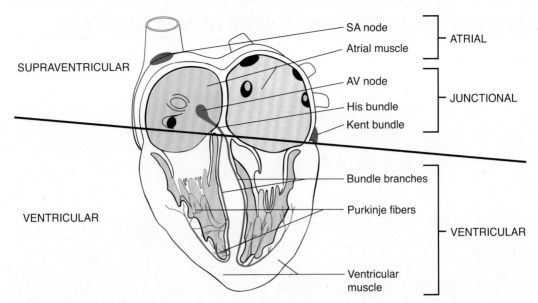

FIGURE 15.2. The anatomic parts of the supraventricular and ventricular areas are indicated. Note the *wide red band* connecting the left atrium and left ventricle on the epicardial surface, which represents a Kent bundle. AV, atrioventricular; SA, sinoatrial. (Modified from Netter FH. *The Ciba Collection of Medical Illustrations.* Vol 5: *Heart.* Summit, NJ: Ciba-Geigy; 1978:49, with permission)

When a PB follows every normal beat, the term *bigeminy* is used; when a PB follows every second normal beat, the term *trigeminy* is used. PBs may originate from any part of the heart other than the sinoatrial (SA) node. They are generally classified as *supraventricular premature beats* (SVPBs) or *ventricular premature beats* (VPBs; Fig. 15.2). This distinction is useful because beats originating from anywhere above the branching of the common bundle (SVPBs) are capable of producing a normal or abnormal QRS complex depending on whether they are conducted normally or *aberrantly* through the intraventricular conduction system. PBs originating from beyond the branching of the common bundle (VPBs), however, can produce only an abnormally prolonged QRS complex of ≥ 0.12 second because they do not have equal access to both the right and left bundle branches. It should be emphasized that VPBs are always abnormally prolonged, but SVPBs are not always of normal duration.

SVPBs may be either *atrial premature beats* (APBs) or *junctional premature beats* (JPBs). The term "junctional" is used instead of "nodal" because it is impossible to distinguish beats originating within the atrioventricular (AV) node from those originating in another structure located between the atria and the ventricles. Normally, the AV junction consists of only the AV node and the common bundle. Abnormally, however, an accessory AV conduction pathway (Kent bundle) is also a part of the AV junction as shown in Figure 15.2.

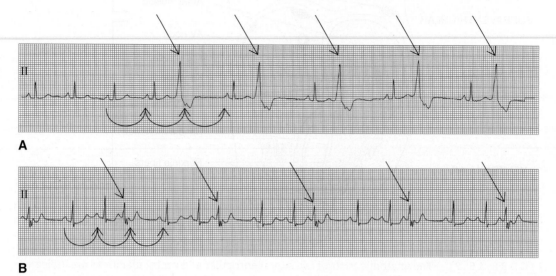

FIGURE 15.3. The *straight arrows* indicate the premature wide QRS complexes in **A** and **B**. The *curved arrows* marking the baseline PP interval indicate that the P waves after the PBs occur "on time" (at twice the normal PP interval) in **A** but not on time (at less than twice the normal PP interval) in **B**. Note that in **A**, the P waves following the PB occurs at the same time as the *curved arrows*, but in **B**, the P wave following the PB occurs before the time as the *curved arrows*.

When SVPBs produce abnormally prolonged or wide QRS complexes (>0.12 second), identification of their supraventricular versus a ventricular origin may be facilitated by observing the effect on the regularity of the underlying sinus rhythm (Fig. 15.3). A VPB typically does not disturb the sinus rhythm, because it is not conducted retrogradely through the slowly conducting AV node into the SA node (see Fig. 15.3A). Although the SA node discharges on time, its impulse cannot be conducted antegradely into the ventricles because of the refractoriness following the VPB. The pause between the VPB and the following conducted beat is termed a *compensatory pause* because it compensates for the prematurity of the VPB. The interval from the sinus beat prior to the VPB to the sinus beat following the VPB is equal to two sinus cycles.

In contrast to a VPB (see Fig. 15.3B), an SVPB does disturb the sinus rhythm. Unlike the VPB, the SVPB can be conducted retrogradely into the SA node, discharging it ahead of schedule and causing the following cycle to also occur ahead of schedule. The pause between the SVPB and the following sinus beat is therefore less than compensatory. This is apparent because the interval from the sinus beat before the SVPB to the sinus beat after the SVPB is less than the duration of two sinus cycles. However, when the SVPB prematurely discharges the SA node, it occasionally suppresses SA nodal automaticity. This *overdrive suppression* may delay the formation of the next sinus impulse for so long that the resulting pause is compensatory, or even longer than compensatory. Thus, the compensatory pause must not be relied upon as the sole indicator of ventricular origin of a wide PB.

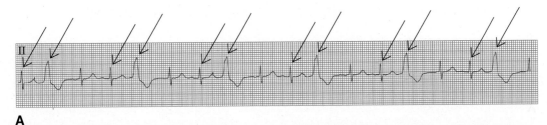

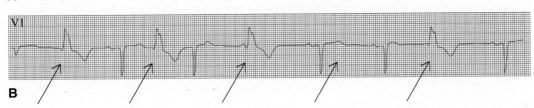

FIGURE 15.4. The *arrows* in the rhythm strips indicate the VPBs coupled to preceding normal beats **(A)** and related to each other **(B)**. In **B**, the *fourth arrow* indicates where a VPB would have occurred had the ventricles been receptive rather than refractory, as indicated by the presence of the T wave.

PBs may be caused by the two mechanisms indicated in Chapter 14: reentry or automaticity. It is usually difficult to determine the mechanism of PBs unless two or more occur in succession. Fortunately, the mechanism of a PB is usually not clinically important unless consecutive abnormal beats are present. When identification of the mechanism for a PB is considered clinically important, the following observations of the *coupling intervals* between beats may be helpful (Fig. 15.4): Reentry produces a constant relationship between normal and PBs (see Fig. 15.4A), whereas automaticity produces a varying relationship between normal and abnormal beats but a constant relationship between abnormal beats (see Fig. 15.4B) as in Table 15.2.

Table 15.2.	
Keys to Diagnosis of Premature Beat (PB) Mechanism	
Observations	Mechanism
There are identical coupling intervals between each PB and the preceding normal beat (see Fig. 15.4A)	Reentry
There are not identical coupling intervals between PBs and normal beats, but there are identical intervals between consecutive PBs (see Fig. 15.4B)	Enhanced automaticity
There are neither identical coupling intervals between PBs and normal beats nor between consecutive PBs	Either

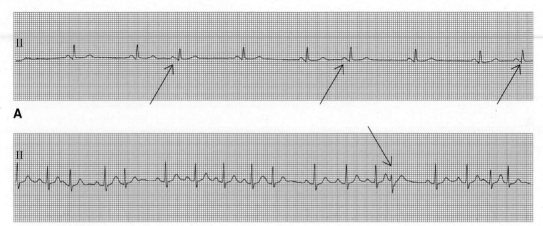

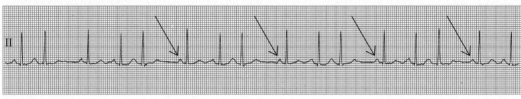

FIGURE 15.5. Three-lead II rhythm strips. *Arrows* indicate normal-appearing premature P waves in **A**, the aberrant QRS resulting from the earliest of the three APBs in **B**, and the timing of the fully compensatory pause resulting from the early APBs in **C**.

The usual APB has three features:

1. A premature and abnormal-appearing P wave.
2. A QRS complex similar to that of the normal sinus beats.
3. A following interval that is less than compensatory because of the retrograde activation of the SA node.

Usually, all of these characteristics are obvious, but "deceptions" occur (particularly when the APB is most premature) so that no one characteristic is completely reliable. In Figure 15.5A, the premature P waves appear normal; in Figure 15.5B, the premature QRS complexes are not always similar to those of the normal sinus beats. Some common ECG deceptions in recognizing APBs are:

1. The P wave may be unrecognizable because it occurs during the previous T wave (see Fig. 15.5B, C).
2. The QRS complex may show aberrant ventricular conduction (see Fig. 15.5B).
3. The pause between the APB and the following P wave is compensatory, probably because of the extreme earliness of the APB (see Fig. 15.5C).

It is extremely rare to have all three of these deceptions appear at the same time. Therefore, with care, one usually has no difficulty in identifying an APB.

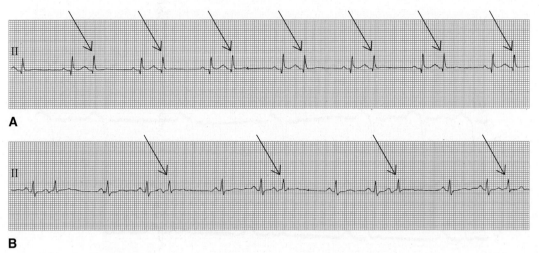

A

B

FIGURE 15.6. In **A**, every normal sinus beat, and in **B**, every second normal sinus beat is coupled through constant PP intervals to APBs. The QRS complexes resulting from these APBs are indicated by the *arrows* in the lead II rhythm strips.

When an APB follows every sinus beat, the result is atrial bigeminy (Fig. 15.6A); when it follows every two consecutive sinus beats, the result is atrial trigeminy (see Fig. 15.6B).

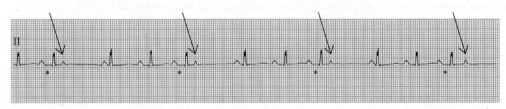

FIGURE 15.7. Nonconducted premature P waves are indicated by *arrows*, but even some on-time P waves have some conduction delay as indicated by prolonged PR intervals (*asterisks*).

When APBs occur very early (a short coupling interval), some parts of the heart may not have had time to complete their recovery from the preceding normal activation. This may result in failure of the premature atrial activation to cause any ventricular activation. Indeed, the most common cause of an unexpected atrial pause is a nonconducted APB (Fig. 15.7). It is better to refer to such beats as "nonconducted" rather than "blocked" because, by definition, "block" implies an abnormal condition. APBs fail to be conducted only because they occur so early in the cycle that the AV node is still in its normal refractory period. It is important to differentiate normal (physiologic) from abnormal (pathologic) nonconduction to avoid mistakenly initiating an antiarrhythmia treatment.

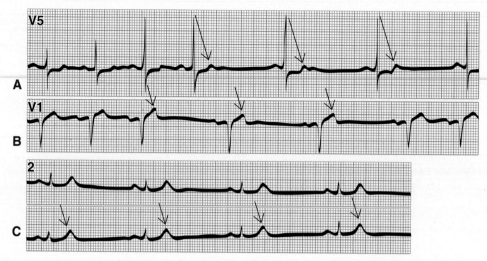

FIGURE 15.8. **A and B.** T waves preceding the pauses (*arrows*) appear different from usual. **C.** There are suspicious peaks on the T waves (*arrows*), but there are no "usual" T waves available for comparison.

Nonconducted APBs that occur in a bigeminal pattern are particularly difficult to identify (Fig. 15.8). If the premature P waves are obscured by the T waves of the preceding normal beats, and if the earlier T waves during the regular sinus rhythm are not available for comparison, then the rhythm is often misdiagnosed as sinus bradycardia.

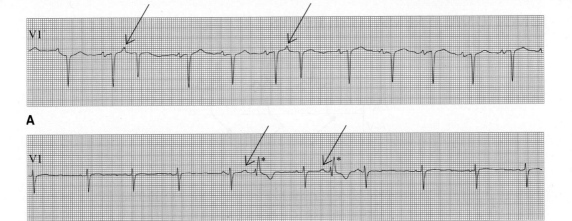

A

B

FIGURE 15.9. Recordings of lead V1 illustrate other varieties of physiologic conduction delays that may occur when the AV node alone **(A)** or both the AV node and the right bundle branch **(B)** have not had time to fully recover from their preceding normal activation. *Arrows* indicate prolonged AV nodal conduction in **A** and **B**, and *asterisks* indicate RBB aberrancy in **B**.

When APBs occur very early in the cardiac cycle of normal beats, they may have other effects on conduction to the ventricles (Fig. 15.9). In Figure 15.9A, there is prolonged AV conduction, whereas in Figure 15.9B there is both slightly prolonged AV conduction and also aberrant intraventricular conduction. In Figure 15.9B, there are varying coupling intervals (*PP intervals*) between normal sinus beats and APBs. When the PP interval is long, the premature PR interval is normal, but when the PP interval is short, the premature PR interval is prolonged. This inverse relationship occurs because of the uniquely long relative refractory period of the AV node: The longer the duration from its most recent activation, the better is the node able to conduct the following impulse and vice versa. This concept is vital to use of the ECG to differentiate a nodal versus Purkinje location of AV block.

When an early APB traverses the AV junction but encounters persistent normal refractoriness in one of the bundle branches or fascicles, aberrant ventricular conduction occurs (see Fig. 15.9B). The morphology of the QRS complex is altered, and its duration may be so prolonged that it resembles a VPB. Detection of the preceding P wave and/or finding that the pause between the APB and the next sinus beat is less than compensatory usually establishes the diagnosis of an APB.

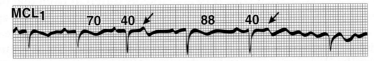

FIGURE 15.10. *Arrows* indicate two early APBs with PP intervals of 0.40 second (40 milliseconds). The first PP interval is longer than half the preceding PP interval of 0.70 second (70 milliseconds), but the second is shorter than half the preceding PP interval of 0.88 second (88 milliseconds), initiating an atrial reentrant tachyarrhythmia (see Chapter 17).

APBs may occur so early that even parts of the atria have not completed their refractory periods. During this time (the *vulnerable period*), the APB may initiate a reentrant atrial tachyarrhythmia (Fig. 15.10). In this instance, the APB becomes the first beat of atrial flutter/fibrillation (see Chapter 17). Killip and Gault[1] developed the rule that when the PP interval is <50% of the previous PP interval, an APB is quite likely to initiate atrial flutter/fibrillation.

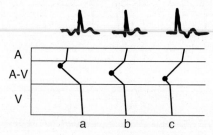

FIGURE 15.11.   Three impulses (*a*, *b*, *c*) are formed within the AV junction (AV) as illustrated in the ECG recordings and explained in the ladder diagrams. In the ladder diagram, the anatomic site of impulse formation (*solid circle*) varies, but the AV nodal conduction velocity is constant, resulting in the varying P–QRS relationships.

PBs arising in the AV junction may retrogradely activate the atria before, during, or after ventricular activation, and the retrograde P wave may therefore be seen preceding or following the QRS complex or may be lost within the QRS complex. These variations are illustrated in Figure 15.11.

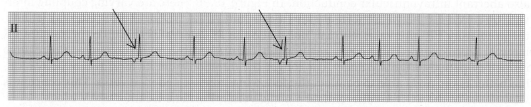

FIGURE 15.12.   The contrasting appearances of P waves originating from the sinus node and the AV junction (*arrows*) are illustrated in this lead II rhythm strip.

The diagnosis of junctional origin of PBs is easiest when a premature normal QRS complex is closely accompanied by an inverted P wave (Fig. 15.12). As expected, the morphology of the P waves associated with JPBs is markedly different from that of the P waves of normal sinus rhythm. The polarity of the P waves associated with JPBs is approximately opposite that of the P waves of normal sinus rhythm, as is best seen in a lead with base-to-apex orientation, such as lead II. A P wave originating from the AV junction is also inverted in the other inferiorly oriented leads (e.g., aVF), is upright in superiorly oriented leads aVR and aVL, and is almost flat in leftward-oriented leads I and V5.

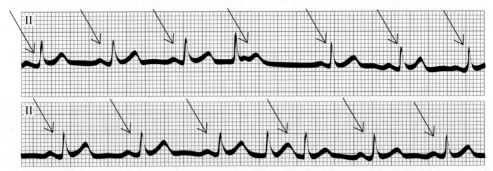

FIGURE 15.13. **Top** and **bottom** panels are recordings of lead II from the same individual. Note that the regular sinus rhythm (*arrows*) "marches through" or is "not reset" by the PBs.

A JPB may be confused with an APB when a premature normal QRS complex is not closely accompanied by an abnormal P wave (Fig. 15.13). In the top panel, the normally appearing and normally timed P wave after the premature normal QRS complex indicates a JPB. In the bottom panel, there are no accompanying P waves to provide clues to a junctional versus atrial origin of the PBs. Differentiation of these two sites of origin requires observation of the influence of the PB on the regularity of the underlying sinus rhythm. The sinus rhythm is typically reset by an APB but may or may not be reset by a JPB. The pause following a JPB is usually fully compensatory.

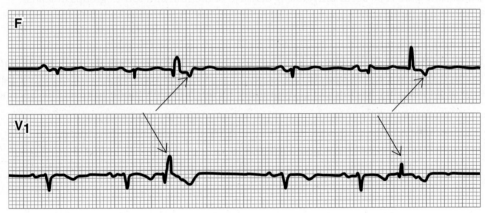

FIGURE 15.14. The long-axis (base-to-apex) orientation of lead aVF (F) provides the best view of the inverted P waves (*arrows*) in this case of JPBs with RBB aberration, and the short-axis (right versus left) orientation of lead V1 provides the best view of the varying amounts of RBB aberrancy (*arrows*). The combined contributions of both leads confirm the junctional origin of the PBs.

A JPB may be confused with a VPB when the premature QRS complex is wide (≥0.12 second). The various principles presented in Chapters 19 and 20 for differentiating supraventricular beats with aberrant intraventricular conduction from ventricular beats may be applied. Figure 15.14 shows JPBs with differing degrees of right bundle branch (RBB) aberration. The retrograde atrial activation is apparent from the P waves following the premature QRS complexes. Although the first PB in each ECG strip cannot be distinguished from a VPB, the fact that the second PB manifests a lesser degree of RBB block is a strong point for aberrant conduction from a JPB.

VENTRICULAR PREMATURE BEATS

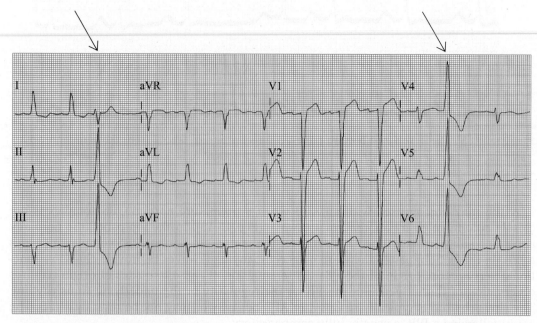

FIGURE 15.15. The views of typical VPBs (*arrows*) from multiple, simultaneously recorded ECG leads. Note that VPBs occur only during displays of the first and fourth groups of leads.

The characteristic VPB (Fig. 15.15) is not preceded by a premature P wave and is represented by a wide and bizarre QRS complex. It is followed by a compensatory pause because of its inability to conduct retrogradely through the AV node to reset the SA node.

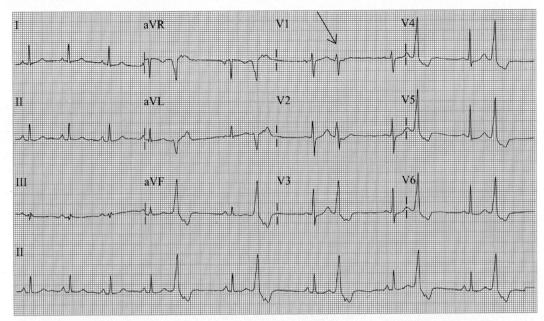

FIGURE 15.16. Multiple VPBs are obvious in many ECG leads. However, in lead V1 (*arrow*), the QRS complexes of the VPBs coincidentally appear very similar to those of the normal sinus beats. If only a lead V1 recording was available, the erroneous diagnosis of APBs might be made.

The following exceptions to all of these characteristics may occur, thereby confounding the distinction of a ventricular from a supraventricular origin of the PB.

1. Regarding a preceding premature P wave, a VPB may be preceded by a premature P wave if both an APB and a VPB are present.
2. Regarding the appearance of the QRS complex, a VPB, although typically ≥0.12 second, may appear to have a normal duration in any single lead because its initial or terminal component is isoelectric. A VPB may even, by coincidence, appear similar to the normal beats in a single lead, as illustrated in lead V1 in Figure 15.16. It is important to consider two or even three simultaneously recorded leads in determining the origin of a PB.
3. Regarding the pause following the VPB, if there is marked variation in the underlying sinus regularity because of sinus arrhythmia, it cannot be determined whether or not a pause is compensatory. When the sinus rhythm is regular, however, there are rare occurrences of a VPB that lacks a following compensatory pause.

A VPB that lacks a compensatory pause occurs for one of two reasons: (a) the VPB is interpolated between consecutive sinus beats or (b) the VPB resets the sinus rhythm. Examples of these two possibilities are seen in Figures 15.17 and 15.18.

The Ventricular Premature Beat Is Interpolated between Consecutive Sinus Beats

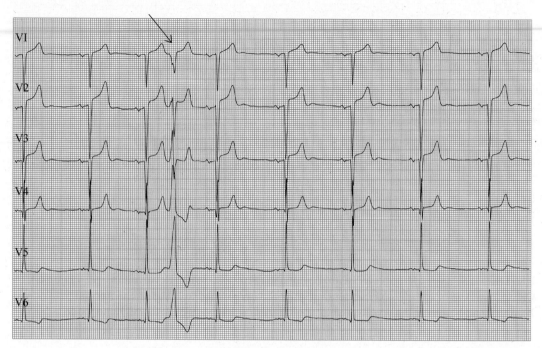

FIGURE 15.17. A single interpolated VPB occurs (*arrow*) between the third and fourth sinus beat. Note the slight sinus irregularity (sinus arrhythmia).

When a VPB is extremely premature (close to the time of the preceding sinus impulse), it cannot be conducted retrogradely through the still refractory AV node. However, when the sinus rate is slow, such a VPB occurs long before the following sinus impulse, and there is ample time for the AV node and ventricles to complete their refractory periods before the next normal sinus impulse is conducted anterogradely. The VPB is therefore *interpolated* between sinus beats, and there is no pause (Fig. 15.17).

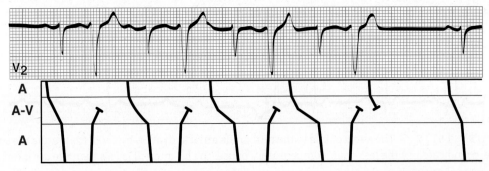

FIGURE 15.18. The ladder diagram indicates the relationships between the P waves and QRS complexes when both anterograde and retrograde activation prevent full recovery of the AV node.

The PR interval of the sinus beat following the VPB is prolonged when the AV node is still partly refractory from its retrograde activation by the VPB. This is an example of "concealed conduction," because the absence of both a retrograde P wave and resetting of the sinus rhythm indicates that the impulse produced by the VPB never reached the atria. The continued bombardment of the AV node from both anterograde and retrograde directions prevents its complete recovery. If there is a recurrence of early VPBs, there may be progressively longer PR intervals (Fig. 15.18) until there is complete failure of conduction. Only then is the AV node able to completely recover, as indicated by the normal PR interval of the next sinus cycle. As was discussed with regard to APBs, this represents a physiologic case of nonconduction in contrast to pathologic AV block.

The Ventricular Premature Beat Resets the Sinus Rhythm

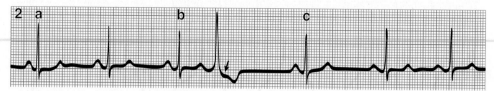

FIGURE 15.19. The *arrow* points to the retrograde atrial activation by a VPB that resets the sinus node, as indicated by the less-than-compensatory pause (the *b-c* interval is less than the *a-b* interval).

When a VPB is only slightly premature (close to the time of the next sinus impulse), it can pass retrogradely through the AV node because this structure has recovered from the anterograde conduction of the previous sinus beat. The VPB can then enter the SA node and reset it in much the same way as does an APB. The retrograde P wave caused by this is usually obscured in the T wave of the VPB, but it may be detected in the ST segment of the VPB (Fig. 15.19). The pause until the next sinus beat is therefore less than compensatory.

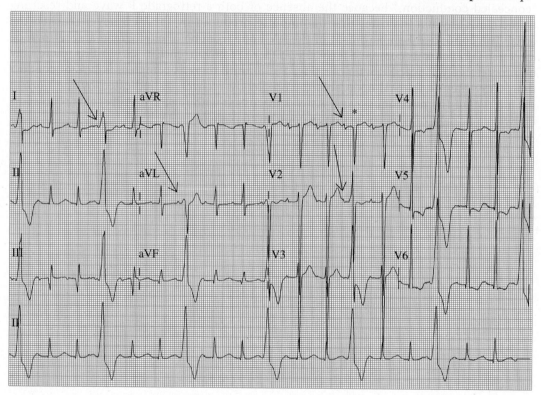

FIGURE 15.20. The VPBs in this ECG recording occur so late in the cycle that they follow the P waves of the normal sinus beats (*arrows*). Note, as in Figure 15.16, that the VPBs appear similar to the normal sinus beats in lead V1 (*asterisk*).

When a VPB occurs so late that the next sinus P wave has already appeared (Fig. 15.20), the compensatory pause is not really a pause at all. Only the short PR interval provides a clue that the wide QRS complex is indeed from a VPB. If the PR interval were normal, the incorrect diagnosis would most likely be intermittent bundle-branch block. The pattern of a normal P wave, short PR interval, and wide QRS complex could also be produced by ventricular preexcitation (see Chapter 7).

THE RULE OF BIGEMINY

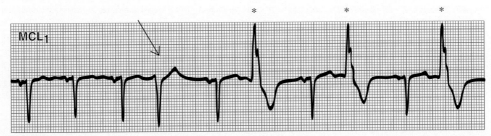

FIGURE 15.21. The use of lead MCL$_1$ provides identification of the ventricle of origin of the VPBs. The *arrow* shows the initial VPB (from the RV) producing a long cycle that precipitates another VPB (from the LV), which is shown by the *asterisk*. This pattern continues, resulting in a bigeminal rhythm.

The occurrence of a long cardiac cycle (or pause) tends to precipitate reentry after the next normal beat. As discussed in Chapter 3, the ventricular recovery time, as estimated by the QT interval, varies with the heart rate. Therefore, the normal beat that follows a compensatory pause has a longer recovery time than other normal beats. This longer recovery time increases the likelihood that adjacent myocardial cells are at different stages of the repolarization process. This greater difference in the cells' electrical potentials creates the possibility for a current to "reenter" a recently recovered cell and to thus initiate another VPB.[2] A bigeminal pattern occurs, with every normal beat followed by a VPB and with constant coupling intervals between each pair of normal sinus and VPBs (Fig. 15.21). Preventing only the first VPB prevents all subsequent VPBs.

RIGHT- VERSUS LEFT-VENTRICULAR PREMATURE BEATS

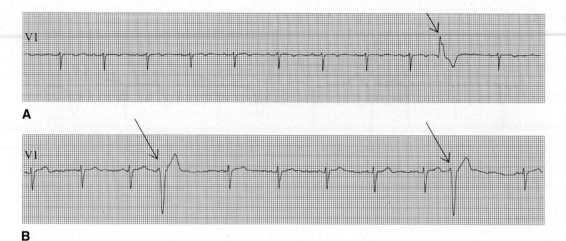

A

B

FIGURE 15.22. The contrasting appearances of V1-positive (left ventricular) **(A)** and V1-negative (right ventricular) **(B)** VPBs (*arrows*).

Figure 15.22 illustrates the contrast between VPBs originating in the right ventricle (*right VPBs*) and those originating from the left ventricle (*left VPBs*). The ventricle of origin of ectopic beats can best be recognized in lead V1, which is oriented to differentiate right- versus left-sided cardiac activity (see Chapter 1). If the VPB in lead V1 is predominantly positive (V1 positive), the impulse must be traveling anteriorly and rightward from its origin in the posteriorly located left ventricle (see Fig. 15.22A). If the VPB in lead V1 is predominantly negative (V1 negative), the impulse must be traveling posteriorly and leftward, usually from its origin in the anteriorly located right ventricle (see Fig. 15.22B).[3] However, myocardial infarctions may produce left ventricular reentrant tachyarrhythmias with *V1-negative* morphology (see Chapter 19).

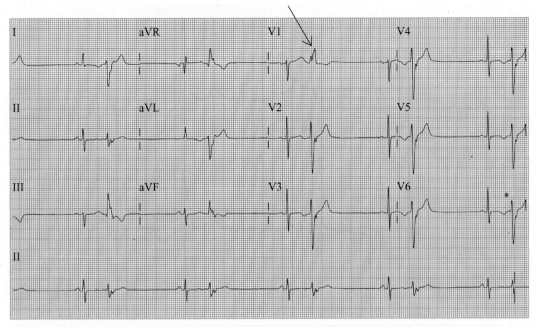

FIGURE 15.23. The monophasic V1 R wave (*arrow*) and diphasic V6 rS wave (*asterisk*) appearances that typify a left VPB. However, note that the first "rabbit ear" is atypically shorter than the right in the VPB in lead V1.

The differentiation between a right- and left-ventricular origin of VPBs is clinically useful for the following reasons:

> 1. Left VPBs are more often associated with heart disease, whereas right VPBs are commonly seen in individuals with normal hearts.[4,5]
> 2. Left VPBs are more likely than right VPBs to precipitate ventricular fibrillation.

A study of >1,000 consecutive patients found no instances of ventricular fibrillation in the 249 patients who manifested only VPBs with a right-ventricular pattern in lead MCL$_1$. Patients with VPBs with a left-ventricular pattern, however, developed ventricular fibrillation 10.4% of the time (82 of 787 patients).

Morphologic features of left VPBs are:

> 1. Usually a monophasic (R) or diphasic (qR) complex in lead V1 and a diphasic (rS) or monophasic (QS) complex in lead V6 (Fig. 15.23).
> 2. An often greater amplitude of the first peak of a two-peaked ("rabbit ears") QRS complex in lead V1. This is illustrated in Figures 15.21 and 15.22A.[6]

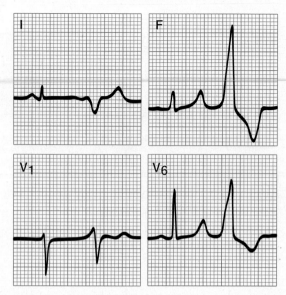

FIGURE 15.24. Typical morphology of a VPB originating from the right ventricle viewed from limb leads I and aVF (F) and precordial leads V1 and V6.

Morphologic features of right VPBs are:

1. An often typically positive morphology in lead V6 but a right-axis deviation in the frontal plane and a wide (>0.04 second) initial R wave in lead V1 (Fig. 15.24).[5,7]
2. A deeper rS or qS complex in lead V4 than in lead V1.[7]

MULTIFORM VENTRICULAR PREMATURE BEATS

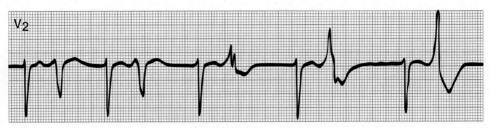

FIGURE 15.25. This lead V2 rhythm strip reveals ventricular bigeminy with constant coupling intervals but continually varying (multiform) VPB morphology.

When VPBs manifest different QRS complex morphologies in the same lead (Fig. 15.25), they are termed *multiform VPBs*. Because such VPBs are assumed to arise from different foci, they are also called *multifocal VPBs*. It is possible, however, that the variation in QRS complex morphology produced by VPBs may result from varying intraventricular conduction rather than from varying sites of origin. Indeed, varying patterns of VPBs have been produced from the same artificially stimulated focus.[8] Therefore, "multiform" is a more appropriate term than "multifocal" for VPBs showing different QRS complex morphology.

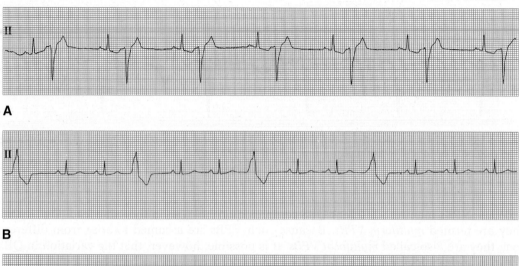

FIGURE 15.26. The contrasting appearances of the different sequences of VPBs in lead II rhythm strips.

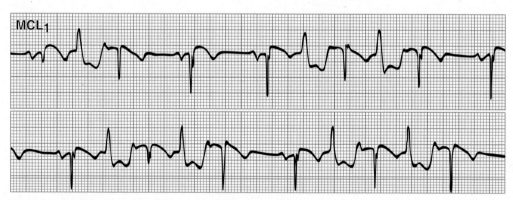

FIGURE 15.27. A continuous recording of lead MCL$_1$. The ventricular rate varies from 110 to 140 beats per minute during the "tachycardia."

The definitions of the various groupings of VPBs was provided earlier in this chapter. Figure 15.26 illustrates the typical appearances of ventricular bigeminy (see Fig. 15.26A), trigeminy (see Fig. 15.26B), and *couplets* (see Fig. 15.26C) of VPBs.

In the typical form of bigeminy (see Fig. 15.26A), a VPB is substituted for every alternate sinus beat, and each VPB is followed by a compensatory pause. However, when the VPBs are interpolated, a tachyarrhythmia with a bigeminal pattern is produced (Fig. 15.27).

VENTRICULAR PREMATURE BEATS INDUCING
VENTRICULAR FIBRILLATION

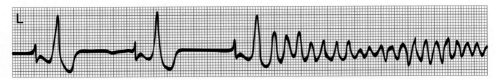

FIGURE 15.28. A lead aVL (L) rhythm strip reveals a bigeminal rhythm produced by very closely coupled VPBs. The VPB that triggers the ventricular flutter has the same coupling interval and morphology as the other VPBs.

When VPBs occur so early that they interrupt the peak of the preceding T wave (Fig. 15.28), they may be considered dangerous.[9] During this early phase of ventricular recovery, there is such inhomogeneity of receptiveness and refractoriness of conduction that the premature impulse may continue to encounter a receptive pathway. The impulse may repetitively reenter, thereby producing a tachyarrhythmia, which has been termed "ventricular tachycardia of the vulnerable period," "ventricular flutter," and "coarse ventricular fibrillation." The tachyarrhythmia may terminate spontaneously or progress to typical ventricular fibrillation.

The peak of the T wave coincides with the vulnerable period in the cardiac cycle. In a series of 48 patients who developed ventricular fibrillation outside the hospital, the initiating beat was an "R-on-T VPB" in more than two thirds.[10] However, other studies have questioned the threat of R-on-T VPBs as compared with later VPBs.[11] One study that carefully documented the VPBs that initiated fibrillation in 20 consecutive patients demonstrated that in more than half, the culpable VPBs occurred after completion of the T wave.[12] Therefore, ventricular fibrillation can even be initiated by late VPBs. Surawicz[13] summarizes the situation by concluding that R-on-T VPBs pose a risk of inducing ventricular fibrillation only in the early stages of myocardial infarction, in hypokalemia, and in the presence of a long QT interval.

Table 15.3.	
Lown's Grading System of Ventricular Premature Beats (VPBs)	
Grade	Description of VPBs
0	None
1	<30/hr
2	≥30/hr
3	Multiform
4A	Two consecutive
4B	≥3 consecutive
5	R-on-T

VPBs are ubiquitous. Most people have them more or less frequently, and even continuous ventricular bigeminy is sometimes found in people with apparently normal hearts. Usually, VPBs are a benign nuisance. During the acute phase of infarction, they appear in 80% to 90% of patients but are also found in the majority of actively employed middle-aged men.[14] Benign VPBs commonly disappear when the sinus rate increases, such as during exercise. The prognostic significance of exercise-induced VPBs is uncertain. VPBs have been reported to occur more readily with isometric than with isotonic (dynamic) exercise.[15]

Many studies have been directed at evaluating the prognostic significance of VPBs during and after acute myocardial infarction. In patients who have survived myocardial infarction, complex VPBs (multiform, couplets, etc.) have been shown to increase the risk of sudden death.[16,17] This is in marked contrast with the prognostic importance of similarly appearing VPBs outside the setting of myocardial infarction. In a 7-year follow-up of 72 asymptomatic subjects with frequent and complex VPBs, none died, although a number had angiographically proven significant coronary disease.[18]

Lown's grading system for VPBs[19,20] (Table 15.3) has become a popular frame of reference for gauging the risk of death after myocardial infarction. There is increased risk as the numerical grade advances from 0 to 5. A subsequent study found that consecutive VPBs (grade 4) were associated with a worse prognosis than were early, single VPBs (grade 5).[21]

Moss[22] has proposed a simplified, two-level system for grading the prognostic significance of VPBs after acute myocardial infarction as follows:

Uniform morphology and late cycle	Low risk	(2-year mortality, 10%)
Multiform and/or early cycle	High risk	(2-year mortality, 20%)

A study by Califf et al[23] documented the relationship between VPBs and left-ventricular function in patients with ischemic heart disease. A subsequent study by these same authors failed to find a subgroup of patients with VPBs of any description and good left-ventricular function that had a high risk of sudden death.[24] Therefore, VPBs do not appear to be independent predictors of a high risk of mortality in patients with ischemic heart disease.

GLOSSARY

Aberrantly: being conducted abnormally (usually through the ventricular conduction system).

Atrial premature beat (APB): a P wave produced by an impulse that originates in the atria and appears before the expected time of the next P wave generated from the sinus node.

Bigeminy: a rhythm pattern in which every sinus beat is followed by a PB.

Compensatory pause: the long cycle length (pause) following a PB completely "compensates for" the short cycle length preceding the PB. This is identified when the interval between the beginning of the P waves of the sinus beats preceding and following a PB is equal to two PP intervals of sinus beats not associated with PBs.

Couplet: two consecutive PBs.

Coupling intervals: the periods between normal sinus beats and PBs. With APBs, the PP' is the coupling interval, and with JPBs and VPBs, the QRS-QRS' is the coupling interval.

Ectopic beat: a beat arising in any location other than the sinus node.

Interpolated: occurring between normal beats.

Junctional premature beat (JPB): a P wave and QRS complex produced by an impulse that originates in the AV node or His bundle and appears before the expected time of the next P wave and QRS complex generated from the sinus node.

Left VPBs: PBs originating from the left ventricle, usually with a V1-positive morphology but sometimes with a V1-negative morphology when associated with ischemic heart disease.

Multifocal VPBs: VPBs originating from two or more different ventricular locations.

Multiform VPBs: VPBs with two or more different morphologies in a single ECG lead.

Overdrive suppression: a decrease in the rate of impulse formation resulting from premature activation of the pacemaking cells.

Palpitation: the physical awareness of a heartbeat.

PP interval: the interval between consecutive P waves.

Right VPBs: PBs originating from the right ventricle, always with a V1-negative morphology.

R-on-T VPB: a VPB that occurs so prematurely that it occurs during the T wave of the previous beat.

Supraventricular premature beat (SVPB): either an APB or a JPB.

Trigeminy: a rhythm pattern in which every second sinus beat is followed by a PB.

Ventricular premature beat (VPB): a QRS complex produced by an impulse originating from the ventricles and appearing before the expected time of the next QRS complex generated from the sinus node or other basic underlying rhythm.

Vulnerable period: the time in the cardiac cycle, before complete repolarization, when a reentrant tachyarrhythmia may be induced by the introduction of a premature impulse.

REFERENCES

1. Killip T, Gault JH. Mode of onset of atrial fibrillation in man. *Am Heart J.* 1965;70:172.
2. Langendorf R, Pick A, Winternitz M. Mechanisms of intermittent ventricular bigeminy. I. Appearance of ectopic beats dependent upon length of the ventricular cycle, the "rule of bigeminy." *Circulation.* 1955;11:422–430.
3. Kaplinsky E, Ogawa S, Kmetzo J, et al. Origin of so-called right and left ventricular arrhythmias in acute myocardial ischemia. *Am J Cardiol.* 1978;42:774–780.
4. Lewis S, Kanakis C, Rosen KM, et al. Significance of site of origin of premature ventricular contractions. *Am Heart J.* 1979;97:159–164.
5. Rosenbaum MB. Classification of ventricular extrasystoles according to form. *J Electrocardiol.* 1969;2:289–297.
6. Gozensky C, Thorne D. Rabbit ears: an aid in distinguishing ventricular ectopy from aberration. *Heart Lung.* 1974;3:634–636.
7. Swanick EJ, LaCamera F Jr, Marriott HJL. Morphologic features of right ventricular ectopic beats. *Am J Cardiol.* 1972;30:888–891.

8. Booth DC, Popio KA, Gettes LS. Multiformity of induced unifocal ventricular premature beats in human subjects: electrocardiographic and angiographic correlations. *Am J Cardiol.* 1982;49:1643–1653.

9. Smirk FH, Palmer DDG. A myocardial syndrome, with particular reference to the occurrence of sudden death and of premature systoles interrupting antecedent T waves. *Am J Cardiol.* 1960;6:620.

10. Adgey AJ, Devlin JE, Webb SW, et al. Initiation of ventricular fibrillation outside hospital in patients with ischemic heart disease. *Br Heart J.* 1982;47:55.

11. Engel TR, Meister SG, Frankl WS. "The R-on-T" phenomenon; an update and critical review. *Ann Intern Med.* 1978;88:221–225.

12. Lie KI, Wellens HJ, Downar E, et al. Observations on patients with primary ventricular fibrillation complicating acute myocardial infarction. *Circulation.* 1975;52:755–759.

13. Surawicz B. R-on-T phenomenon: dangerous and harmless. *J Appl Cardiol.* 1986;1:39.

14. Hinkle LE Jr, Carver ST, Stevens M. The frequency of asymptomatic disturbances of cardiac rhythm and conduction in middle-aged men. *Am J Cardiol.* 1969;24:629–650.

15. Atkins JM, Matthews OA, Blomqvist CG, et al. Incidence of arrhythmias induced by isometric and dynamic exercise. *Br Heart J.* 1976;38:465–471.

16. Moss AJ, Davis HT, DeCamilla J, et al. Ventricular ectopic beats and their relation to sudden and nonsudden cardiac death after myocardial infarction. *Circulation.* 1979;60:998–1003.

17. Ruberman W, Weinblatt E, Goldberg JD, et al. Ventricular premature beats and mortality after myocardial infarction. *N Engl J Med.* 1977;297:750–757.

18. Horan MJ, Kennedy HL. Characteristics and prognosis of apparently healthy patients with frequent and complex ventricular ectopy: evidence for a relative benign syndrome with occult myocardial and/or coronary disease. *Am Heart J.* 1981;102:809–810.

19. Lown B, Wolf M. Approaches to sudden death from coronary heart disease. *Circulation.* 1971;44:130–142.

20. Lown B, Graboys TB. Management of patients with malignant ventricular arrhythmias. *Am J Cardiol.* 1977;39:910–918.

21. Bigger JT, Weld FJ. Analysis of prognostic significance of ventricular arrhythmias after myocardial infarction. Shortcomings of the Lown grading system. *Br Heart J.* 1981;45:717–724.

22. Moss AJ. Clinical significance of ventricular arrhythmias in patients with and without coronary artery disease. *Prog Cardiovasc Dis.* 1980;23:33–52.

23. Califf RM, Burks JM, Behar VS, et al. Relationships among ventricular arrhythmias, coronary artery disease, and angiographic and electrocardiographic indicators of myocardial fibrosis. *Circulation.* 1978;57:725–732.

24. Califf RM, McKinnis RA, Burks J, et al. Prognostic implications of ventricular arrhythmias during 24 hour ambulatory monitoring in patients undergoing catheterization for coronary artery disease. *Am J Cardiol.* 1982;50:23–31.

16

Accelerated Automaticity

GALEN S. WAGNER

INTRODUCTION TO ACCELERATED AUTOMATICITY

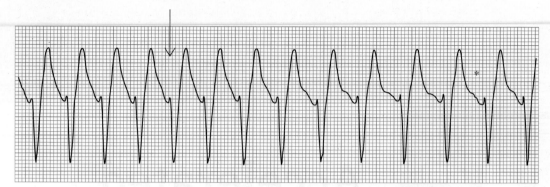

FIGURE 16.1. Lead V1 rhythm strip. *Arrow* indicates the time at which exercise was stopped, and *asterisk* indicates the P wave emerging from the T wave. (From Wagner GS, Waugh RA, Ramo BW. *Cardiac Arrhythmias.* New York, NY: Churchill Livingstone; 1983:145, with permission.)

The arrhythmias presented in this chapter have gradual onsets and terminations because they result from acceleration of automaticity in the cells of the pacemaking and conduction system. This is apparent on the electrocardiogram (ECG) as a gradual decrease in the interval between cardiac cycles (the *PP interval*) during the period of onset and a gradual increase during the period of termination of a tachyarrhythmia. In Figure 16.1, there is a tachyarrhythmia during exercise at a rate of 140 beats per minute, with no visible P waves and wide (V1-negative) QRS complexes (0.14 second). When the exercise is stopped, the rate gradually slows and P waves emerge from the ends of each of the T waves, indicating that the rhythm is sinus tachycardia with left-bundle-branch block (LBBB).

Cells termed *pacemakers* (see Chapter 1)—located in the sinoatrial (SA) node, at various sites in the atria, and throughout the His–Purkinje network—have the capacity for spontaneous depolarization. Atrial and ventricular muscle cells and atrioventricular (AV) nodal cells do not have pacemaking capabilities. The rate of impulse formation by pacemaker cells is determined by the rate of their spontaneous depolarization, and the more superior the location of the pacemaking cell, the more rapidly this depolarization occurs. Accelerated automaticity is considered to be a tachyarrhythmia only when the heart rate exceeds the arbitrary limit of 100 beats per minute. Because the upper limit of normal automaticity of the SA nodal and atrial cells is 100 beats per minute, any acceleration in the rate of automaticity of these cells is considered a tachyarrhythmia. The upper limit of normal automaticity is 60 beats per minute in the common bundle and 50 beats per minute in the bundle branches. The rhythm produced is called an *accelerated rhythm* until it reaches 100 beats per minute (Table 16.1).

Table 16.1.

Sites, Terms, and Rates of Pacemaker Tachyarrhythmias

Site	Term	Rate Range (beats/min)
Sinus node	Sinus tachycardia	100–200
Atria	Atrial tachycardia	100–200
Common bundle	Accelerated junctional rhythm (AJR)	60–130
Bundle branches	Accelerated ventricular rhythm (AVR)	50–110

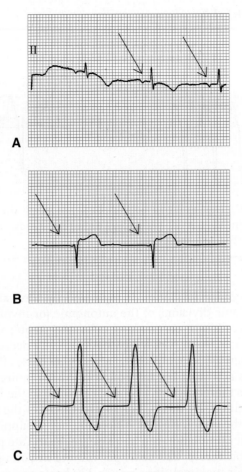

FIGURE 16.2. Lead II rhythm strips with *arrows* indicating abnormally directed P waves **(A)** and absence of P waves **(B and C)**.

Examples of arrhythmias due to accelerated atrial, junctional, and ventricular automaticity are presented in Figure 16.2. In Figure 16.2A, the *accelerated atrial rhythm* (*AAR*) is apparent from the frequent, regular (evenly spaced), but "different from sinus" P waves. In Figure 16.2B, the *accelerated junctional rhythm* (*AJR*) is apparent from the frequent, regular, narrow QRS complexes not preceded by P waves. In Figure 16.2C, the *accelerated ventricular rhythm* (*AVR*) is apparent from the frequent, regular, wide QRS complexes not preceded by P waves.

Usually, the cardiac rhythm is controlled by the SA node. However, there are several reasons why the rhythm becomes dominated by the accelerated pacing activity from a nonsinus site. These include:

1. A pharmacologic agent that selectively increases automaticity in lower pacemakers.
2. Blockage of sinus impulses in the AV conduction system, permitting an escape focus in the common bundle to control the ventricular rhythm.
3. Local pathology (especially ischemia) that induces automaticity in lower areas with pacemaking capability.
4. Local pathology that decreases automaticity within the SA node.

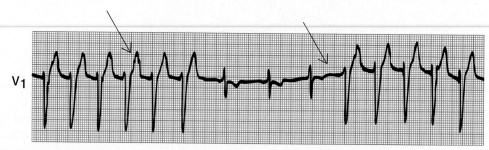

FIGURE 16.3. Lead V1 rhythm strip with *arrows* indicating the beginning and ending of carotid sinus massage. (From Wagner GS, Waugh RA, Ramo BW. *Cardiac Arrhythmias*. New York, NY: Churchill Livingstone; 1983:140, with permission.)

The rate of cardiac impulse formation is regulated by the balance between the parasympathetic and sympathetic divisions of the autonomic (or involuntary) nervous system. The more superior the location of pacemaking cells, the greater is the degree of their autonomic regulation. An increase in parasympathetic activity decreases the rate of impulse formation, whereas an increase in sympathetic activity increases the rate. The sympathetic nervous system becomes activated by any condition that requires "flight or fight." Sinus tachycardia that results is therefore a physiologic response to the body's needs rather than a pathologic cardiac condition. By this principle, treatment of the tachyarrhythmia should be directed at correcting the underlying condition and not at suppression of the SA node itself. Maximal sympathetic stimulation can increase the heart rate produced by the SA node to 200 beats per minute or, rarely, 220 beats per minute in younger individuals. The generally accepted formula for maximal sinus rate is 220 beats per minute subtracted by age. The rate rarely exceeds 160 beats per minute in nonexercising adults.

In sinus tachycardia, there is normally one normal P wave for every QRS complex, but coexisting abnormalities of AV conduction may alter this relationship. The PR interval is shorter than during normal sinus rhythm because the increased *sympathetic tone* that produces the sinus tachycardia also speeds AV nodal conduction. The QRS complex is usually normal in appearance but can be abnormal either because of a fixed intraventricular conduction disturbance (such as bundle-branch block, hypertrophy, or myocardial infarction) or because the rapid rate of activation does not permit time for full recovery of the intraventricular conduction system before the arrival of the next impulse (see Chapter 6). Figure 16.3 demonstrates sinus tachycardia with LBBB. Conduction block is proven to be due to rate-related aberrancy when it disappears during *carotid sinus massage*–induced sinus slowing or AV block and returns when the rate gradually increases following the massage.

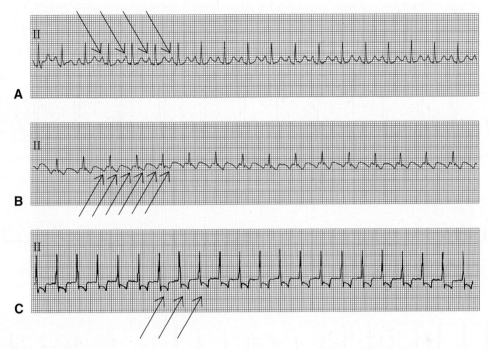

FIGURE 16.4. Lead II rhythm strips with *arrows* indicating sinus P waves **(A)**, flutter waves **(B)**, and retrograde P waves **(C)**. (From Wagner GS, Waugh RA, Ramo BW. *Cardiac Arrhythmias*. New York, NY: Churchill Livingstone; 1983:176, with permission.)

Although the other tachyarrhythmias caused by accelerated automaticity and discussed in this chapter do not mimic sinus tachycardia, a common clinical problem is the differentiation of sinus tachycardia from various reentrant tachyarrhythmias that are discussed in later chapters. If discrete P waves (with anterograde orientation), a short PR interval, and a normal QRS complex duration are present, the diagnosis of sinus tachycardia is most likely. True sinus tachycardia is shown in Figure 16.4A, and two reentrant supraventricular tachyarrhythmias that have a similar appearance to sinus tachycardia are shown in Figure 16.4B and C. When apparent sinus tachycardia is associated with a prolonged PR interval, one should suspect that it is not really a sinus tachycardia. Figure 16.4B presents an example of the reentrant atrial tachyarrhythmia of typical sawtooth-like atrial flutter (see Chapter 17) with only every other flutter wave conducted to the ventricles (2:1 AV conduction). An abnormal limb lead P-wave axis also suggests a nonsinus origin of the tachyarrhythmia. Figure 16.4C presents an example of reentrant junctional tachycardia (see Chapter 18) with inverted P waves following each QRS complex and long PR interval.

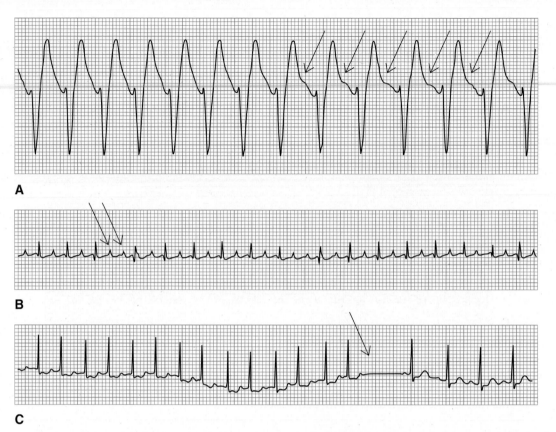

FIGURE 16.5. Lead II rhythm strips with *arrows* indicating gradual emergence of P waves from T waves **(A)**, sudden appearance of consecutive flutter waves **(B)**, and sudden termination of the tachyarrhythmia **(C)**. (From Wagner GS, Waugh RA, Ramo BW. *Cardiac Arrhythmias*. New York, NY: Churchill Livingstone; 1983;144:179, with permission.)

When the appearance of atrial activity fails to provide the foregoing clinical differentiation of the source of a tachyarrhythmia, it may be necessary to observe the onset and termination of the tachyarrhythmia: A gradual change in rate establishes the diagnosis of sinus tachycardia (Fig. 16.5A). The sudden block in AV conduction allows visualization of the typical sawtooth-like atrial activity of flutter (see Fig. 16.5B). The sudden termination of the tachyarrhythmia establishes the diagnosis of reentrant junctional tachycardia (see Fig. 16.5C). If the beginning or ending of the tachyarrhythmia does not occur spontaneously, a diagnostic maneuver or pharmacologic intervention to increase parasympathetic nervous activity, such as a *vagal maneuver* or adenosine administration, may be necessary. The absence of any change in the ECG during the vagal maneuver does not permit any diagnostic conclusion. A transesophageal or intra-atrial recording may be required when no diagnosis can be made from surface ECG recordings (see Fig. 14.9). A summary of the steps toward the diagnosis of an unknown tachyarrhythmia includes the following:

1. Note the P-wave morphology and the PR and QRS intervals in the ECG.
2. Observe either the onset or the termination of the tachyarrhythmia in the ECG.
3. Perform a maneuver to increase parasympathetic activity.
4. Record the atrial activity from the esophagus or right atrium.

Accelerated Atrial Rhythm and Paroxysmal Atrial Tachycardia with Block

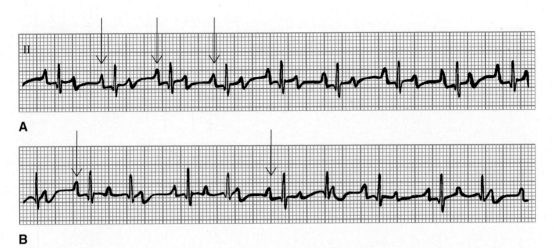

FIGURE 16.6. Lead II rhythm strips from a 75-year-old woman with heart failure treated with digitalis and diuretics. **A.** A "paroxysmal atrial tachycardia" caused by digitalis toxicity in the presence of hypokalemia (K^+ = 3.1 mEq/L). The atrial rate is 180 beats per minute (*arrows*) and there is 2:1 AV block. **B.** Digitalis was withheld and potassium given (K^+ = 4.6 mEq/L), resulting in the slowing of the atrial rate to 168 beats per minute. (From Wagner GS, Waugh RA, Ramo BW. *Cardiac Arrhythmias.* New York, NY: Churchill Livingstone; 1983:138, with permission.)

Enhanced automaticity causes three varieties of atrial tachyarrhythmias: AAR, *paroxysmal atrial tachycardia (PAT) with block,* and *multifocal atrial tachycardia (MAT).*

Normal individuals may have periods when a lower atrial pacing site dominates the SA node, producing an AAR. The presence of AAR is apparent when the morphology of the QRS complex is normal in the presence of a ventricular rate in the range of 60 to 130 beats per minute and there are preceding abnormal P waves caused by the origination of the atrial activation in a site other than the SA node (see Fig. 16.2A). The PR interval may be normal or decreased depending on the distance from the atrial pacing site to the AV node.

The term *paroxysmal* is actually inaccurate with regard to PAT with block because it implies the sudden onset and termination of a cardiac rhythm. Because *digitalis toxicity* is the most common cause, this rhythm is now rare. The atrial rate gradually accelerates as digitalis is added (or potassium is depleted) and then gradually decelerates when the digitalis is withheld (or potassium is replaced; Fig. 16.6).[1,2] Digitalis has a parasympathetic effect on both the SA and AV nodes, resulting in sinus slowing and AV block. However, digitalis has a sympathetic effect on other sites with pacemaking capability and thereby enhances automaticity. If the site of this enhancement is above the AV node, the result is the combination of atrial tachycardia with AV block, which has been incorrectly termed "PAT with block."

Multifocal Atrial Tachycardia

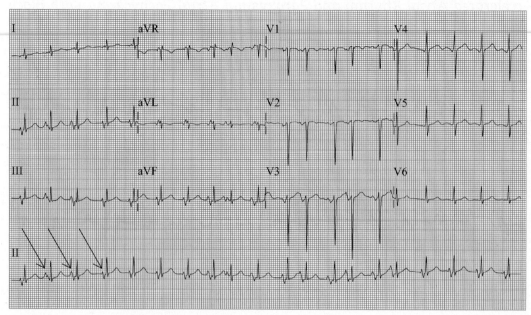

FIGURE 16.7. A 12-lead ECG and lead II rhythm strip from a 53-year-old woman with severe pulmonary emphysema. *Arrows* indicate marked variation in P-wave morphology in the rhythm strip.

MAT is a rapid, irregular atrial tachyarrhythmia with multiple, differently appearing P waves that has also been termed *chaotic atrial tachycardia*[3] (Fig. 16.7). It almost always occurs with pulmonary disease. In contrast to the atrial acceleration that occurs with digitalis toxicity, there is no enhancement of the parasympathetic effect on the AV node in MAT, therefore every P wave is conducted to the ventricles (1:1 AV conduction). MAT is typically a transitional arrhythmia between frequent atrial premature beats (APBs) and atrial flutter/fibrillation. In a series of 31 patients reported by Lipson and Naimi,[3] 20 had preceding APBs and 17 progressed to atrial flutter/fibrillation.

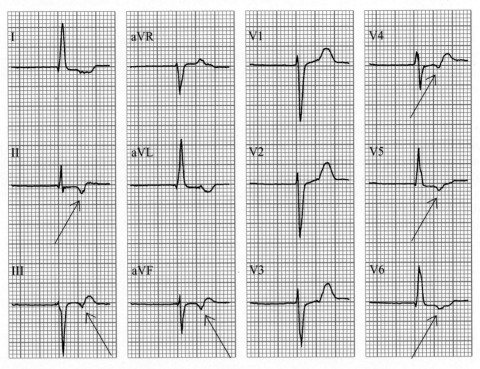

FIGURE 16.8. A 12-lead ECG from a healthy 51-year-old woman. *Arrows* indicate retrograde P waves associated with junctional beats.

AJR is produced by enhanced automaticity in common bundle (His) of the ventricular Purkinje system. As in AAR, acceleration of impulse formation in the AV junction occurs in AJR as a normal variation in cardiac rhythm. The presence of AJR is easily diagnosed when the morphology of the QRS complex is normal, the ventricular rate is in the range of 60 to 130 beats per minute, and there are no preceding P waves (see Fig. 16.2B). Retrogradely conducted atrial activation is present during or after anterograde ventricular activation, but the inverted P waves may be obscured by the larger QRS complexes or may be hidden in T waves (Fig. 16.8). When inverted P waves are visible but the heart rate is rapid, it is difficult to determine whether the P wave is associated with the preceding QRS complex (AJR) or with the following QRS complex (sinus tachycardia with a prolonged PR interval). If P waves can be seen clearly on a 12-lead ECG, their direction in the frontal plane should provide differentiation of these conditions.

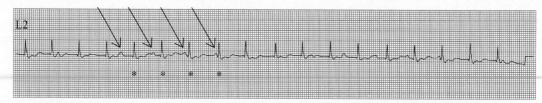

FIGURE 16.9. A lead II (*L2*) rhythm strip from a 72-year-old woman with digitalis toxicity. *Arrows* indicate the anterograde (sinus) P waves dissociated from the junctional beats (*asterisks*).

Other forms of AJR may produce normal P waves before the QRS complexes, but with varying PR intervals, because the SA node is activating the atrium and an accelerated junctional pacing site is activating the ventricles. This is an example of dissociation between atrial and ventricular activity (Fig. 16.9). It may be necessary to observe a long rhythm strip to document this AV dissociation because the atrial and ventricular rates may be similar (isorhythmic) with a constant PR interval.

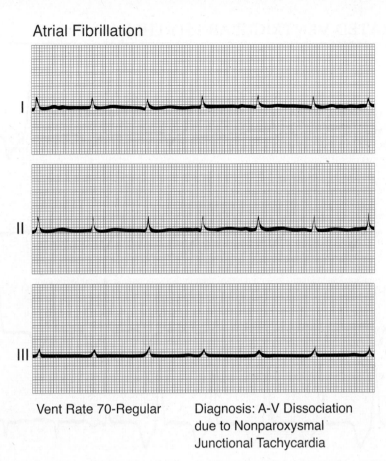

Atrial Fibrillation

I

II

III

Vent Rate 70-Regular   Diagnosis: A-V Dissociation
                              due to Nonparoxysmal
                              Junctional Tachycardia

FIGURE 16.10. Simultaneous recording of three ECG leads showing the slightly undulating baseline of atrial fibrillation dissociated from the regular narrow QRS complexes of AJR. "Nonparoxysmal junctional tachycardia" is another term used for AJR. (From Wagner GS, Waugh RA, Ramo BW. *Cardiac Arrhythmias.* New York, NY: Churchill Livingstone; 1983:149, with permission.)

A regular ventricular rate of >60 beats per minute with normal-appearing QRS complexes in the presence of atrial fibrillation (see Chapter 17) is diagnostic of AJR. This is another example of AV dissociation, with one tachyarrhythmia resulting from reentry above the AV node and another tachyarrhythmia resulting from accelerated automaticity below the AV node (Fig. 16.10). This combination of decreased conduction in the AV node and enhanced automaticity in the common bundle is usually caused by digitalis toxicity (see Chapter 24). If this condition is unrecognized, additional digitalis further accelerates the AJR.

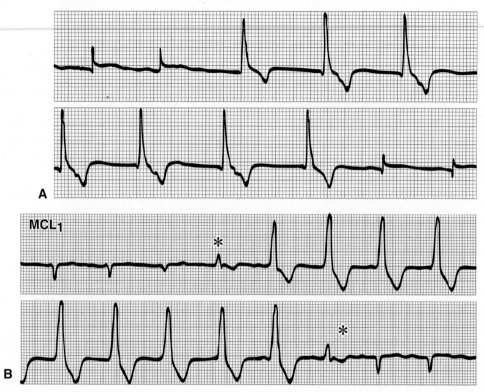

FIGURE 16.11. The contrasting appearances of the onset of an AVR that results from an increased discharge rate of the ventricular pacemaker **(A)** and its termination that results from slight acceleration of the sinus rate **(B)**. *Asterisk*, fusion.

AVR is produced by enhanced automaticity in the bundle branches or fascicles of the ventricular Purkinje system. As in AAR and AJR, this acceleration of impulse formation in the ventricles occurs as a normal variation in cardiac rhythm. The presence of AVR is easily diagnosed when the morphology of the QRS complex is abnormal in the presence of a heart rate in the range of 50 to 110 beats per minute and there are no preceding P waves (see Fig. 16.2C). In AVR, retrogradely conducted atrial activation is present during or after anterograde ventricular activation, but the inverted P waves may be obscured by the larger QRS complexes or T waves.

AVR is often given other names, such as accelerated idioventricular rhythm or *slow ventricular tachycardia*. Because the pacing rate of the cells causing AVR that are located at the distal end of the pacemaking and conduction system is normally very slow, AVR is diagnosed when the ventricular rate is >50 beats per minute. The most rapid rate of AVR is 110 beats per minute, and the heart rate in this condition is rarely >100 beats per minute. AVR most commonly occurs following reperfusion of an acute myocardial infarction, with reported incidences ranging from 8% to 46%. Its occurrence has been shown to indicate less than optimal reperfusion.[4] AVR is also a common manifestation of digitalis toxicity.

AVR occurs either because the sinus rhythm slows and permits the AVR to reveal itself or because the ventricular rhythm accelerates so much that it usurps control from a normally functioning SA node (Fig. 16.11A). These precipitating sources of AVR can therefore be differentiated by observing the pattern of sinus rhythm preceding the onset of the AVR.

When AVR is present, the rates of sinus and ventricular impulse formation are usually similar. The dominance of the ventricular pacemaker may begin and terminate (see Fig. 16.11B) with one or more QRS complexes formed partly by a sinus-originated impulse and partly by a ventricular-originated impulse (fusion beats).

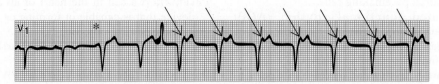

FIGURE 16.12. In this ECG, AVR appears after two beats of sinus rhythm. It is initially dissociated from the atrial activity (*asterisk*), and the causative impulse is then conducted retrogradely to capture the atrial rhythm (*arrows*).

AVR, like AJR, commonly occurs when atrial fibrillation is accompanied by decreased AV nodal conduction. These combined effects often result from digitalis toxicity. Once the AVR caused by these effects begins, it usually proceeds as a regular rhythm, although it sometimes shows progressive acceleration or progressive slowing until it spontaneously ceases.

In some instances of AVR, there is retrograde conduction to the atria (Fig. 16.12) rather than dissociation between the atria and ventricles. AVR is usually benign, even when multiform, and neither affects the blood pressure nor leads to more serious ventricular arrhythmias.[5,6] However, because the normal sequence of atrial and ventricular activation is absent, and there is loss of the normal atrial contribution to ventricular filling, AVR may be accompanied by a feeling of weakness.

GLOSSARY

Accelerated atrial rhythm (AAR): tachyarrhythmia caused by an increase of automaticity in atrial pacemaking cells.

Accelerated junctional rhythm (AJR): tachyarrhythmia caused by an increase of automaticity in the pacemaking cells of the His bundle.

Accelerated rhythm: an increase in a particular cardiac rhythm above its normal limit.

Accelerated ventricular rhythm (AVR): tachyarrhythmia caused by an increase of automaticity in pacemaking cells of the bundle branches and their fascicles.

Carotid sinus massage: manual stimulation of the area of the neck that overlies the bifurcation of the carotid artery to increase parasympathetic nervous activity.

Chaotic atrial tachycardia: another term used for MAT.

Digitalis toxicity: an arrhythmia produced by digitalis.

Multifocal atrial tachycardia (MAT): a rapid rhythm produced by increased automaticity in pacemaking cells located at multiple sites within the atria.

Pacemaker: a cell in the heart or an artificial device that is capable of forming or generating an electrical impulse.

Paroxysmal: a term referring to an arrhythmia of sudden occurrence.

Paroxysmal atrial tachycardia (PAT) with block: a tachyarrhythmia, commonly caused by digitalis toxicity, in which a rapid atrial rhythm is accompanied by failure of some of the atrial impulses to be conducted through the AV node to the ventricles.

Slow ventricular tachycardia: another term used for an AVR.

Sympathetic tone: the relative amount of sympathetic nervous activity as compared with the amount of parasympathetic activity.

Vagal maneuver: an intervention that increases parasympathetic activity in relation to the amount of sympathetic activity.

REFERENCES

1. Lown B, Wyatt NF, Levine HD. Paroxysmal atrial tachycardia with block. *Circulation*. 1960;21:129–143.
2. Geer MR, Wagner GS, Waxman M, et al. Chronotropic effect of acetylstrophanthidin infusion into the canine sinus nodal artery. *Am J Cardiol*. 1977;39:684–689.
3. Lipson MJ, Naimi S. Multifocal atrial tachycardia (chaotic atrial tachycardia): clinical associations and significance. *Circulation*. 1970;42:397–407.
4. Engelen DJ, Gressin V, Krucoff MW, et al. Usefulness of frequent arrhythmias after epicardial recanalization in anterior wall acute myocardial infarction as a marker of cellular injury leading to poor recovery of left ventricular function. *Am J Cardiol*. 2003;92(10):1143–1149.
5. Denes P, Kehoe R, Rosen KM. Multiple reentrant tachycardias due to retrograde conduction of dual atrioventricular bundles with atrioventricular nodal-like properties. *Am J Cardiol*. 1979;44:162–170.
6. Epstein ML, Stone FM, Benditt DG. Incessant atrial tachycardia in childhood: association with rate-dependent conduction in an accessory atrioventricular pathway. *Am J Cardiol*. 1979;44:498–504.

17

Reentrant Atrial Tachyarrhythmias— The Atrial Flutter/ Fibrillation Spectrum

GALEN S. WAGNER AND
DAVID G. STRAUSS

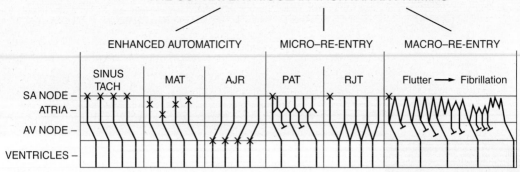

THE SUPRAVENTRICULAR TACHYARRHYTHMIAS

ENHANCED AUTOMATICITY   MICRO–RE-ENTRY   MACRO–RE-ENTRY

FIGURE 17.1. In the ladder diagrams, *X* indicates the site of impulse formation, a *vertical line* indicates normal conduction through atria or ventricles, a *diagonal line* indicates normal conduction though the atrioventricular (AV) node and conduction around a re-entry circuit, and a *short perpendicular line* indicates the site of block of impulse conduction. AJR, accelerated junctional rhythm; MAT, multifocal atrial tachycardia; PAT, paroxysmal atrial tachycardia; RJT, reentrant junctional tachycardia; SA, sinoatrial; TACH, tachycardia. See Animations 17.1–17.4.

The supraventricular tachyarrhythmias in the *atrial flutter/fibrillation spectrum* are caused by the continuing reentry of an electrical impulse within the atrial myocardium. Figure 17.1 schematically contrasts this mechanism with the tachyarrhythmias caused by accelerated automaticity as described in Chapter 16 and those caused by junctional reentry as described in Chapter 18. Because the reentrant circuit includes a large area of atrial myocardium, the reentry mechanism responsible for atrial flutter/fibrillation should be considered macro–re-entry (see Chapter 14). (Atrial micro–re-entrant tachyarrhythmias also occur but are very uncommon; they are also diagrammed in Figure 17.1.)

Atrial flutter and *atrial fibrillation* are at the two extremes of a spectrum. At the flutter end of the spectrum, the causative reentering impulse cycles around a single circuit (usually within the right atrium), producing slower, regular, uniform, and sharp ("sawtooth-like") waves (*F waves*). At the fibrillation end of the spectrum, the causative reentering impulse cycles around multiple circuits, producing more rapid, irregular, multiform, and rounded waves (*f waves*). As a result of the macro–re-entry mechanism responsible for both atrial flutter and fibrillation, P waves are replaced either by F waves, representing the continuous activation within the flutter circuit, or by f waves, representing the continuous activation within the fibrillation circuits.

Animation 17.1   Animation 17.2   Animation 17.3   Animation 17.4

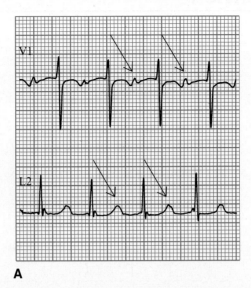

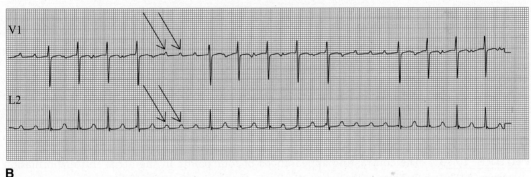

FIGURE 17.2. Lead II (L2) and V1 rhythm strips from a woman presenting with shortness of breath who was found to have idiopathic cardiomyopathy. *Arrows* indicate similar-appearing P waves in L2 and V1 in the presenting condition **(A)** and during carotid sinus massage **(B)**.

Although atrial micro–re-entrant tachycardia (paroxysmal atrial tachycardia [PAT]) occurs rarely, it is useful to present an example because of its clearly identifiable characteristics (Fig. 17.2). In Figure 17.2A, a micro–re-entrant tachycardia masquerades as a typically appearing sinus tachycardia (110 beats per minute) with first-degree atrioventricular (AV) block (0.26 second). However, in Figure 17.2B, the true atrial rate of 220 beats per minute is revealed by the vagal stimulation provided by carotid sinus massage. This atrial tachyarrhythmia could possibly be atrial flutter, but the discrete P waves rather than a sawtooth-like morphology in both leads V1 and L2 (II) makes flutter unlikely. In the patient presented in Figure 17.2, sinus rhythm emerged after electrical cardioversion, confirming the reentrant mechanism of the tachycardia. The similar P-wave morphologies observed during PAT and sinus rhythm indicate that the micro–re-entrant circuit was in or near the sinus node, high in the right atrium.

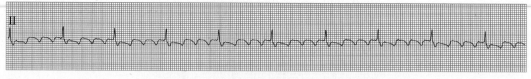

A

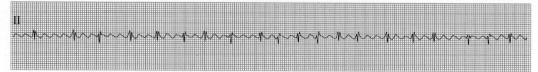

B

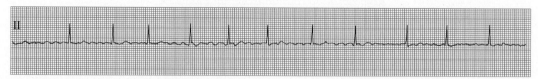

C

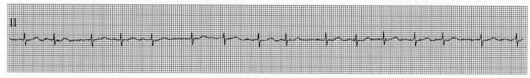

D

FIGURE 17.3. The contrasting appearances of four points in the atrial flutter/fibrillation spectrum. **A.** Flutter. **B.** Flutter-fibrillation. **C.** Coarse fibrillation. **D.** Fine fibrillation.

The F waves of atrial flutter typically occur at rates between 200 and 350 beats per minute (Fig. 17.3A).[1,2] At an atrial rate of >350 beats per minute, either the atrial waves have some characteristics of both flutter and fibrillation at a single point in time (see Fig. 17.3B) or there are alternations between F and f waves, with the appropriate term being *atrial flutter-fibrillation.* Fibrillation varies from coarse to fine. In *coarse fibrillation,* prominent f waves are clearly visible in many leads of the electrocardiogram (ECG; see Fig. 17.3C); in *fine fibrillation,* either there are small f waves or no visible atrial activity (see Fig. 17.3D).

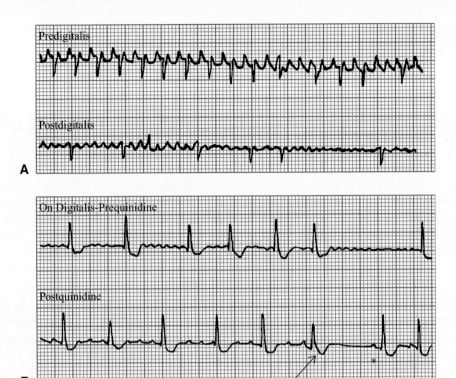

FIGURE 17.4. The effect of digitalis **(A)** and quinidine **(B)** on the atrial flutter/fibrillation spectrum in two patients. The *arrow* in **B** indicates the quinidine-induced termination of atrial reentry, and the *asterisk* indicates the onset of sinus rhythm. (From Wagner GS, Waugh RA, Ramo BW. *Cardiac Arrhythmias.* New York, NY: Churchill Livingstone; 1983:159, with permission.)

Some patients' atrial tachyarrhythmias may spontaneously undergo a change from flutter to fibrillation, whereas others have such variation only when certain drugs are administered. Digitalis increases the atrial rate toward the fibrillation end of the spectrum by shortening the refractory periods of atrial myocardial cells within the re-entry circuit (Fig. 17.4A). Conversely, drugs such as quinidine and procainamide (Vaughn Williams class IA) and flecainide (class IC) decrease the atrial rate toward the flutter end of the spectrum by lengthening the refractory periods of the atrial myocardial cells (see Fig. 17.4B).

VENTRICULAR RATE AND REGULARITY IN ATRIAL FLUTTER/FIBRILLATION

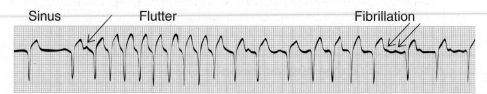

FIGURE 17.5. A lead V1 rhythm strip from an elderly woman with chronic heart failure and a history of recurrent "rapid heartbeats." The first *arrow* indicates the APB that initiates the atrial reentrant tachycardia, and the second and third *arrows* indicate the f waves when the ventricular rate slows. (From Wagner GS, Waugh RA, Ramo BW. *Cardiac Arrhythmias*. New York, NY: Churchill Livingstone; 1983:155, with permission.)

Atrial flutter produces a ventricular rhythm that varies from precisely regular to *irregularly irregular*; however, fibrillation always produces an irregularly irregular ventricular rhythm. Therefore, when atrial fibrillation is accompanied by a regular ventricular rate, there is dissociation between the atrial and ventricular rhythms. A pacemaking Purkinje cell in the common bundle or bundle branches is initiating the regular ventricular rhythm.

Because the atrial rate may vary dramatically within the flutter/fibrillation spectrum, the ventricular rate may also vary. At times, it may change abruptly from rapid and regular to slow and irregular, incorrectly suggesting a change in the basic underlying atrial rhythm (Fig. 17.5). After two beats of sinus rhythm, an atrial premature beat (APB) initiates a supraventricular tachyarrhythmia that is initially regular and then becomes irregular. The regular phase is most likely caused by flutter at a rate of 200 beats per minute with 1:1 AV conduction, after which the irregular phase occurs because the atrial rate accelerates into the flutter/fibrillation spectrum at 300 beats per minute, with a resultant slower, irregular ventricular rate.

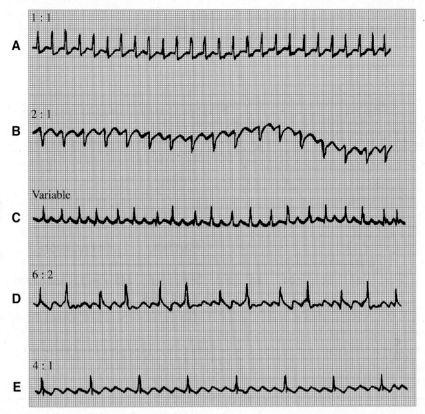

FIGURE 17.6. Lead II rhythm strips from five patients with atrial flutter. Various typical patterns of AV conduction in atrial flutter are shown. **A.** There is 1:1 conduction with a rate of 200 beats per minute. **B.** The atrial rate is 250 beats per minute and there is a regular ventricular rate of 125 beats per minute with a constant relationship between the flutter waves and the QRS complexes. **C.** The atrial rate is 300 beats per minute (note the typical flutter waves during periods of increased AV block), and there is a variable, irregular ventricular response. **D.** The atrial rate is 270 beats per minute, and there is a regularly irregular ventricular response in a pattern of six flutter waves for every two QRS complexes. **E.** The atrial rate is 240 beats per minute, and there is a 4:1 ventricular response, again with a constant relationship between atrial activity and each ventricular complex. (From Wagner GS, Waugh RA, Ramo BW. *Cardiac Arrhythmias.* New York, NY: Churchill Livingstone; 1983:156, with permission.)

During atrial flutter, the ratio of atrial to ventricular waveforms may vary from 1:1 to 2:1 to 6:2 to 4:1 (Fig. 17.6A–E) so that the ventricles may or may not have a rapid rate. The ratio of atrial-to-ventricular waveforms depends on the capability of the slowly conducting AV node to transport the atrial impulses to the common bundle. When ratios of atrial-to-ventricular waveforms of 1:1, 2:1, or 4:1 remain constant (see Fig. 17.6A, B, and E), the ventricular rhythm is regular. When the ratio is 6:2 (because the atrial impulses are blocked at two levels within the AV node), the ventricular rhythm is regularly irregular. When the AV conduction ratio is variable (e.g., switching between 2:1 and 6:2 conduction), the ventricular rhythm is irregularly irregular.

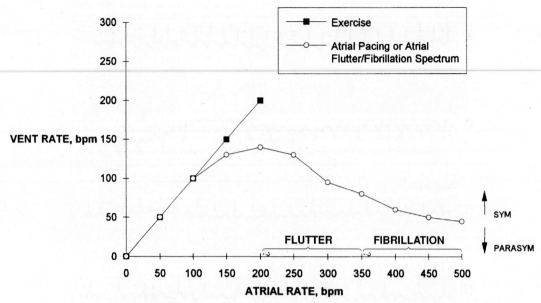

FIGURE 17.7. Ventricular rate regulation by the balance between sympathetic (SYM) and parasympathetic (PARASYM) tone is indicated by *arrows*. Note that the ventricular rate follows the atrial rate to about 100 beats per minute regardless of the mechanism of increase in atrial rate as indicated by the *open squares*. (From Wagner GS, Waugh RA, Ramo BW. *Cardiac Arrhythmias*. New York, NY: Churchill Livingstone; 1983:9, with permission.)

When atrial fibrillation is present, the innumerable f waves compete for penetration of the AV node, making it most difficult for any impulse to reach the common bundle. Therefore, the ventricular rhythm is slower at the fibrillation end of the flutter/fibrillation spectrum (Fig. 17.7).[3-5] Typically, a 1:1 AV relationship persists to the upper limit of the atrial rate during exercise or with other conditions that enhance sympathetic stimulation. However, when the atrial rate increases through other mechanisms (such as artificial atrial pacing or a reentrant tachyarrhythmia), the 1:1 AV relationship persists only until the atrial rate reaches 150 to 160 beats per minute. Above this atrial rate, the physiologic delay in AV nodal conduction prevents some atrial impulses from reaching the ventricles. As the atrial rate increases further, the ventricular rate decreases because of the competition within the AV node. The nonconducted atrial impulses are blocked only after they have been able to penetrate some distance into the node. This *concealed conduction* depolarizes a part of the AV node, making it refractory to the following atrial impulse.[6] Changes in the sympathetic-to-parasympathetic balance can either facilitate (sympathetic) or further inhibit (parasympathetic) AV nodal conduction, as indicated by the directions of the arrows at the right side of the figure.

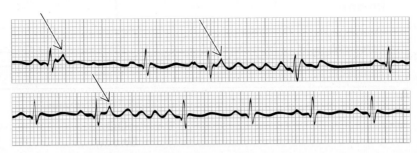

FIGURE 17.8. A lead II (2) continuous rhythm strip from a patient with complaint of recurrent "palpitations." *Arrows* indicate three APBs, two of which initiate brief runs of atrial flutter.

Both spontaneous and electrically induced atrial flutter/fibrillation may typically be produced when APBs occur within a narrow range of the atrial refractory period. Thus, flutter/fibrillation is typically sudden in onset, as are all reentrant arrhythmias (Fig. 17.8).

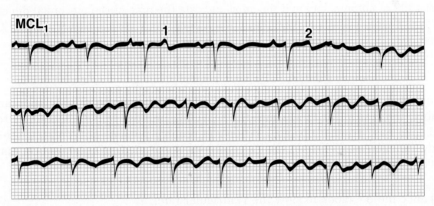

FIGURE 17.9. A lead MCL$_1$ recording from an elderly woman with pulmonary emphysema. The 1 indicates the APB occurring just outside and the 2 indicates the APB occurring just inside the atrial vulnerable period.

Like the ventricles, the atria have a vulnerable period: a point in the atrial cycle at which an APB is most likely to precipitate atrial flutter/fibrillation (Fig. 17.9). Killip and Gault[7] have formulated the situation as follows: If the interval from the normal P wave to the premature P wave is less than half of the preceding interval between normal P waves, the premature P wave is within the atrial vulnerable period and may induce flutter/fibrillation.

TERMINATION OF ATRIAL FLUTTER/FIBRILLATION

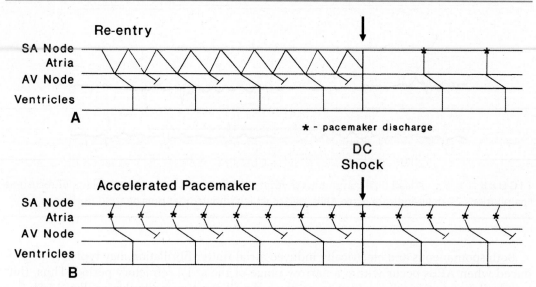

FIGURE 17.10. Ladder diagrams used to contrast the expected responses of tachyarrhythmias caused by atrial macro–re-entry **(A)** with those caused by enhanced atrial automaticity **(B)**. *Asterisks* indicate the site of automaticity and the *arrow* indicate the time of the precordial direct-current shock. (From Wagner GS, Waugh RA, Ramo BW. *Cardiac Arrhythmias.* New York, NY: Churchill Livingstone; 1983:25, with permission.) See Animation 17.5.

As illustrated in Figure 17.8, atrial flutter/fibrillation may terminate spontaneously. Presumably, the reason for this is that the recycling impulse fails to encounter receptive cells and thus has "nowhere to go." When the reentry persists and creates either acute cardiac dysfunction or a chronic clinical problem, some medical intervention may be required. There are two possible treatment strategies:

1. Enhance the AV block to slow the ventricular rate.
2. Terminate the flutter/fibrillation.

Terminating or "breaking" this atrial reentrant tachycardia may be accomplished either with drugs or through electrical stimulation. A drug can effect termination of a tachyarrhythmia either by increasing the speed of the recycling impulse so that it encounters only cells that are still refractory or by prolonging the refractory periods of the involved cells. No drugs yet exist that both speed conduction and prolong the refractory period. The primary therapeutic effect of available drugs is prolongation of refractoriness. An electrical stimulation can terminate a tachyarrhythmia by suddenly depolarizing all cardiac cells that are not already in the depolarized state (Fig. 17.10A). This eliminates the receptivity to reentry that is required to maintain the tachyarrhythmia. As illustrated in Figure 17.10B, such an electrical stimulation cannot "break" a tachyarrhythmia produced by accelerated automaticity; instead, the rapidly discharging site continues to maintain the tachyarrhythmia after a brief interruption.

Animation 17.5

Characteristics of the Atrial Flutter/Fibrillation Spectrum at the Various Atrial Rates

Atrial rate	200	220	300	360	400	≥500
Ventricular rate	200	180	150	120	100	70
Ventricular rhythm	Regular	Regularly irregular	Regular	Regularly irregular	Irregularly irregular	Irregular
		⌣		⌣	⌣	
Name		Flutter		Flutter-fibrillation		Fibrillation
Digitalis decreases AV conduction		Seldom		Sometimes		Usually
DC shock terminates		Low energy		Intermediate energy		High energy
Pacing terminates		Usually		Sometimes		Almost never

Modified from Wagner GS, Waugh RA, Ramo BW. *Cardiac Arrhythmias.* New York, NY: Churchill Livingstone; 1983:154, with permission.

When the atrial re-entry is orderly, as at the flutter end of the flutter/fibrillation spectrum, it can be suddenly terminated by intra-atrial electrical stimulation from a pacemaker. Maintenance of the orderly reentry of the impulse requires that areas of atrial myocardium have completed their refractory periods and are receptive to the advancing wave of depolarization. A properly timed stimulus, delivered via a pacing electrode, produces premature activation of receptive areas, and the advancing wavefront encounters no cells that it can depolarize.

When the reentry is disorderly, as at the fibrillation end of the spectrum, it cannot be terminated by intra-atrial stimulation because no particular areas of atrial myocardium are essential for maintenance of the reentry. Therefore, electrical termination requires that stimuli be applied simultaneously to the entire atrial myocardium (see Fig. 17.10A). Such premature activation of all potentially receptive areas leaves the advancing wavefronts with nothing available to depolarize. A body surface electrical shock (*electrical cardioversion*) can terminate tachyarrhythmias in the entire flutter/fibrillation spectrum.

Table 17.1 summarizes many of the characteristics of the atrial flutter/fibrillation spectrum.

ATRIAL FLUTTER

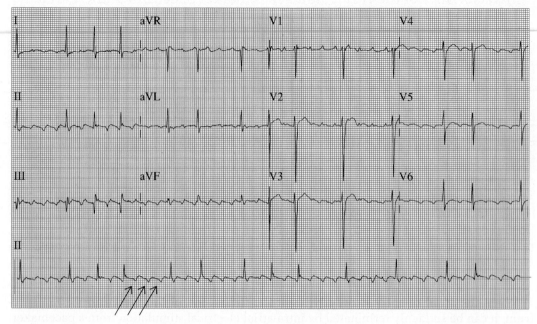

FIGURE 17.11. Twelve-lead ECG and lead II rhythm strip from a 68-year-old man 1 day after cholecystectomy. The patient had a long history of poorly treated hypertension. *Arrows* indicate the typical "sawtooth" appearance of F waves in the lead II rhythm strip.

Atrial flutter is much less common in adults than is atrial fibrillation. It is most often found in patients with *ischemic heart disease* and is particularly rare in *mitral valve disease*. Flutter may complicate any form of heart disease, may be precipitated by any acute illness, and often occurs transiently after cardiac surgery. In the first few years of life, flutter is much more common than fibrillation, presumably because fibrillation requires a greater mass of atrial muscle.

In the usual variety of atrial flutter, the sawtooth pattern of F waves is best seen in the inferiorly oriented leads of the ECG (Fig. 17.11). Indeed, the F-wave deflections are positive in leads V1 and V2 and negative in leads V5 and V6, and there may be no evidence of atrial activity in the laterally oriented leads such as I and aVL. In leads V1 and V2, the F waves commonly mimic discrete P waves.

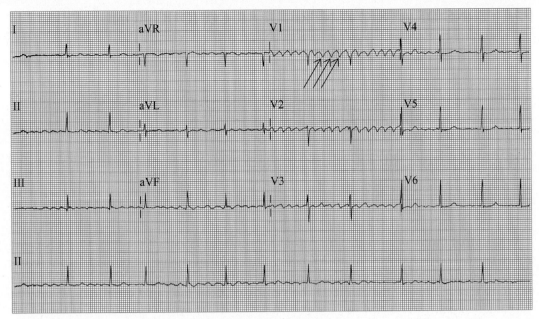

FIGURE 17.12. Twelve-lead ECG and lead II rhythm strip from an elderly woman during a routine health evaluation. No cardiac-related symptoms were present. *Arrows* indicate the "sawtooth" appearance of the F waves in lead V1.

In a rare variety of atrial flutter, however, the F waves may be inconspicuous in the limb leads and seen clearly only in precordial leads V1 to V3 (Fig. 17.12).

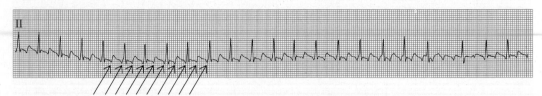

FIGURE 17.13. A lead II rhythm strip from a patient with mitral valve disease who presented with acute shortness of breath. *Arrows* indicate the F waves during 2:1 conduction, which then became obvious during later 3:1 conduction.

When atrial flutter is untreated, the usual AV conduction ratio is 2:1 (Fig. 17.13) because of the normal refractoriness in the AV node. This rhythm should be termed "atrial flutter with 2:1 conduction" rather than "2:1 block," because the AV node is in its normal physiologic role as a "shield" that protects the ventricles from the rapid atrial rate. It may be difficult to recognize either of the F waves in each cardiac cycle because one of the waves is masked by the QRS complex and the other is masked by the T wave. The diagnosis becomes obvious only when an increase in the AV nodal block slows the ventricular rate to unmask F waves (see Fig. 17.13).

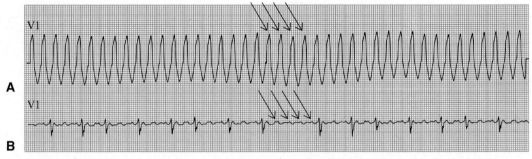

FIGURE 17.14. Lead V1 rhythm strips from a woman who had undergone repair of an atrial septal defect as a child and who presented to the hospital emergency department with profound dyspnea and weakness. No atrial activity is visible during the presenting wide QRS complex tachyarrhythmia **(A)**, but *arrows* indicate the flutter waves in **B** occurring at the identical rate as the QRS complexes in **A**, recorded after several days of intensive treatment of congestive heart failure.

Odd-numbered AV conduction ratios (1:1, 3:1, etc.) are rare. Figure 17.14 presents an example of 1:1 conduction with both atrial and ventricular rates of about 250 beats per minute. Such abnormally rapid AV conduction is rarely possible unless an accessory pathway is present (see Chapter 7). In a patient with such conduction, the regular wide QRS complexes without obvious atrial activity often lead to an erroneous diagnosis of ventricular tachycardia (see Chapter 19).

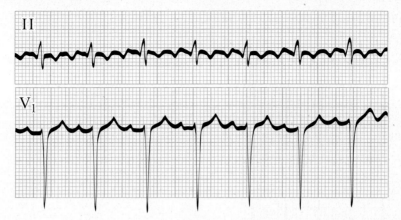

FIGURE 17.15. A two-channel rhythm strip (II and V1) from a woman with chronic obstructive lung disease.

Figure 17.15 presents atrial flutter with the rare 3:1 AV ratio. The diagnosis is obvious in lead II, but the recording in lead V1 has the appearance of sinus tachycardia. Instead of one P wave, there are three F waves during each cardiac cycle. The first F wave mimics a P wave, the second is obscured by the QRS complex, and the third appears as a peak in the T wave.

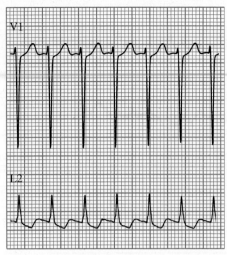

A

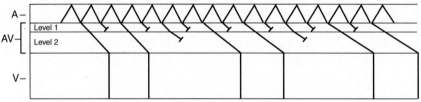

B

FIGURE 17.16. Leads V1 and II (L2) rhythm strips from a patient who presented to the emergency department with weakness and a feeling of his "heart fluttering" **(A)** and after β-adrenergic–blocking treatment was begun **(B)**. No atrial activity is visible in **A**, but *arrows* indicate the locations of the F waves in **B**. The ladder diagram beneath the rhythm strip in **B** illustrates 2:1 conduction in level 1 of the AV node and 3:2 conjunction in level 2. The size of the diagram has been increased to approximately twice that of the rhythm strip in **B** to enhance clarity.

An interesting feature of atrial flutter is the variety of conduction patterns that may develop because of the interplay at various levels within the AV node.[6] These may produce a regularly irregular ventricular rhythm with a bigeminal pattern. Although all of the atrial impulses enter the AV node, as indicated by the ladder diagram, only two of every three reach the ventricles. A supraventricular tachyarrhythmia (Fig. 17.16A) is proven to be atrial flutter with a 2:1 AV conduction ratio by pharmacologic sympathetic blockade (see Fig. 17.16B). The intervention causes a second level of block within the node. The regularly irregular ventricular rhythm has six F waves for every two QRS complexes (6:2 AV conduction ratio).

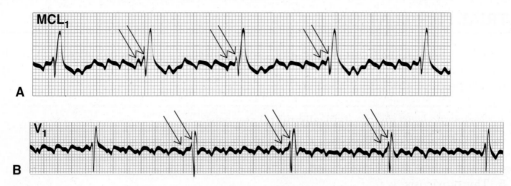

FIGURE 17.17. A QRS complex with RSR' configuration in lead MCL$_1$ in **A** is due to right-bundle-branch block and that in lead V1 in **B** is due to an escape focus in the left bundle branch. *Arrows* in **A** indicate constant F-to-QRS interval intervals and in **B** indicate varying intervals.

Conduction ratios of ≥ 6:1 are sometimes produced when atrial flutter is accompanied by an AV nodal conduction abnormality (Fig. 17.17). In this situation, it may be difficult to distinguish between some AV conduction (termed "second-degree block") and no AV conduction (termed "third-degree block"; see Chapter 22). Some AV conduction may be assumed when, as in Figure 17.17A, a constant ventricular rate (RR intervals) is accompanied by a constant relationship between atria and ventricles (FR intervals). In contrast, the rhythm strip shown in Figure 17.17B presents an example of atrial flutter with complete (third-degree) AV block, as indicated by constant RR intervals accompanied by varying FR intervals.

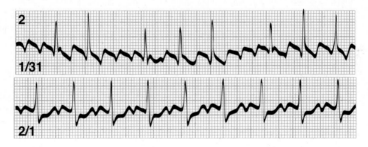

FIGURE 17.18. Lead II rhythm strips from an elderly man receiving chronic digitalis therapy for heart failure before (January 31) and 1 day after quinidine therapy was begun in an attempt to convert the patient's cardiac rhythm to sinus rhythm.

The atrial rate in the flutter/fibrillation spectrum may be greatly influenced by drugs. The rate may be accelerated by digitalis and decelerated by quinidine, procainamide (class IA), and flecainide (class IC). In Figure 17.18, the top strip was taken on a day when the patient was receiving digitalis alone. The bottom strip was obtained 1 day later, 24 hours after quinidine was begun. The atrial rate slowed from 270 to 224 beats per minute, but the ventricular rate increased from 96 to 108 beats per minute. This inverse relationship between atrial and ventricular rates (see Fig. 17.7) occurs because the more beats that enter the AV node, the fewer are able to completely traverse it and reach the ventricles.

ATRIAL FIBRILLATION

Atrial fibrillation may complicate any cardiac disease and is sometimes seen in the absence of any apparent cardiac disease (*lone fibrillation*).[8] The five most common conditions that produce atrial fibrillation are[9,10]:

1. *Rheumatic heart disease* (typically mitral stenosis);
2. Ischemic heart disease;
3. Hypertensive heart disease;
4. Heart failure of any cause; and
5. Thyrotoxicosis.

Advancing age and increased left-atrial size are also related to the development of atrial fibrillation.[11,12] Chronic atrial fibrillation in the elderly often conceals an underlying sick sinus node, and such patients may have postmortem evidence of narrowing of the sinus node artery with atrophy of the sinus node cells.[13] It is not known whether dysfunction of the sinus node leads to the atrial fibrillation, or whether disuse of the sinus node during chronic atrial fibrillation leads to its dysfunction.

Chronic atrial fibrillation, unless therapeutically terminated, usually lasts for life. However, it may occasionally revert to sinus rhythm after surgical replacement of a stenotic mitral valve.[14] Atrial fibrillation appears during two stages of ischemic heart disease: acute myocardial infarction and chronic heart failure.

CHARACTERISTICS OF THE f WAVES OF ATRIAL FIBRILLATION

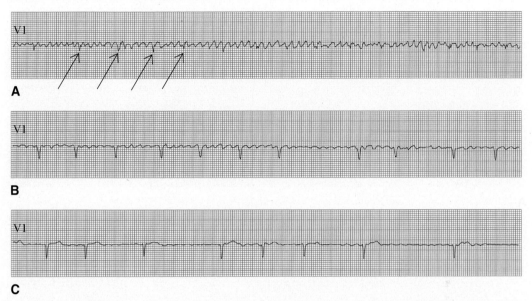

FIGURE 17.19. **A–C.** Lead V1 rhythm strips from three patients with atrial fibrillation. *Arrows* indicate the hidden QRS complexes in **A**.

Atrial fibrillation is recognized by irregular undulation of the ECG baseline, with an irregularly irregular ventricular rhythm. The undulation may be gross and distinct (Fig. 17.19A), intermediate in form (see Fig. 17.19B), or barely perceptible (see Fig. 17.19C). For descriptive purposes, the fibrillation may be coarse, medium, or fine, respectively. Although the size of the f waves in atrial fibrillation has not been found to correlate with the size of the atria or the type of the heart disease,[15] large f waves are unlikely to occur in the presence of a normal-sized left atrium.[16]

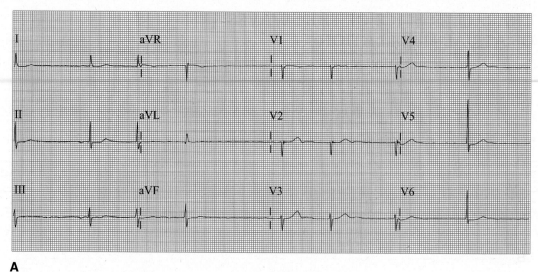

A

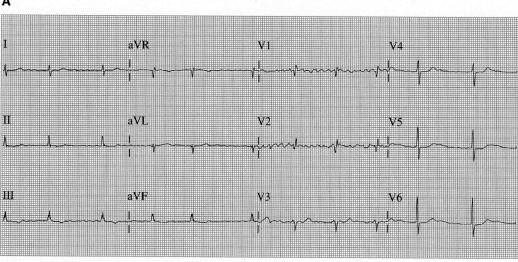

B

FIGURE 17.20. Twelve-lead ECGs from a patient with a previous anterior myocardial infarction **(A)** and a 57-year-old woman with chronic obstructive pulmonary disease **(B)**.

When there is no recognizable deflection of the baseline, atrial fibrillation may be inferred from an irregularly irregular ventricular rhythm (Fig. 17.20A). In fine fibrillation, some baseline undulation may be present in leads V1 to V3 (see Fig. 17.20B).

PATTERNS OF ATRIOVENTRICULAR CONDUCTION

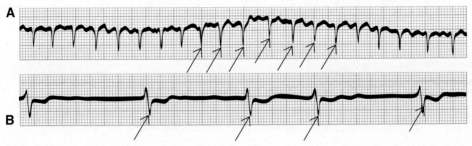

FIGURE 17.21. **A and B.** Lead V1 rhythm strips from two patients with atrial fibrillation. *Arrows* indicate irregularly irregular ventricular rhythm.

The ventricular rate during atrial fibrillation is variable. If the AV node is normal and its conduction has not been suppressed by digitalis, a β-adrenergic receptor blocker, or a *calcium antagonist*, rates as high as 200 beats per minute may develop (Fig. 17.21A). However, if the AV node is diseased or markedly suppressed by drugs, the ventricular rate may be markedly reduced (see Fig. 17.21B).

Unlike the slower, more orderly atrial flutter, atrial fibrillation is not capable of producing a regular ventricular rhythm. Therefore, when both atrial fibrillation and a regular ventricular rhythm coexist, they are independent of each other. Such AV dissociation may occur for two reasons:

1. There is excessive AV block, which creates the need for emergence of impulse formation from a site in the ventricular Purkinje system (see Chapter 22).
2. There is normal AV conduction, but interference has developed from enhanced automaticity in the ventricular Purkinje system (see Chapter 16).

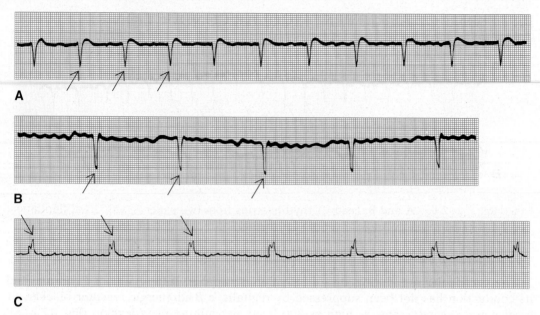

FIGURE 17.22. Lead V1 rhythm strips from three patients with atrial fibrillation. *Arrows* indicate regular ventricular rhythms.

In Figure 17.22, the ventricular rhythm is regular and the rate varies from accelerated (65 beats per minute; see Fig. 17.22A) to within the typical escape range (50 beats per minute; see Fig. 17.22B) to a rate in the slow escape range (40 beats per minute; see Fig. 17.22C). The proper terminology for each of these conditions would be atrial fibrillation with (a) AV dissociation owing to high-degree AV block and accelerated junctional rhythm (AJR; see Fig. 17.22A), (b) complete AV block with right-ventricular escape rhythm (see Fig. 17.22B), and (c) complete AV block with left-ventricular escape rhythm (see Fig. 17.22C). At times, the escape site may be below the branching of the common bundle, producing a widened QRS complex.

Whenever atrial fibrillation is accompanied by a regular ventricular rate and the patient is receiving digitalis, one should consider the possibility of digitalis toxicity.[17] Additional digitalis could cause acceleration of the junctional or ventricular rhythm, producing an AJR or accelerated ventricular rhythm (AVR; see Chapter 16). In this situation, the atrial fibrillation is accompanied by a regular ventricular rhythm at an accelerated rate. The proper terminology would be "atrial fibrillation with AV dissociation due to AJR or AVR."

ATRIAL FLUTTER/FIBRILLATION WITH VENTRICULAR PREEXCITATION

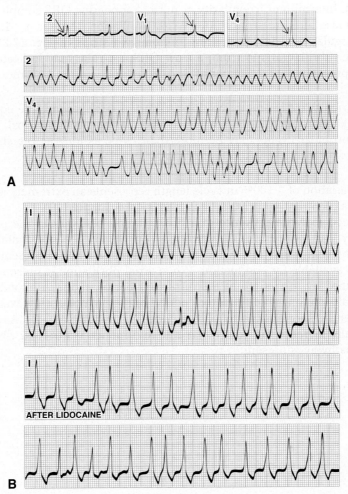

FIGURE 17.23. ECG recordings from two teenage patients evaluated in the emergency department with complaints of palpitations and weakness. A previous ECG during sinus rhythm **(A)** documented ventricular preexcitation (leads 2, V1, and V4). Leads II (2) and V4 rhythm strips in **A** and lead I rhythm strips in **B** document the rapid, irregularly irregular wide QRS tachycardias. Note the marked slowing of the ventricular rate following lidocaine administration in **B**.

Normally, the AV node is the only electrical pathway connecting the atria and the ventricles. However, as discussed in Chapter 7, some individuals have the congenital abnormality of an accessory AV conduction pathway (bundle of Kent). Because this pathway is composed of myocardial cells, these individuals have a bypass of the AV nodal protection that is so important when atrial flutter/fibrillation occurs. The normal inverse relationship between the atrial and ventricular rates illustrated in Figure 17.7 is lost. Instead, the pre-excitation pathway permits a direct relationship between the two rates and thereby allows for particularly rapid ventricular rates at the fibrillation end of the spectrum. The refractory period of the accessory pathway determines the ventricular rate, and rates as high as 300 beats per minute may occur (Fig. 17.23A, B).[18,19] There is a serious risk of ventricular fibrillation, either because the impulse arrives during the vulnerable phase of the ventricular cycle or because the rapid ventricular rate causes such a low cardiac output and causes myocardial ischemia.

It can be extremely difficult, and sometimes impossible, to differentiate atrial flutter/fibrillation with preexcitation from a ventricular tachycardia. At the flutter end of the spectrum, there is often a 1:1 AV ratio and a regular ventricular rhythm (see Figs. 17.14 and 17.23A, B, top). Intermittent irregularity or normal-appearing QRS complexes (second strip in Fig. 17.23B) also indicate atrial flutter. With fibrillation, there is a <1:1 ratio accompanied by an irregular ventricular rhythm (bottom two strips in Fig. 17.23A). Throughout the atrial flutter/fibrillation spectrum, a slow QRS upstroke may indicate the delta wave of ventricular preexcitation. When atrial fibrillation and ventricular preexcitation coexist:

1. The ventricular cycle length may be as short as 0.20 second, the equivalent of a rate of 300 beats per minute (see Fig. 17.23A, B, top rhythm strips).
2. Some ventricular cycles may be more than twice as long as the shortest cycles (bottom two rhythm strips in Fig. 17.23A).

This latter variation of >100% in cycle length represents an extremely unusual degree of irregularity in a reentrant ventricular tachycardia (see Chapter 19).

Failure to recognize the presence of a preexcitation pathway in the presence of atrial fibrillation may lead to a serious therapeutic error. This is because digitalis has the opposite effect on the ventricular rate when a preexcitation pathway is present than when only the AV node is available for conduction. When atrial fibrillation is present, the ventricular rate is determined by the length of the refractory period of the AV conduction pathway. As noted, digitalis prolongs the refractory period of the AV node. However, as discussed in Chapter 13, digitalis shortens the refractory period of myocardial cells. As a result, digitalis can paradoxically increase the ventricular rate and induce ventricular fibrillation when a preexcitation pathway is present.[20]

GLOSSARY

Atrial fibrillation: the tachyarrhythmia at the rapid end of the flutter/fibrillation spectrum; it is produced by macro–re-entry within multiple circuits in the atria and is characterized by irregular multiform f waves.

Atrial flutter: the tachyarrhythmia at the slow end of the flutter/fibrillation spectrum; it is produced by macro–re-entry within a single circuit in the atria and is characterized by regular uniform F waves.

Atrial flutter-fibrillation: the tachyarrhythmia in the middle of the flutter/fibrillation spectrum; it has some aspects of flutter and some of fibrillation.

Atrial flutter/fibrillation spectrum: a range of tachyarrhythmias caused by macro–re-entry in the atria and which extends from flutter, with an atrial rate of 200 beats per minute, through flutter-fibrillation and coarse fibrillation to fine fibrillation without atrial activity detectable on the body surface.

Calcium antagonist: a drug that diminishes calcium entry into cells and slows conduction through the AV node.

Coarse fibrillation: fibrillation marked by prominent f waves in some of the ECG leads.

Concealed conduction: nonconducted atrial impulses that depolarize part of the AV node and thereby make it refractory to following impulses.

Electrical cardioversion: use of transthoracic electrical current to terminate a reentrant tachyarrhythmia, such as those in the atrial flutter/fibrillation spectrum.

F waves: the regular, uniform, sawtooth-like atrial activity characteristic of flutter.

f waves: the irregular, multiform atrial activity characteristic of fibrillation.

Fine fibrillation: either minute f waves or no atrial activity at all in any of the ECG leads.

Irregularly irregular: a term describing an irregular rhythm with no discernible pattern to the sequence of ventricular beats.

Ischemic heart disease: a cardiac abnormality caused by decreased blood flow to the myocardium, usually because of atherosclerosis with or without superimposed thrombosis in the coronary arteries.

Lone fibrillation: atrial fibrillation occurring in an individual who shows no evidence of cardiac disease.

Mitral valve disease: a condition marked either by an abnormally tight (stenotic) or leaky (insufficient) valve between the left atrium and left ventricle.

Rheumatic heart disease: active or inactive disease of the heart resulting from rheumatic fever and characterized by inflammatory changes in the myocardium or by scarring of the valves that reduces the functional capacity of the heart.

REFERENCES

1. Waldo AL, Henthorn RW, Plumb VJ. Atrial flutter—recent observations in man. In: Josephson ME, Wellens HJJ, eds. *Tachycardias: Mechanisms, Diagnosis, Treatment.* Philadelphia, PA: Lea & Febiger; 1984:113–127.

2. Wells JL Jr, MacLean WAH, James TN, et al. Characterization of atrial flutter: studies in man after open heart surgery using fixed atrial electrodes. *Circulation.* 1979;60: 665–673.

3. Langendorf R, Pick A, Catz LN. Ventricular response in atrial fibrillation: role of concealed conduction in the atrioventricular junction. *Circulation.* 1965;32:69–83.

4. Lau SH, Damato AN, Berkowitz WD, et al. A study of atrioventricular conduction in atrial fibrillation and flutter in man using His bundle recordings. *Circulation.* 1969;40:71–78.

5. Moore EN. Observations on concealed conduction in atrial fibrillation. *Circ Res.* 1967; 21:201–211.

6. Besoain-Santander M, Pick A, Langendorf R. A-V conduction in auricular flutter. *Circulation.* 1950;2:604.

7. Killip T, Gault JH. Mode of onset of atrial fibrillation in man. *Am Heart J.* 1965;70:172.

8. Peter RH, Gracey JG, Beach TB. A clinical profile of idiopathic atrial fibrillation. *Ann Intern Med.* 1968;68:1296–1300.

9. Kannel WB, Abbott RD, Savage DD. Coronary heart disease and atrial fibrillation: the Framingham study. *Am Heart J.* 1983;106:389–396.

10. Morris DC, Hurst JW. Atrial fibrillation. *Curr Probl Cardiol.* 1980;5:1–51.

11. Henry WL, Morganroth J, Pearlman AS, et al. Relation between echocardiographically determined left atrial size and atrial fibrillation. *Circulation.* 1976;53:273–279.

12. Probst P, Goldschlager N, Selzer A. Left atrial size and atrial fibrillation in mitral stenosis: factors influencing their relationship. *Circulation.* 1973;48:1282–1287.

13. Davies MJ, Pomerance A. Pathology of atrial fibrillation in man. *Br Heart J.* 1972; 34:520–525.

14. Zimmerman TJ, Basta LL, January LE. Spontaneous return of sinus rhythm in older patients with chronic atrial fibrillation and rheumatic mitral valve disease. *Am Heart J.* 1973;86:676–680.

15. Morganroth J, Horowitz LN, Josephson ME, et al. Relationship of atrial fibrillatory wave amplitude to left atrial size and etiology of heart disease. *Am Heart J.* 1979;97:184–186.

16. Bartall H, Desser KB, Benchimol A, et al. Assessment of echocardiographic left atrial enlargement in patients with atrial fibrillation. An electrovectorcardiographic study. *J Electrocardiol.* 1978;11:269–272.

17. Kastor JA. Digitalis intoxication in patients with atrial fibrillation. *Circulation.* 1973;47:888–896.

18. Klein GJ, Bashore TM, Sellers TD, et al. Ventricular fibrillation in the Wolff-Parkinson-White syndrome. *Circulation.* 1976;11:187.

19. Grant RP, Tomlinson FB, Van Buren JK. Ventricular activation in the pre-excitation syndrome (Wolff-Parkinson-White). *Circulation.* 1958;18:355.

20. Sellers TD Jr, Bashore TM, Gallagher JJ. Digitalis in the pre-excitation syndrome. Analysis during atrial fibrillation. *Circulation.* 1977;56:260–267.

18 Reentrant Junctional Tachyarrhythmias

MARCEL GILBERT, GALEN S. WAGNER,
AND DAVID G. STRAUSS

INTRODUCTION TO REENTRANT JUNCTIONAL
TACHYARRHYTHMIAS

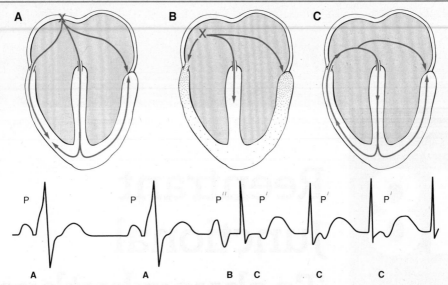

FIGURE 18.1. Formation and conduction of the cardiac impulse during sinus rhythm **(A)** and an APB **(B)** and impulse conduction through the various parts of the heart during a sustained tachyarrhythmia **(C)** are shown anatomically **(top)** and electrocardiographically **(bottom)**. The P waves are designated as P in sinus rhythm, as P′ during the RJT, and as P″ for the APB that initiates the RJT. Sites of impulse formation are indicated by x, the directions of impulse conduction by *arrows*, the AV node by an *open channel* at the summit of the ventricular septum, the Kent bundle by an *open channel* between the right atrium and ventricle, and persistent refractoriness in the ventricles and Kent bundle by *stippling*. (Modified from Wagner GS, Waugh RA, Ramo BW. *Cardiac Arrhythmias.* New York, NY: Churchill Livingstone; 1983:13, with permission.) See Animation 18.1.

The *reentrant junctional tachyarrhythmias* (RJTs) usually occur in young people without underlying heart disease. An alternative term for "reentrant RJT" is "reciprocating RJT." If conduction proceeds homogeneously, there can only be entry into the structures ahead and no reentry into structures behind. However, the presence of nonhomogeneous conduction leads to reentry from the distal end of one pathway into the distal end of another pathway.

Reentry in the atrioventricular (AV) junction can occur entirely within the AV node when differences in refractoriness cause nonhomogeneous conduction or when an accessory AV pathway provides a site for reentry from the ventricles back to the atria as illustrated in Figure 18.1.

Reentry within the AV junction can result in a single junctional premature beat or in sustained RJT (see Fig. 18.1C). These tachyarrhythmias may be more difficult to understand and identify than those originating in the atria and ventricles because the AV junction is not represented by any waveform in the ECG.

In the normal heart, the only electrically conducting structures of the junction between the atria and ventricles are the AV node and the common (His) bundle. However, congenitally anomalous accessory AV (Kent) bundles, either located centrally in the region of the AV node and His bundle or peripherally, may serve as part of the circuit of RJTs. Usually, the accessory pathway is identified by ECG evidence of ventricular preexcitation during sinus rhythm (see Chapter 7). The combination of ventricular pre-excitation and RJT is called the Wolff-Wolff–Parkinson–White syndrome (see Chapter 7; Fig. 18.1).[1] The younger the individual with RJT, the more likely that an accessory AV conduction pathway is present. The definitions of the P, P′, and P″ symbols appearing in Figure 18.1 are presented in Table 18.1.

Animation 18.1

Table 18.1.		
Characteristic Atrial Activity		
Arrhythmia	Atrial Activity	Symbol
Sinus tachycardia	Discrete anterograde P waves	P
Ectopic atrial tachycardia	Discrete modified P waves	P″
Atrial flutter	Regular undulating waves	F
RJTs	Discrete retrograde P waves	P′

RJT, re-entrant junctional tachyarrhythmias.

In most individuals, the accessory pathway is capable of conduction in both the antero-grade and retrograde directions. However, the accessory pathway may be capable of conduction only in one direction, causing either ventricular preexcitation or RJT:

1. If only anterograde conduction is possible along an accessory AV pathway, there is preexcitation during sinus rhythm.
2. If only retrograde conduction is possible along an AV accessory pathway, there is no preexcitation during sinus rhythm but there is the potential for RJT. In this instance, a *concealed fast AV-bypass pathway* is present.

Natural History of the Reentrant Junctional Tachyarrhythmias

There have been several follow-up studies of children and young adults with RJT, both with and without evidence of ventricular preexcitation.[2,3] A high percentage of neonates with RJT have evidence of ventricular preexcitation, but many of these spontaneously lose their accessory pathway during the first year of life. Some lose only the capability for anterograde conduction through their accessory AV pathway but retain the capability for retrograde conduction, as evident from recurrent episodes of RJT. There is a decreasing incidence of evidence of preexcitation among progressively older individuals with RJT.

One study reported that 85% of adults with RJT did not have evidence of an accessory pathway and that those without accessory pathways were older than those with pathways (a mean of 55 versus 40).[4] There was also a much higher incidence of underlying heart disease in adults without accessory pathways (50% versus 10%).

Terms That Characterize the Reentrant Junctional Tachyarrhythmias

Many different terms used to characterize an RJT fall into three categories:

1. Those that apply to the clinical behavior of the RJT: paroxysmal, persistent, permanent, incessant, sustained, nonsustained, chronic, relapsing, and repetitive;
2. Those that describe the site of origin of the RJT: supraventricular, atrial, AV nodal, AV bypass, and junctional; and
3. Those that describe the mechanism of the RJT: reentrant, reciprocating, circus movement, slow–fast, fast–slow, orthodromic, and antidromic.

VARIETIES OF REENTRANT JUNCTIONAL TACHYARRHYTHMIAS

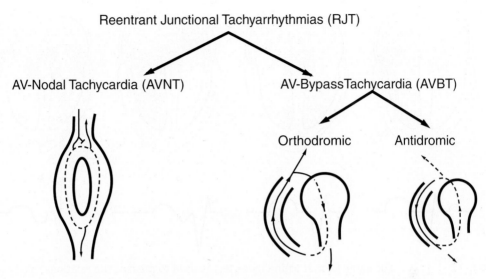

FIGURE 18.2. The typical forms of the three varieties of RJT are illustrated. *Arrows* indicate the direction of conduction and *dashed* versus *solid* lines indicate the speeds of conduction in the AV node (slow) and myocardium (fast). The ⊥ symbol indicates blocked conduction. See Animation 18.2.

The mechanism that produces RJT may be either micro–re-entry occurring totally within the AV node (*AV nodal tachycardia*; Fig. 18.2A) or macro–re-entry involving one atrium, an accessory pathway, one ventricle, and the AV node (*AV-bypass tachycardia*; see Fig. 18.2B). The AV node is the slowest conducting structure with the longest refractory period in the heart. If an impulse entering from the atria encounters a part of the node that has not yet completed its refractory phase, the condition for AV nodal reentry occurs as shown in Figure 18.2A and may lead to either single premature atrial contractions or to AV nodal tachycardia. The presence of an accessory AV conduction pathway creates the potential for the development of re-entry circuits in which the impulses travel in either the normal or reverse direction through the AV node and ventricular Purkinje system. Although its re-entry circuit also includes atrial and ventricular myocardium, AV-bypass tachycardia is included as an RJT because its existence depends on the presence of a congenital anomaly in the junction between the atria and ventricles. The term *orthodromic (AV-bypass) tachycardia* is used when the impulse proceeds in the normal direction, and the term *antidromic (AV-bypass) tachycardia* is used when the impulse proceeds in the reverse direction. (This reverse impulse direction results from a premature beat that occurs in close proximity to the AV node and therefore finds the node still in its refractory phase.) The AV node also must be far away from the accessory pathway as seen with the left-side pathway. A *concealed AV-bypass pathway* is capable only of participating in an orthodromic tachycardia.

Animation 18.2

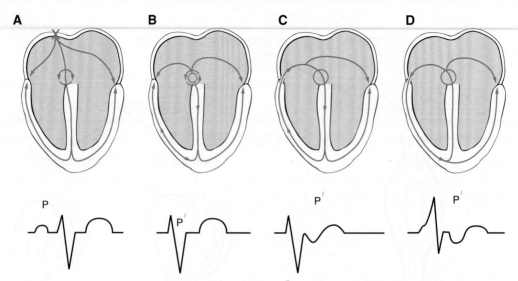

FIGURE 18.3. The same format as in Figure 18.1 is used to present the relationships between intracardiac impulse conduction and the surface ECG during sinus rhythm **(A)**, AV nodal reentrant tachycardia **(B)**, orthodromic AV-bypass tachycardia **(C)**, and antidromic AV-bypass tachycardia **(D)**. The *circle* above the summit of the interventricular septum represents the AV node, and the small *circle* within this larger circle in **B** represents the micro–re-entry circuit shown in Figure 18.2A. See Animation 18.3.

Because the AV junction is distal to the atria, RJT produces *retrograde atrial activation* (P′) resulting in inversion of the P waves in the ECG (see Fig. 18.1). The P′ waves are therefore negative in the limb leads (e.g., lead II).

Two of the varieties of RJT—AV nodal tachycardia (Fig. 18.3B) and orthodromic AV-bypass tachycardia (see Fig. 18.3C)—produce anterograde ventricular activation that can result in normal-appearing QRS complexes, and these two varieties of RJT are therefore considered supraventricular tachyarrhythmias. Like all supraventricular tachyarrhythmias, however, an RJT can result in abnormal QRS complexes if it encounters "aberrant conduction" within the bundle branches or fascicles. Conversely, antidromic AV-bypass tachycardia can produce only abnormal QRS complexes because the impulses have "aberrant conduction" to the ventricles via the accessory pathway (see Fig. 18.3D). Note the normal P-wave appearance and timing in Figure 18.3A, the absence of a P′ wave because atrial activation occurs during the QRS complex in Figure 18.3B, the inverted P′ wave immediately following the QRS complex in Figure 18.3C, and the inverted P′ wave following the wide QRS complex in Figure 18.3D.

Animation 18.3

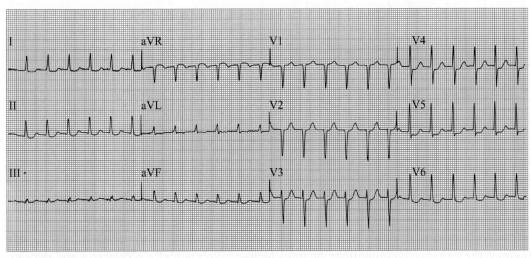

FIGURE 18.4. Twelve-lead ECG recording from a 20-year-old woman who presented to the emergency department with a sudden onset of weakness and palpitations.

When the QRS complex is normal, RJT superficially resembles sinus tachycardia, ectopic atrial tachycardia, and flutter (with a 2:1 AV conduction ratio). If atrial activity is visible in the ECG, its appearance should be diagnostic because it differs markedly in RJT, sinus tachycardia, ectopic atrial tachycardia, and flutter (Table 18.1).

However, there may be no visible atrial activity in any of the ECG leads, as in the example shown in Figure 18.4. The ventricular rate may also be diagnostically helpful because sinus tachycardia rarely exceeds 150 beats per minute in a nonexercising adult, whereas RJT almost always exceeds this rate (about 155 beats per minute in Fig. 18.4).

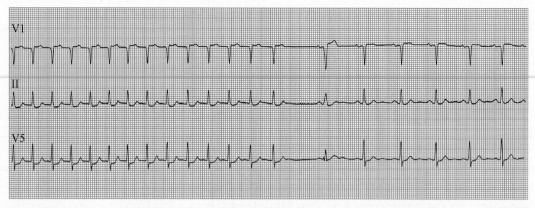

FIGURE 18.5. A three-lead rhythm strip from the patient in Figure 18.4 during spontaneous termination of the tachyarrhythmia.

Observance of the onset or termination should differentiate sinus tachycardia from RJT because the enhanced automaticity of sinus tachycardia gradually accelerates and decelerates in contrast with the abrupt behavior of reentrant tachyarrhythmias. This characteristic, however, does not differentiate RJT from ectopic atrial tachycardia or flutter with 2:1 AV conduction because the ventricular rates in these arrhythmias are similar. Further observation of the rhythm may, however, help in differentiating these three arrhythmias because the 2:1 conduction pattern of ectopic atrial tachycardia or flutter tends to be unstable with variable AV block, thereby providing a clear view of the P″ or F waves. However, no differentiating features among ectopic atrial tachycardia, atrial flutter with 2:1 conduction and RJT may be apparent even on a 12-lead ECG, as shown in Figure 18.4. Figure 18.5 illustrates typical abrupt termination of an RJT. Note, however, that there may be slight slowing of the tachyarrhythmia just before the abrupt termination. The period of asystole following termination of the reentry is quickly ended by reemergence of the normal sino-atrial node pacemaker. In this instance, an escape pacemaker also emerges so that the initial QRS complex after the RJT is a fusion beat. This coincidental occurrence masquerades as ventricular preexcitation, but the subsequent sinus beats have no delta wave.

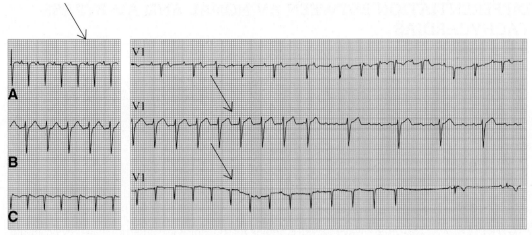

FIGURE 18.6. Lead V1 rhythm strips from three patients with various supraventricular tachyarrhythmias. All three appear as undifferentiated SVT at the left and then differentiated as a particular entity at the right. *Arrows* above the rhythm strips indicate the onset of carotid sinus massage in these typical examples of the responses of paroxysmal atrial tachycardia (**A**), atrial flutter (**B**), and RJT (**C**).

When an arrhythmia fails to terminate spontaneously, a vagal maneuver may provide the differential diagnosis. A classic review by Lown and Levine[5] provides a comprehensive review of the techniques for safely and effectively performing this intervention. The typical responses of paroxysmal atrial tachycardia, atrial flutter, and RJT to vagal maneuvers are presented in Figure 18.6. All three tachyarrhythmias have a supraventricular appearance (QRS complex duration <0.12 second), with atrial activity either apparent after the T waves (see Fig. 18.6A, B) or absent (see Fig. 18.6C). The paroxysmal atrial tachycardia (see Fig. 18.6A) and the atrial flutter (see Fig. 18.6B) are unaffected by the maneuver, but the diagnosis is provided by the increased AV nodal block. The abrupt termination of the arrhythmia seen in Figure 18.6C is a typical response of RJT. The increase in parasympathetic activity terminates RJT by prolonging the AV nodal refractory period, thereby eliminating the receptive pathway for the recycling impulse. When the arrhythmia fails to respond to the parasympathetic stimulation, the diagnosis remains uncertain; a pharmacologic intervention with adenosine, intravenous (IV) β-blockers, or IV calcium antagonists may be used.

When the QRS complex is abnormal because of aberrant conduction via the accessory pathway in antidromic AV-bypass tachycardia or via the Purkinje system in either orthodromic AV-bypass tachycardia or AV nodal tachycardia, the differential diagnosis becomes more difficult because ventricular tachycardia must also be considered. Clues to this differentiation are presented in Chapters 19 and 20.

DIFFERENTIATION BETWEEN AV NODAL AND AV-BYPASS TACHYCARDIAS

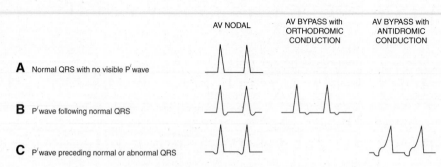

FIGURE 18.7. The three P wave to QRS complex relationships are illustrated as they occur during the three re-entrant junctional tachycardias.

The differentiation between AV nodal and AV-bypass tachycardias becomes most important when the arrhythmia is resistant to conservative treatment and catheter ablation is being considered. The diagnosis of antidromic AV-bypass tachycardia is made obvious by the presence of delta waves at the onset of the QRS complexes in the ECG, because the impulses causing this type of tachycardia enter the ventricles via the accessory pathway, as illustrated by the slow QRS upstroke in Figure 18.7C.

The relationship of the P wave to the QRS complex is helpful in distinguishing AV nodal from orthodromic AV-bypass tachycardia. Because the micro–re-entry circuit of AV nodal tachycardia is contained within the AV node, the P waves and QRS complexes must occur either completely or almost simultaneously. Among the AV nodal tachycardias, about two thirds have no visible P waves (see Fig. 18.7A), one third have P' following the QRS (see Fig. 18.7B), and only a very few have P' waves preceding the QRS complex (see Fig. 18.7C). Because the macro–re-entry circuit in orthodromic AV-bypass tachycardia includes both an atrium and a ventricle, the P waves and QRS complexes cannot occur simultaneously, and because of the direction of the re-entry circuit, the P wave cannot immediately precede the QRS complex. Therefore, differentiation between AV nodal tachycardia and orthodromic AV-bypass tachycardia is only difficult when P waves immediately follow the QRS complexes (see Fig. 18.7B). However, the retrograde P wave in AV nodal tachycardia typically appears as a "pseudo-S wave" of the QRS complex in leads II, III, and aVF or pseudo-R' wave in lead V1. In contrast, the normal QRS complex and the retrograde P wave in orthodromic AV-bypass tachycardia (see Fig. 18.7B) and the retrograde P wave and abnormal QRS complex in antidromic AV bypass tachycardia (see Fig. 18.7C) are identified.

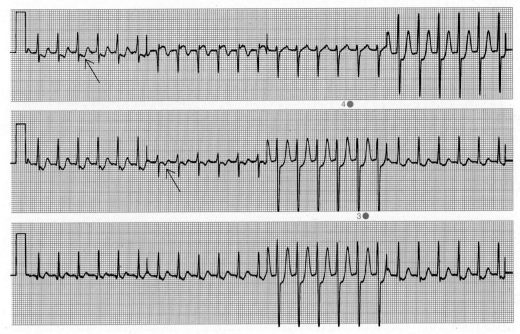

FIGURE 18.8. A standard 12-lead ECG in a patient with symptomatic RJT and left-sided preexcitation.

The differentiation between AV nodal tachycardia and orthodromic AV-bypass tachycardia is more challenging. Orthodromic AV-bypass tachycardia may be assumed when there has been preexcitation during sinus rhythm (see Fig. 18.1A). However, the accessory pathway may be concealed during sinus rhythm if the bypass pathway is incapable of anterograde conduction. The diagnosis of orthodromic AV-bypass tachycardia is facilitated by observing the following characteristics, which are uniquely present because of the location of the macro–re-entry circuit[6]:

1. A negative P wave in leads I and aVL, which suggests that both the left atrium and a left-sided accessory pathway are components of a   rcuit[8] (Fig.   18.8).

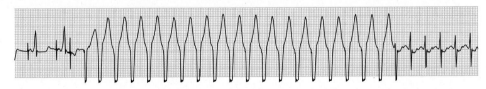

FIGURE 18.9. Lead II ECG of a patient before ablation of left lateral pathway.

2. A sudden decrease in the rate of the tachycardia coincident with the development of aberrant conduction. This suggests that both the bundle branch in which the aberrancy has occurred and an accessory pathway on the same side of the heart are components of a macro–re-entry circuit (Fig. 18.9). The first two atrial-paced beats produce ventricular preexcitation. The paced atrial premature beat causes RJT with left-bundle-branch block morphology. The end of the recording shows normalization of the QRS complex.

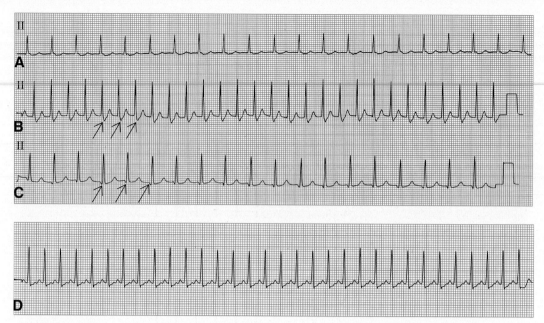

FIGURE 18.10. The contrasting P-wave-to-QRS-complex relationships during the three varieties of AV nodal tachycardia, presented in the same order as in Figure 18.7 **(A–C)**, and the P-wave-to-QRS-complex relationship in orthodromic AV-bypass tachycardia **(D)**. *Arrows* indicate the retrograde P waves appearing as pseudo-S waves **(B)**, pseudo-Q waves **(C)**, and notched T waves **(D)**.

Figure 18.10 presents examples of the three varieties of the relationship between the P wave and QRS complex in AV nodal tachycardia (see Fig. 18.10A–C) and the typical relationship of the P′ wave and QRS complex in orthodromic AV-bypass tachycardia (see Fig. 18.10D). Lead II rhythm strips have been selected for illustrating these examples because this frontal plane view provides the inverted appearance of the retrogradely conducted atrial activation (P′ waves). Note that these P′ waves could be mistaken for either the S wave (see Fig. 18.10B) or Q wave (see Fig. 18. 10C) of the QRS complex.

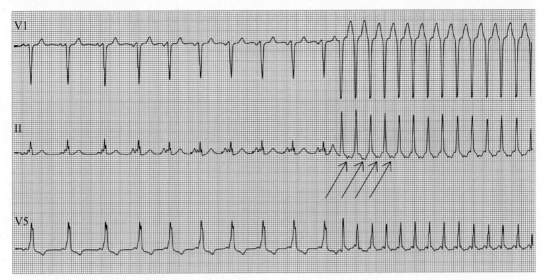

FIGURE 18.11. A three-lead ECG rhythm strip during sinus rhythm and the abrupt onset of orthodromic AV-bypass tachycardia. *Arrows* indicate the retrograde P waves visible in lead II.

Because of the decreased duration of the QT interval during a tachyarrhythmia (see Chapter 3), the following retrograde P wave may be concealed in the T wave during orthodromic AV-bypass tachycardia (Fig. 18.11). The multiple views provided by simultaneous ECG leads may be required for recognition of the P waves when they occur simultaneously with the T waves. In Figure 18.11, the diagnosis of orthodromic AV-bypass tachycardia is clearly established by the presence of delta waves during the baseline sinus rhythm, and abrupt onset of the arrhythmia initiated by an inverted P wave in lead V5. However, of the three leads presented, the P waves during the tachycardia are clearly visible only in lead II.

THE TWO VARIETIES OF AV NODAL TACHYCARDIA

Typical AV Nodal Tachycardia (Slow–Fast)

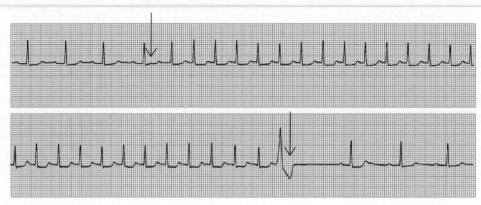

FIGURE 18.12. Continuous recording in lead II of a 52-year-old woman before slow pathway ablation. Typical AV nodal RT with no visible P wave (hidden by the QRS). APB (*arrow*) unmasks the slow pathway (prolonged PR) and initiates the RT. PVB (*arrow*) terminates the tachycardia by a concealed penetration of the AV node.

The typical form of AV nodal tachycardia, sometimes termed "slow–fast," is common in adults. It may be congenital but more often results either from diseases or drugs that impair AV nodal conduction. The AV nodal reentry is usually initiated by an APB associated with a prolonged PR interval (Fig. 18.12). The premature impulse finds the faster pathway still refractory but the slower pathway available for its conduction to the ventricles. By the time the impulse reaches the distal AV node, the fast pathway has completed its refractory period and reentry is possible. This process may result in a single junctional premature beat (an *echo beat*) or in *slow–fast Av nodal tachycardia*. The retrograde P wave is often hidden by the QRS complex because activation of the atria occurs via the fast pathway at the same time that activation of the ventricles occurs via the Purkinje system. The P' wave is either invisible, as in Figure 18.7A, or is seen just emerging from the terminal part of the QRS complex, as in Figure 18.7B and Figure 18.12.

Atypical AV Nodal Tachycardia (Fast–Slow)

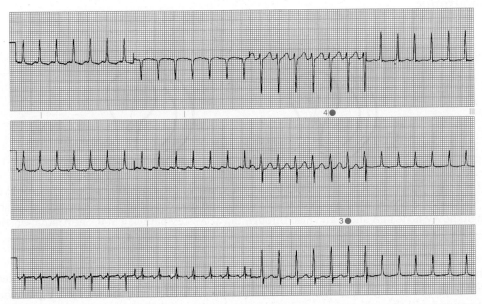

FIGURE 18.13. A standard 12-lead ECG from a young woman with a long history of paroxysmal tachycardia.

The atypical form of AV nodal tachycardia is sometimes referred to as "fast–slow" AV nodal tachycardia, as presented in Figure 18.13. This form is extremely rare in children and adults. Because it occurs only intermittently, it is not associated with tachycardia-induced cardiomyopathy.

THE THREE VARIETIES OF AV-BYPASS TACHYCARDIA

Orthodromic

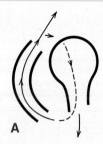 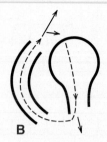

A   **B**

FIGURE 18.14. Typical (slow–fast) **(A)** and atypical (slow–slow) **(B)** orthodromic AV-bypass tachycardia. *Arrows* indicate the direction of conduction and *dashes* indicate similarly slow speed through the AV node in **A** and **B** and also through the accessory pathway in **B**. See Animation 18.4.

The typical form of orthodromic AV-bypass tachycardia has been previously presented in Figure 18.2. The retrograde (ventriculoatrial [VA]) conduction via the accessory pathway is much more rapid than the anterograde (AV) conductions, as would be expected for myocardial versus AV nodal tissue. However, there is an atypical form in which the retrograde conduction is much slower because the accessory pathway has AV nodal–like function. The typical form could be termed slow–fast, and the atypical form termed "slow-slow" (Fig. 18.14).

The atypical form of orthodromic AV bypass tachycardia was first described by Coumel et al[9] and is currently known as "permanent" RJT.[10,11] The majority of these accessory pathways are localized in the right posterior septum zone near the orifice of the coronary sinus. Patients with the permanent form of RJT, mostly children, are at risk of developing tachycardia-induced cardiomyopathy. This atypical form of AV-bypass tachycardia must be differentiated from AV nodal tachycardia by intracavitary electrophysiologic studies.

Animation 18.4

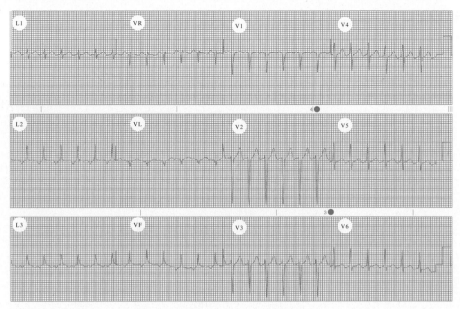

FIGURE 18.15. The 12-lead ECG of a patient admitted for near-syncope episode.

The hallmarks of the 12-lead ECG include an inverted, wide P wave (P') in leads II, III, and aVF in the frontal plane and in leads V2 through V6 in the transverse plane (Fig. 18.15). These P' waves are wide and negative because the accessory pathway delivers the retrograde conduction initially into the right atrium.

This tachycardia must be differentiated from ectopic atrial tachycardia either by using pharmacologic or vagal intervention or by observing a period when the tachycardia temporarily interrupts.

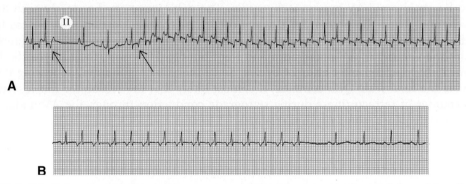

FIGURE 18.16. **A.** An infant with permanent RJT and congestive heart failure. Note the end of the episode (*arrow*) with retrograde P wave (P') and the beginning of another episode without PR prolongation (*arrow*). **B.** A patient with permanent RJT prior to right-side atrial posteroseptal ablation above the coronary sinus.

Permanent RJT initiation is commonly related to critical shortening of the atrial cycle length without following prolongation of AV conduction, as shown in Figure 18.16. This permanent RJT ends with a retrograde P wave (P') ruling out ectopic atrial tachycardia. Most often, however, termination of permanent RJT is associated with a block in the slowly conducting accessory pathway, as seen in Figure 18.16B.

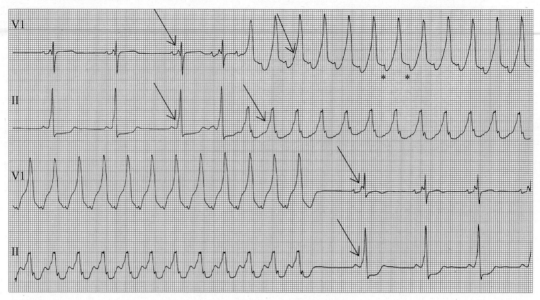

FIGURE 18.17. Continuous two-lead (V1 and II) rhythm strips from a patient with pre-excitation who developed a wide QRS complex tachycardia **(top)** that could have been ectopic atrial tachycardia with 1:1 conduction, or antidromic AV-bypass tachycardia. *Arrows* indicate delta waves present before, during, and after the tachycardia. *Asterisks* indicate abnormally appearing P waves preceding each wide QRS complex.

Figure 18.17 shows the sudden onset and offset of a wide QRS tachyarrhythmia that is typical for antidromic AV-bypass tachycardia. The delta wave can be clearly seen during sinus rhythm. Then the premature P wave originates from a location with access to the Kent bundle, initiating orthodromic conduction around a reentry circuit that sequentially includes the ventricles, AV node, atria and Kent bundle. However, the tachycardia is not sustained, stopping abruptly after 24 cycles. Since there is no abnormal appearing P wave following the final wide QRS complex, it is most likely that the reason for the cessation is the encounter of refractoriness during retrograde conduction through the AV node. After an appropriate pause, sinus rhythm resumes.

GLOSSARY

Antidromic tachycardia: an RJT of the AV-bypass variety produced by macro–re-entry in which the causative impulse recycles sequentially through an accessory AV-bypass pathway, a ventricle, the AV node, and an atrium.

AV-bypass tachycardia: an RJT produced by macro–re-entry, which includes the AV node along with an atrium, a ventricle, and an accessory AV-bypass pathway.

AV nodal tachycardia: an RJT produced by micro–re-entry within the AV node.

Concealed AV-bypass pathway: a Kent bundle that is capable only of VA conduction and is therefore incapable of producing ventricular preexcitation.

Echo beat: an APB produced by reentry within the AV node.

Fast–slow accessory pathway tachycardia: refers to the permanent (another term is "incessant") form of reciprocating junctional tachycardia.

Fast–slow AV nodal tachycardia: an RJT of the AV nodal variety produced by micro–re-entry in which the impulse travels down the fast pathway and up the slow pathway.

Orthodromic tachycardia: an RJT of the AV-bypass variety produced by macro–re-entry in which the impulse recycles sequentially through the AV node, a ventricle, an accessory AV-bypass pathway, and an atrium.

Reentrant junctional tachyarrhythmias (RJTs): any of the tachyarrhythmias (RJTs) produced by continual recycling of an impulse through structures that are present either normally or abnormally between the atria and the ventricles.

Retrograde atrial activation: spread of an activating impulse from the AV junction through the atrial myocardium and toward the sinoatrial node.

Slow–fast AV nodal tachycardia: an RJT of the AV nodal variety produced by micro–re-entry in which the impulse travels down the slow pathway and up the fast pathway.

Slow–slow AV-bypass tachycardia: the permanent form of AV junctional tachycardia.

REFERENCES

1. Wolff L. Syndrome of short P-R interval with abnormal QRS complexes and paroxysmal tachycardia (Wolff-Parkinson-White syndrome). *Circulation.* 1954;10:282.
2. Lundberg A. Paroxysmal tachycardia in infancy. Follow-up study of 47 subjects ranging in age from 10 to 26 years. *Pediatrics.* 1973;51:26–35.
3. Giardinna ACV, Ehlers KH, Engle MA. Wolff-Parkinson-White syndrome in infants and children. *Br Heart J.* 1972;34:839–846.
4. Wu D, Denes P, Amat-y-Leon F, et al. Clinical, electrocardiographic and electrophysiologic observations in patients with paroxysmal supraventricular tachycardia. *Am J Cardiol.* 1978;41:1045–1051.
5. Lown B, Levine SA. The carotid sinus: clinical value of its stimulation. *Circulation.* 1961;23:766.
6. Farre J, Wellens HJJ. The value of the electrocardiogram in diagnosing site of origin and mechanism of supraventricular tachycardia. In: Wellens HJJ, Kulbertus HE, eds. *What's New in Electrocardiography.* Boston, MA: Martinus Nijhoff; 1981:131.
7. Sung RJ, Castellanos A. Supraventricular tachycardia: mechanisms and treatment. *Cardiovasc Clin.* 1980;11:27–34.
8. Puech P, Grolleau R. L'onde P retrograde negative en D1, signe de faisceau de Kent postero-lateral. *Arch Mal Coeur.* 1977;70:48.
9. Coumel P, Cabrol C, Fabiato A, et al. Tachycardia permanente par rythme reciproque. *Arch Mal Coeur.* 1967;60:1830–1864.
10. Gallagher JJ, Sealy WG. The permanent form of junctional reciprocating tachycardia. *Eur J Cardiol.* 1978;8:413–430.
11. Gaita F, Haissaguerre M, Giustetto C, et al. Catheter ablation of permanent junctional reciprocating tachycardia with radiofrequency current. *J Am Coll Cardiol.* 1995;25:648–654.

19 Reentrant Ventricular Tachyarrhythmias

MARCEL GILBERT, GALEN S. WAGNER, AND DAVID G. STRAUSS

VARIETIES OF VENTRICULAR TACHYARRHYTHMIAS

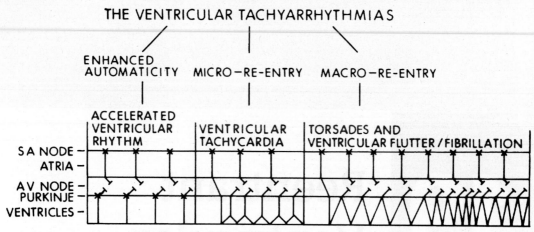

FIGURE 19.1. In the ladder diagrams, an X indicates the site of impulse formation, a *vertical line* indicates normal conduction through the atria or ventricles, a *diagonal line* indicates conduction through the AV node and conduction around a re-entry circuit, and a *short perpendicular line* indicates the site of block. (Modified from Wagner GS, Waugh RA, Ramo BW. *Cardiac Arrhythmias.* New York, NY: Churchill Livingstone; 1983:189, with permission.) See also Figure 17.1 and Animations 17.1 to 17.4, in Chapter 17: *Reentrant Atrial Tachyarrhythmias--The Atrial Flutter/Fibrillation Spectrum.*

A ventricular tachyarrhythmia can result from enhanced automaticity in Purkinje cells (see Chapter 16) or from reentry occurring either in a localized area (micro–re-entry) or in a wider area of myocardium (macro–re-entry).[1-5] Only the most extremely accelerated ventricular rhythm (AVR) caused by enhanced automaticity can achieve a rate >100 beats per minute and thereby actually qualify for the term "tachyarrhythmia." Therefore, the great majority of the true ventricular tachyarrhythmias are caused by reentry (see Chapter 14).

Figure 19.1 presents ladder diagrams that illustrate the mechanisms of the different ventricular tachyarrhythmias. The arrhythmia commonly called *ventricular tachycardia* (VT) is analogous to the atrioventricular (AV) nodal variety of junctional tachyarrhythmia (see Fig. 17.1) in that it originates from a re-entry circuit so small that it is not represented on the electrocardiogram (ECG). VT can be easily differentiated from AVR on the basis of rate (>120 beats per minute versus <120 beats per minute, respectively). In contrast, the macro–re-entry mechanism of *ventricular flutter/fibrillation* is analogous to that of the atrial flutter/fibrillation spectrum presented in Chapter 17. This mechanism produces neither discrete QRS complexes nor T waves, just as the atrial flutter/fibrillation mechanism produces no discrete P waves. *Torsades de pointes* is an atypical form of reentrant ventricular tachyarrhythmia that is difficult to classify. In this chapter, torsades is considered a separate form of ventricular tachyarrhythmia rather than a variety of VT. There is no analogy to this tachyarrhythmia occurring in other parts of the heart. Torsades de pointes is probably caused by macro–re-entry: "macro-" because the ECG shows no discernible QRS complexes or T waves, and "re-entry" because the arrhythmia both appears and terminates abruptly.

Animation 17.1   Animation 17.2   Animation 17.3   Animation 17.4

DESCRIPTION

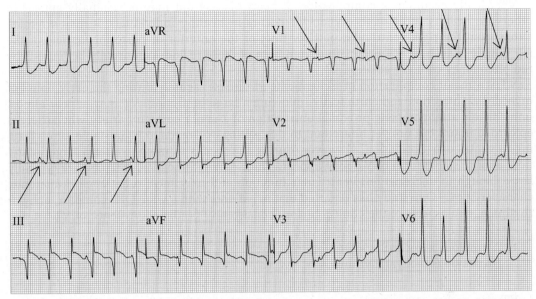

FIGURE 19.2. A 12-lead ECG from a young girl with a viral myocarditis. Note that the QRS duration of the VT is slightly <0.12 second because of the patient's age. *Arrows* indicate the P waves occurring without a fixed relationship to the QRS complexes. The P waves are clearly visible only in leads II, III, and V1 to V4.

By definition, VT consists of at least three consecutive QRS complexes originating from the ventricles and recurring at a rapid rate (>120 beats per minute). Like other tachyarrhythmias, VT is considered either nonsustained or sustained, depending on whether it persists for a specified time, as defined below. The rhythm of VT is either regular or only slightly irregular.

In this chapter, the term "the ventricles" refers to any area distal to the branching of the common bundle (bundle of His) and includes both the Purkinje cells of the pacemaking and conduction system and the ventricular myocardial cells. The re-entry circuit in VT is confined to a localized region, and the remainder of the myocardium receives the electrical impulses, just as it would if they were originating from an automatic (pacemaking) focus (Fig. 19.2). The QRS complexes and T waves that appear on the ECG in VT are generated from the regions of ventricular myocardium not involved in the re-entry circuit.

ETIOLOGIES

VT usually occurs as a complication of heart disease but may occasionally appear in otherwise healthy individuals. When VT occurs in healthy individuals, it may originate either from the right-ventricular outflow tract or the anterior or posterior fascicle of the left bundle branch.[6-13] VT originating from both of these regions can usually be "cured" by radiofrequency catheter ablation.[14]

VT is a major complication of ischemic heart disease, acutely during the early hours of myocardial infarction and chronically following a large infarction. VT may appear almost immediately after complete proximal obstruction of a major coronary artery when there is epicardial injury but not yet infarction. In this setting, VT tends to be unstable, often leading to ventricular fibrillation. However, during the weeks to months after a large infarction, a more stable form of VT may appear. These "arrhythmogenic infarcts" are typically large enough to decrease left-ventricular function and may have other typical anatomic characteristics.[15] One study has reported that in patients with a wide QRS complex tachyarrhythmia, two aspects of the clinical history consistently predicted presence of VT.

1. A previous myocardial infarction.
2. No previous tachyarrhythmia.

VT also occurs as a complication of various nonischemic cardiomyopathies,[1] including the "idiopathic dilated," "hypertrophic obstructive," and "arrhythmogenic right-ventricular" forms.

Many of the antiarrhythmic drugs also have proarrhythmic effects that are manifested either by VT or torsades de pointes.[16-18] Drugs that slow conduction (such as flecainide) may prolong the QRS complex and convert nonsustained VT into sustained VT; those that prolong recovery time (such as sotalol) may prolong the QT interval and produce torsades de pointes (see Figure 19.16). VT is most likely to occur as a proarrhythmic effect in patients with poor ventricular function caused by ischemic heart disease.[3]

DIAGNOSIS

The diagnosis of VTs would be easy if the impulses causing all supraventricular tachyarrhythmias (SVTs) were conducted normally through the ventricles. However, aberrant conduction of supraventricular impulses because of either refractoriness in the bundle branches and fascicles or presence of an accessory pathway occurs frequently (see Chapter 20). The importance of differentiating VT from an SVT was emphasized in one study by the adverse responses of VT to the calcium channel–blocking drug verapamil. In this study, half of a group of patients were given verapamil because of an erroneous diagnosis of SVT; as a result, many of these patients promptly deteriorated and some required resuscitation.[19]

It is also commonly believed that VT is associated with a greater alteration of hemodynamics than is SVT, but a study by Morady et al[15] showed this to be a misconception. The main factors that determine a patient's tolerance to a tachyarrhythmia of any origin are the (a) ventricular rate, (b) size of the heart, (c) severity of the underlying clinical problem, and (d) associated conditions, such as drugs.

With the advent of intracardiac recordings, it became possible to distinguish VT from SVT with bundle-branch block and to determine the site of origin of wide-complex tachycardia. This allowed confirmation of some older[20-25] and some more recently defined[26-31] ECG criteria, and it has provided a basis for improving these criteria. Previously, both extremely prolonged QRS duration or extremely deviated frontal plane axis were considered diagnostic of VT. However, because exceptions occur, it is now recommended to use a well-structured, systematic approach to wide QRS tachycardia in a stepwise manner.

To ensure the diagnosis of VT using all available pertinent criteria, the "scan and zoom approach" is suggested. Scanning provides a global view of the 12-lead ECG in both frontal and transverse planes. Zooming provides specific inspection of QRS waveforms in leads such as V1, V2, or V6.

Step 1: Scan the 12-Lead ECG for P Waves

Atrioventricular Dissociation

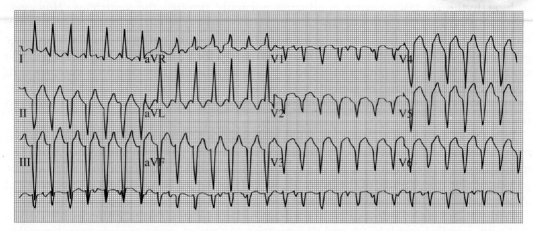

FIGURE 19.3.   A 12-lead ECG from a young patient with a previous myocardial infarction and resultant ventricular aneurysm. Note the QRS duration is slightly <0.12 second because of the patient's age. *Arrows* indicate the P waves occurring without a fixed relationship to the QRS complexes. The P waves are clearly visible only in leads II, III, and V1 to V4.

During VT, the atria may be associated with the ventricles via retrograde activation, or may be dissociated from the ventricles, with their own independent rhythm (usually sinus rhythm; Fig. 19.3).

Because wide QRS complexes or T waves are occurring constantly in both of these situations, the P waves are often lost in the barrage of rapid ventricular cycles. Sometimes, however, the P waves may be recognized as bumps or notches in the vicinity of T waves. One may look in lead V1, where atrial activity tends to be most prominent, or in any lead with low amplitude or isoelectric QRS to improve accuracy.

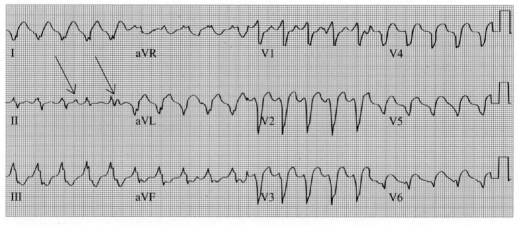

FIGURE 19.4.   A 12-lead ECG from an elderly patient with a dilated cardiomyopathy. *Arrows* indicate consecutive P waves in lead II.

Figure 19.4 is an example in which the low QRS amplitude in lead II facilitates observation of P waves. Presence of AV dissociation is entirely specific but minimally sensitive because of difficulty in finding definitive P waves among the wide QRS complexes and T waves.[31]

Intermittent Irregularity

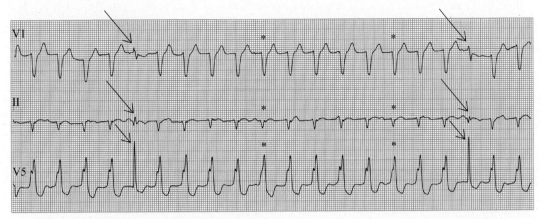

FIGURE 19.5. A three-lead rhythm strip from a 62-year-old man who presented with acute shortness of breath 2 months after an inferior–posterior myocardial infarction. *Arrows* indicate capture beats and *asterisks* indicate fusion beats.

When the ECG waveform morphology of VT is consistent from beat to beat, the term *monomorphic* is applied. When an intermittent on-time narrowing of the QRS complex occurs, the most likely cause is a breakthrough of conduction of the atrial rhythm to the ventricles. If the atrial breakthrough occurs during a QRS complex of the VT, the result is a "fusion beat." If the atrial breakthrough occurs before a QRS complex has begun, the result is a "capture beat," as in beats 5 and 18 in Figure 19.5. Fusion describes a hybrid QRS morphology, in which a portion of the QRS complex represents the areas of the ventricles activated by the VT while the other portion represents the areas activated by a competing atrial impulse, as in Figure 19.5, beats 10 and 15. "Capture" means that the entire QRS complex represents activation of the ventricles by a competing atrial impulse. If either fusion or capture beats are proven to be present, the diagnosis is almost certainly VT. However, fusion and/or capture beats are seldom seen in VT and only at the less rapid rates (<160 beats per minute). Indeed, they appeared in only 4 of a series of 33 reported patients with sustained VT.[26]

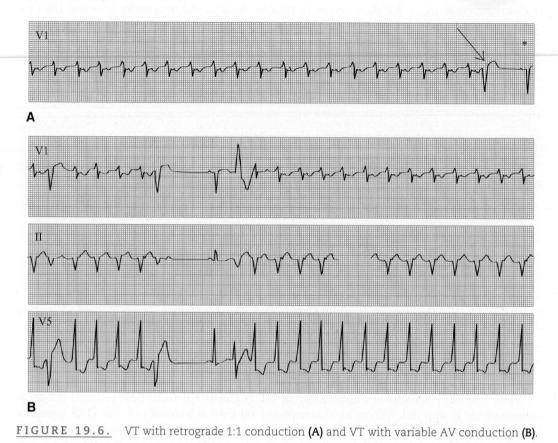

A

B

FIGURE 19.6. VT with retrograde 1:1 conduction **(A)** and VT with variable AV conduction **(B)**.

When atrial and ventricular activation are associated, there is a particular ventricular-to-atrial ratio, such as 1:1, 2:1, or 3:2. In Figure 19.6A, the VT with retrograde 1:1 conduction is terminated by the premature ventricular activation (arrow). This could be either a ventricular premature beat (VPB) or an atrial capture with aberrancy. The termination of the VT is followed by a sinus capture beat with normal QRS morphology (asterisk). In Figure 19.6B, there is initially variable retrograde conduction during nonsustained VT. Then, after the VT resumes, there is 1:1 retrograde conduction.

Step 2: Scan the Precordial Leads for Presence or Absence of RS Morphology

No RS Pattern

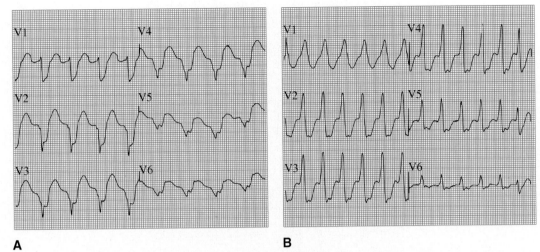

FIGURE 19.7. The ECG recordings in the six precordial leads from a patient with recurrent VT and heart failure **(A)** are contrasted with those of a patient who returned with acute chest pain 1 month after a posterolateral myocardial infarction **(B)**.

Typically, right- or left-bundle-branch block has an RS pattern in at least one of the precordial leads (V1 to V6), and the time from the beginning of the R wave to the nadir of the S is <100 milliseconds (see Chapter 6).

When there is no RS morphology in any of the precordial leads, VT is strongly suggested. However, there is a low sensitivity (21%) as documented by Brugada et al[27]. Scanning all the precordial leads reveals R, qR, or qS QRS complex morphologies (Fig. 19.7).

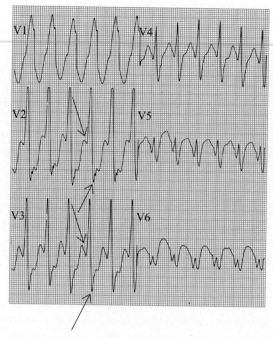

FIGURE 19.8. The six precordial leads of the ECG from a patient illustrating VT with a prolonged interval from onset of the QRS complex to the nadir of the S wave. *Arrows* indicate the period of 0.12 second from QRS onset to S nadir in leads V2 and V3.

An interval >100 milliseconds from the beginning of the R wave to the nadir of the S wave in one precordial lead had a specificity of 0.98 and sensitivity of 0.66.[27] An RS interval >100 milliseconds is difficult to calculate when the QRS merges with the previous T wave, masking the QRS onset during rapid tachycardia. An increased RS interval occurs in SVT with conduction over an accessory pathway and with drugs that prolong QRS duration (Fig. 19.8).

Step 3: Zoom to Specific Precordial Leads for QRS Morphology
Right-Bundle-Branch Block Pattern

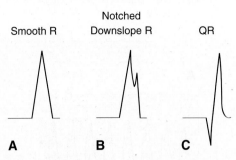

FIGURE 19.9. The three variations in QRS complex morphology in lead V, during "RBBB pattern VT."

FIRST ZOOM TO LEAD V1. Just as the presence of the terminal positive (R or R′) morphology in lead V1 of conducted beats indicates a right-bundle-branch block, this morphology during VT indicates that the RV is activated after the LV. Therefore, the term "right-bundle-branch block pattern" is used to classify VT as left ventricular in origin (Fig. 19.9). The terminal positive wave is preceded in Figure 19.9A and 19.9B by a smooth or notched R wave but by a Q wave in Figure 19.9C. The most commonly occurring variety of the right-bundle-branch block is the notched downslope R.

Wellens and colleagues[20] and Drew and Scheinman[31] analyzed the morphologic features of the ECGs of 122 and 121 patients, respectively, with proven SVT or SVT with aberration established by electrophysiologic studies. These three QRS morphologies were strongly suggestive of VT.

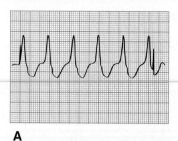

A

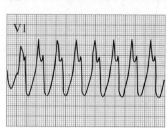

B

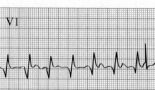

C

FIGURE 19.10. Signs of VT. **A.** Smooth R. **B.** Notched downslope R. **C.** QR pattern.

Monophasic R waves (Fig. 19.10A) are highly suggestive of VT.

Biphasic RR' with the taller first rabbit ear (Marriott sign; see Fig. 19.10B) is by far the most specific criteria for VT, but the sensitivity is low.

A qR pattern (see Fig. 19.10C) can also be associated with SVT with right-bundle-branch block and myocardial infarction.

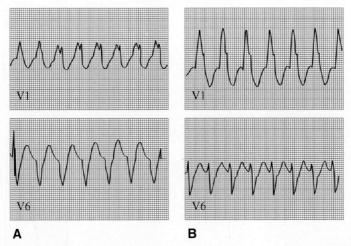

FIGURE 19.11. **A and B.** The QS and RS morphologies of the QRS complex in lead V6 during "RBBB pattern VT" are illustrated.

Observation of a QS morphology in lead V6, illustrated in Figure 19.11A, is valuable in either left- or right-bundle-branch block pattern VTs. The R/S <1 pattern in lead V6 in Figure 19.11B should only be considered indicative of VT when there is left-axis deviation evident in the limb leads.

Left-Bundle-Branch Block Pattern

FIRST ZOOM TO LEADS V1 AND V2

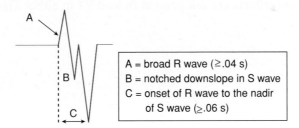

FIGURE 19.12. The three characteristics of the QRS morphology of "LBBB pattern VT" in leads V1 and V2 are illustrated.

Just as the presence of the terminal negative morphology in lead V1 of conducted beats indicates a left-bundle-branch block, this morphology during VT indicates that the RV is activated after the left ventricle. Therefore the term "left-bundle-branch block pattern" is used to classify VT as right ventricular in origin.

The ECG criteria illustrated in the diagram and presented in the box in Figure 19.12 were proposed by Kindwall et al.[30] They evaluated 118 patients with VT or SVT with aberration who underwent intracavitary recording. Predictive accuracy was 96%.

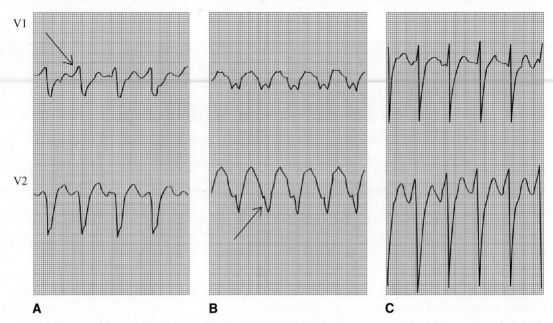

FIGURE 19.13. **A–C.** Each of the three characteristics of "LBBB pattern VT" in leads V1 and V2 are illustrated.

Zooming to leads V1 and V2 for the three ECG examples provides observation of the criteria of Kindwall et al[30] for VT with the LBBB pattern, as indicated by the arrows:

Figure 19.13A: The broad R wave in V1.
Figure 19.13B: The notched S wave downslope in V2.
Figure 19.13C: The prolonged R onset to the S nadir in V2.

Note that the latter two criteria are not present in lead V1 in either Figure 19.13B and C.

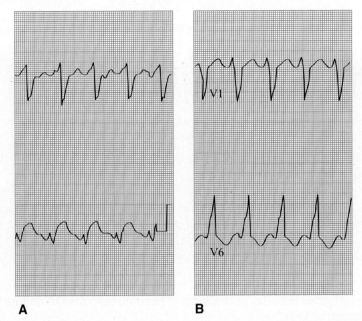

A   **B**

FIGURE 19.14.   **A and B.** The QRS and qR morphologies of the QRS complex in lead V6 during "LBBB pattern VT" are illustrated.

QRS (Fig. 19.14A) and qR (see Fig. 19.14B) in V6 are diagnostic of VT but are seldom seen.

In conclusion, there are limitations with this approach.

Other specific criteria should be applied to patients with other etiology, such as idiopathic left VT (LVT) or right VT (RVT) or VT associated with ventricular dysplasia.

The usefulness of so many criteria is related to a low sensitivity yield (20% to 50%) of each criterion, even though they are associated with a high probability in favor of VT. Consideration of ventricular versus supraventricular with aberrant conduction in the next chapter focuses on this challenge.

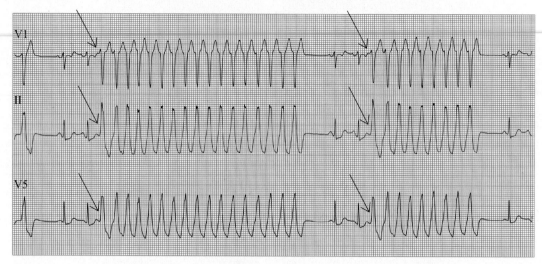

FIGURE 19.15. Simultaneous recording of leads V1, II, and V5 from a 32-year-old woman who presented with palpitations but no other evidence of heart disease. *Arrows* indicate initiation of the episodes of palpitation by VPBs.

VT is usually designated as either *nonsustained VT* or *sustained VT*, depending on whether it persists for >30 seconds.[1] Nonsustained VT has alternatively been defined as VT lasting <1 minute[32] and for <10 beats.[33] Figure 19.15 illustrates two recurrences of VT initiated by VPBs that satisfy most of these definitions of nonsustained VT. Note that the initial episode continues for >10 beats.

Episodes of nonsustained VT may recur chronically over a period of months to years.[34] However, there are striking differences in incidence and prognosis between RVT and LVT.[35] Patients with LVT tend to be older, to be male, and to have heart disease, whereas those with RVT tend to be younger, to be female, and to not have heart disease. RVT is more likely to be induced by particular situations, such as moderate exercise, emotional excitement, upright posture, or smoking.[36,37] LVT, associated with either ischemic or idiopathic cardiomyopathy, has also been shown to be exercise-induced.[38] RVT is commonly associated with arrhythmogenic right-ventricular cardiomyopathy.[1]

VARIATIONS IN THE ELECTROCARDIOGRAPHIC APPEARANCE OF VENTRICULAR TACHYCARDIA: TORSADES DE POINTES

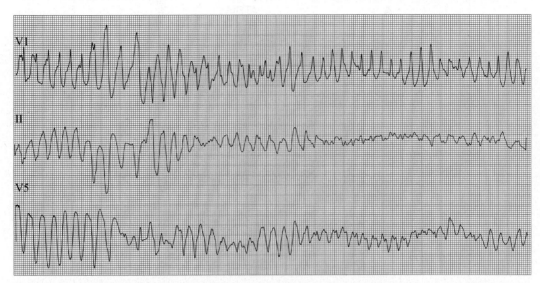

FIGURE 19.16. Simultaneous recordings of leads V1, II, and V5 from a 62-year-old woman receiving diuretic therapy who presented after experiencing a syncopal episode at home. Syncope recurred in the emergency department during this ECG recording. The patient's serum potassium concentration was 2.3 mEq/L.

All of the examples provided in the previous sections have been of *monomorphic VT* with consistency of their QRS complex morphologies. However, torsades de pointes represents a commonly occurring VT with variations in morphology (*polymorphic VT*; Fig. 19.1). This French term translates as "twistings of the points."[39,40] Torsades de pointes VT is characterized by undulations of continually varying amplitudes that appear alternately above and below the baseline. The wide ventricular waveforms are not characteristic of either QRS complexes or T waves, and the rate varies from 180 to 250 beats per minute (Fig. 19.16).[41] Torsades de pointes VT is usually nonsustained; however, it may persist for >30 seconds, satisfying the definition of a sustained tachyarrhythmia. It may also at times evolve into ventricular fibrillation.

Torsades de pointes almost always occurs in the presence of QTc-interval prolongation.[42-44] This may be caused by the proarrhythmic effect of drugs that prolong ventricular recovery time, such as sotalol, phenothiazines, some antibiotics, some antihistamines, and tricyclic antidepressants.[45,46] It also occurs with electrolyte abnormalities such as hypokalemia and hypomagnesemia, insecticide poisoning,[47] subarachnoid hemorrhage, congenital prolongation of the QTc interval,[49] ischemic heart disease,[50] and bradyarrhythmias.[3]

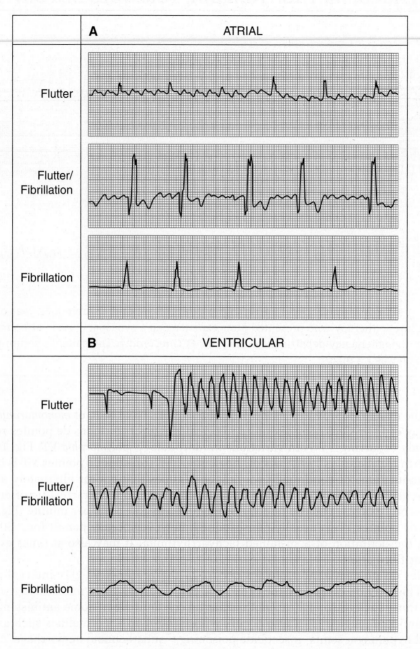

FIGURE 19.17. The atrial flutter/fibrillation spectrum **(A)** is compared with its ventricular counterpart **(B)**. (From Wagner GS, Waugh RA, Ramo BW. *Cardiac Arrhythmias.* New York, NY: Churchill Livingstone; 1983:22, with permission.)

Ventricular flutter/fibrillation is a macro–re-entrant tachyarrhythmia within the ventricular muscle that is analogous to the atrial flutter/fibrillation spectrum discussed in Chapter 17 (Fig. 19.17A). Neither QRS complexes nor T waves are clearly formed, and the rhythm looks similar when viewed right side up or upside down. Immediately after the onset of reentry, a regularly undulating baseline is present (see Fig. 19.17B, top). This *ventricular flutter* looks like a larger version of atrial flutter, but it remains regular and orderly only transiently because the rapid, weak myocardial contractions produce insufficient coronary blood flow (see Fig. 19.17B, middle). As a result, there is prompt deterioration toward the irregular appearance of *ventricular fibrillation* (see Fig. 19.17B, bottom). Ventricular flutter has been given various names, including "VT of the vulnerable period" and "prefibrillation."

Clinical Observations

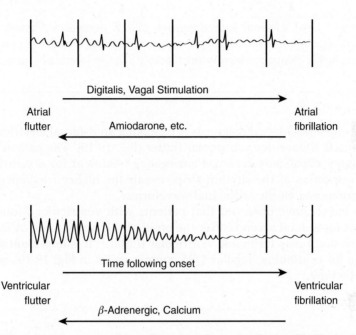

FIGURE 19.18. Movement in either direction along the flutter/fibrillation spectrum in the atria **(A)** and ventricles **(B)**. The *arrows* indicate the direction in which the various factors tend to affect the rate of the reentry process. (From Wagner GS, Waugh RA, Ramo BW. *Cardiac Arrhythmias.* New York, NY: Churchill Livingstone; 1983:23, with permission.) See Animation 19.1.

The various factors capable of creating movement along the flutter/fibrillation spectra in the atria and ventricles are presented in Figure 19.18. When the ventricular reentry is electrically induced during cardiac surgery (to decrease the myocardial energy requirement) and coronary blood flow is maintained by an external pump, slow-coarse ventricular flutter persists until it is electrically terminated at the completion of the surgical procedure. When ventricular flutter/fibrillation occurs spontaneously, it soon deteriorates toward the rapid-fine end of the spectrum, and electrical shock is less effective in its termination. This inverse relationship

between the coarseness of the rhythm and the strength of the electrical current required for termination of ventricular flutter/fibrillation has clinical applicability. β-Adrenergic agents and calcium are commonly used when, during an episode of ventricular fibrillation–induced cardiac arrest, even the maximal output

Animation 19.1   of the electrical defibrillator fails to terminate the reentry process.

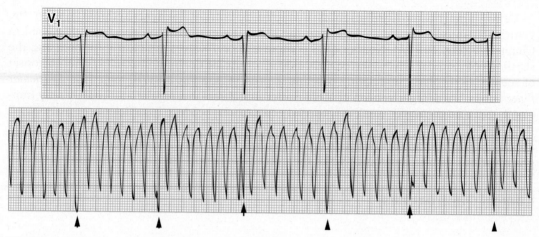

FIGURE 19.19. Lead V1 from a preoperative ECG is used as a reference for the MCL₁ monitoring lead immediately after cholecystectomy in a 72-year-old woman. The *arrows* indicate the regularly occurring higher frequency waveforms representing the locations of the patient's normal QRS complexes.

A common error in ECG-based diagnosis is mistaking an external electrical artifact (e.g., from skeletal muscle tremor) for ventricular flutter (Fig. 19.19). The patient whose ECG is shown in the figure mistakenly received emergency treatment for a ventricular arrhythmia, but close inspection of the rhythm strip reveals the higher frequency, normal QRS complexes superimposed on the artifactual waveforms.

Critical care nurses have observed that patients with ventricular flutter may remain apparently stable for several seconds after the onset of this arrhythmia. A firm blow to the chest ("thump-version") may terminate ventricular flutter.[51] It is important to quickly scan the rhythm strip for continuing, regular QRS complexes (as in Fig. 19.19) before initiating the emergency therapy.

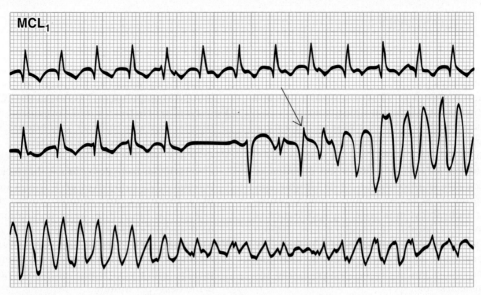

FIGURE 19.20. Continuous bedside recording of lead MCL$_1$ from a 67-year-old man at the onset of a cardiac arrest. An *arrow* indicates the early occurring VPB that initiates the ventricular flutter that rapidly deteriorates into ventricular fibrillation.

Holter recordings that fortuitously capture the onset of "sudden death" have confirmed that the cause is usually ventricular fibrillation (Fig. 19.20). The onset may be preceded by another reentrant ventricular tachyarrhythmia.[52,53] In patients undergoing continuous bed-side monitoring during acute myocardial infarction, the arrhythmias observed just before the onset of ventricular fibrillation have been a single R-on-T VPB, sustained monomorphic VT, nonsustained monomorphic VT with a rate >180 beats per minute, or polymorphic VT.[54] The wide QRS complex tachyarrhythmia (in the top and middle strips of Fig. 19.19) could be either LVT or an SVT with RBB aberrancy. In the ECG shown in Figure 19.20, sinus rhythm resumes after termination of the VT; however, the ensuing lengthened cardiac cycle precipitates an R-on-T VPB. This in turn initiates ventricular flutter that rapidly degenerates into fibrillation in the bottom strip.

Monomorphic: a single appearance of all QRS complexes.

Monomorphic VT: VT with a regular rate and consistent QRS complex morphology.

Nonsustained VT: VT of <30-second duration.

Polymorphic VT: VT with a regular rate but frequent changes in QRS complex morphology.

Sustained VT: VT of ≥30-second duration or requiring an intervention for its termination.

Torsades de pointes: a polymorphic ventricular tachyarrhythmia with the appearance of slow polymorphic ventricular flutter without discernible QRS complexes or T waves. The ventricular activity has constantly changing amplitudes and seems to revolve around the isoelectric line.

Ventricular fibrillation: rapid and totally disorganized ventricular activity without discernible QRS complexes or T waves in the ECG.

Ventricular flutter: rapid, organized ventricular activity without discernible QRS complexes or T waves in the ECG.

Ventricular flutter/fibrillation: the spectrum of ventricular tachyarrhythmias that lack discernible QRS complexes or T waves in the ECG; these tachyarrhythmias produce ECG effects that range from gross undulations to no discernible electrical activity.

Ventricular tachycardia: a rhythm originating distal to the branching of the common bundle, with a ventricular contraction rate of ≥100 beats per minute.

REFERENCES

1. Shenasa M, Borggrefe M, Haverkamp W, et al. Ventricular tachycardia. *Lancet*. 1993;341:1512–1519.

2. Akhtar M, Gilbert C, Wolf FG, et al. Reentry within the His Purkinje system: elucidation of re-entrant circuit using right bundle-branch and His bundle recordings. *Circulation*. 1976;58:295.

3. Ben-David J, Zipes DP. Torsades de pointes and proarrhythmia. *Lancet*. 1993;341:1578–1582.

4. Toboul P. Torsades de pointes. In: Wellens HJJ, Kulbertus HE, eds. *What's New in Electrocardiography*. Boston, MA: Martinus Nijhoff; 1981:229.

5. Welch WJ. Sustained macroreentrant ventricular tachycardia. *Am Heart J*. 1982;104:166–169.

6. Lesch M, Lewis E, Humphries JO, et al. Paroxysmal ventricular tachycardia in the absence of organic heart disease: report of a case and review of the literature. *Ann Intern Med*. 1967;66:950–960.

7. Pedersen DH, Zipes DP, Foster PR, et al. Ventricular tachycardia and ventricular fibrillation in a young population. *Circulation*. 1979;60:988–997.

8. Fulton DR, Chung KJ, Tabakin BS, et al. Ventricular tachycardia in children without heart disease. *Am J Cardiol*. 1985;55:1328–1331.

9. Swartz MH, Teichholz LE, Donoso E. Mitral valve prolapse: a review of associated arrhythmias. *Am J Med*. 1977;62:377–389.

10. Wei JY, Bulkley BH, Schaeffer AH, et al. Mitral-valve prolapse syndrome and recurrent ventricular tachyarrhythmias: a malignant variant refractory to conventional drug therapy. *Ann Intern Med*. 1978;89:6–9.

11. Campbell TJ. Proarrhythmic actions of antiarrhythmic drugs: a review. *Aust N Z J Med*. 1990;20:275–282.

12. The Cardiac Arrhythmia Suppression Trial (CAST) Investigators. Preliminary report: effect of encainide and flecainide on mortality in a randomized trial of arrhythmia suppression after myocardial infarction. *N Engl J Med*. 1989;321:406–412.

13. Bolick DR, Hackel DB, Reimer KA, et al. Quantitative analysis of myocardial infarct structure in patients with ventricular tachycardia. *Circulation*. 1986;74:1266–1279.

14. Tchou P, Young P, Mahmud R, et al. Useful clinical criteria for the diagnosis of ventricular tachycardia. *Am J Med*. 1988;284:53–56.

15. Morady F, Baerman JM, DiCarlo LA Jr, et al. A prevalent misconception regarding wide-complex tachycardias. *JAMA*. 1985;254:2790–2792.

16. Marriott HJ. Differential diagnosis of supraventricular and ventricular tachycardia. *Geriatrics*. 1970;25:91–101.

17. Sandler IA, Marriott HJL. The differential morphology of anomalous ventricular complexes of RBBB-type in V1: ventricular ectopy versus aberration. *Circulation*. 1965; 31:551.

18. Swanick EJ, LaCamera F Jr, Marriott HJL. Morphologic features of right ventricular ectopic beats. *Am J Cardiol*. 1972;30:888–891.

19. Wellens HJJ, Bar FW, Vanagt EJ, et al. Medical treatment of ventricular tachycardia, considerations in the selection of patients for surgical treatment. *Am J Cardiol*. 1982;49:186–193.

20. Wellens HJJ, Bar FW, Lie KI. The value of the electrocardiogram in the differential diagnosis of a tachycardia with a widened QRS complex. *Am J Med*. 1978;64:27–33.

21. Switzer DF. Dire consequences of verapamil administration for wide QRS tachycardia. *Circulation*. 1986;74(suppl 2):105.

22. Dancy M, Camm AJ, Ward D. Misdiagnosis of chronic recurrent ventricular tachycardia. *Lancet*. 1985;2:320–323.

23. Stewart RB, Bardy GH, Greene HL. Wide-complex tachycardia: misdiagnosis and outcome after emergent therapy. *Ann Intern Med*. 1986;104:766–771.

24. Vera Z, Cheng TO, Ertem G, et al. His bundle electrography for evaluation of criteria in differentiating ventricular ectopy from aberrancy in atrial fibrillation. *Circulation*. 1972;45(suppl 2):355.

25. Gulamhusein S, Yee R, Ko PT, et al. Electrocardiographic criteria for differentiating aberrancy and ventricular extrasystole in chronic atrial fibrillation: validation by intracardiac recordings. *J Electrocardiol*. 1985;18:41–50.

26. Gozensky C, Thorne D. Rabbit ears: an aid in distinguishing ventricular ectopy from aberration. *Heart Lung*. 1974;3:634–636.

27. Brugada P, Brugada J, Mont L, et al. A new approach to the differential diagnosis of a regular tachycardia with a wide QRS complex. *Circulation*. 1991;83:1649–1659.

28. Rosenbaum MB. Classification of ventricular extrasystoles according to form. *J Electrocardiol*. 1969;2:289–297.

29. Wellens HJJ. The wide QRS tachycardias. *Ann Intern Med*. 1986;104:879.

30. Kindwall E, Brown JP, Josephson ME. ECG criteria for ventricular and supraventricular tachycardia in wide complex tachycardias with left bundle branch morphology. *J Am Coll Cardiol*. 1987;9:206A.

31. Drew BJ, Scheinman MM. Value of electrocardiographic leads MCL$_1$, MCL$_6$, and other selected leads in the diagnosis of wide QRS complex tachycardia. *J Am Coll Cardiol*. 1991;18:1025–1033.

32. Vandepol CJ, Farshidi A, Spielman SR, et al. Incidence and clinical significance of induced ventricular tachycardia. *Am J Cardiol*. 1980;45:725–731.

33. Josephson ME, Horowitz LN, Farshidi A, et al. Recurrent sustained ventricular tachycardia. I. Mechanisms. *Circulation*. 1978;57: 431–440.

34. Denes P, Wu D, Dhingra RC, et al. Electrophysiological studies in patients with chronic recurrent ventricular tachycardia. *Circulation*. 1976;54:229–236.

35. Pietras RJ, Mautner R, Denes P, et al. Chronic recurrent right and left ventricular tachycardia: comparison of clinical, hemodynamic and angiographic findings. *Am J Cardiol*. 1977;40:32–37.

36. Vetter VL, Josephson ME, Horowitz LN. Idiopathic recurrent sustained ventricular tachycardia in children and adolescents. *Am J Cardiol*. 1981;47:315–322.

37. Wu D, Kou HC, Hung JS. Exercise-triggered paroxysmal ventricular tachycardia: a repetitive rhythmic activity possibly related to afterdepolarization. *Ann Intern Med*. 1981;95:410–414.

38. Mokotoff DM. Exercise-induced ventricular tachycardia: clinical features, relation to chronic ventricular ectopy, and prognosis. *Chest*. 1980;77:10–16.

39. Kossmann CE. Torsade de pointes: an addition to the nosography of ventricular tachycardia. *Am J Cardiol*. 1978;42:1054–1056.

40. Smith WM, Gallagher JJ. "Les torsades de pointes": an unusual ventricular arrhythmia. *Ann Intern Med*. 1980;93:578–584.

41. Kay GN, Plumb VJ, Arcciniegas JG, et al. Torsade de pointes: the long-short initiating sequence and other clinical features: observations in 32 patients. *J Am Coll Cardiol*. 1983;2:806–817.

42. Soffer J, Dreifus LS, Michelson EL. Polymorphous ventricular tachycardia associated with normal and long Q-T intervals. *Am J Cardiol*. 1982;49:2021–2029.

43. Reynolds EW, Vandeer Ark CR. Quinidine syncope and the delayed repolarization syndromes. *Mod Concepts Cardiovasc Dis*. 1976;45:117–122.

44. Roden DM, Thompson KA, Hoffman BF, et al. Clinical features and the basic mechanisms of quinidine-induced arrhythmias. *J Am Coll Cardiol.* 1986;8:73A–78A.

45. Nicholson WJ, Martin CE, Gracey JG, et al. Disopyramide-induced ventricular fibrillation. *Am J Cardiol.* 1979;43:1053–1055.

46. Wald RW, Waxman MB, Colman JM. Torsades de pointes ventricular tachycardia: a complication of disopyramide shared with quinidine. *J Electrocardiol.* 1981;14:301–307.

47. Ludomirsky A, Klein HO, Sarelli P, et al. Q-T prolongation and polymorphous ("Torsades de pointes") ventricular arrhythmias associated with organic insecticide poisoning. *Am J Cardiol.* 1982;49:1654–1658.

48. Carruth JE, Silverman ME. Torsades de pointes: atypical ventricular tachycardia complicating subarachnoid hemorrhage. *Chest.* 1980;78:886–888.

49. Jervell A, Lange-Nielsen F. Congenital deaf-mutism, functional heart disease with prolongation of the Q-T interval and sudden death. *Am Heart J.* 1957;54:59.

50. Krikler DM, Curry PVL. Torsades de pointes, an atypical ventricular tachycardia. *Br Heart J.* 1976;38:117–120.

51. Lown B, Taylor J. Thump-version. *N Engl J Med.* 1978; 283:1223–1224.

52. Kempf FC, Josephson ME. Cardiac arrest recorded on ambulatory electrocardiograms. *Am J Cardiol.* 1984;53: 1577–1582.

53. Panadis IP, Morganroth J. Sudden death in hospitalized patients: cardiac rhythm disturbances detected by ambulatory electrocardiographic monitoring. *J Am Coll Cardiol.* 1983;2:798–805.

54. Bluzhas J, Lukshiene D, Shlapikiene B, et al. Relation between ventricular arrhythmia and sudden cardiac death in patients with acute myocardial infarction: the predictors of ventricular fibrillation. *J Am Coll Cardiol.* 1986;8(suppl 1A): 69A–72A.

20

Ventricular versus Supraventricular with Aberrant Conduction

GALEN S. WAGNER

Having considered all of the commonly occurring tachyarrhythmias, it may help to consider in depth the differential diagnosis of tachyarrhythmias of ventricular origin and tachyarrhythmias of supraventricular origin with aberrant ventricular conduction. The term "ventricular *ectopy*" is useful for indicating a ventricular origin for a given tachyarrhythmia because such arrhythmias range from a single wide premature beats PBs to sustained wide QRS complex tachyarrhythmias. The diagnostic differentiation of ventricular ectopy from aberrant conduction must be made whenever the QRS complex is "wide" (duration ≥120 milliseconds) because aberrancy does not always result in a QRS complex sufficiently wide as to "mimic" an arrhythmia of ventricular origin. Indeed, aberrancy often produces only minor distortion of the normal QRS complex, with little or no prolongation (<120 milliseconds).

In its general consideration, "aberrant" ventricular conduction occurs either intermittently or persistently in individuals with abnormalities of intraventricular conduction (see Chapter 6). Ventricular preexcitation (see Chapter 7) is also technically an aberrancy, but it is not considered again in this chapter. Aberrancy occurs when a supraventricular impulse encounters refractoriness in a part of the ventricular conduction system, usually because of a change in length of the cardiac cycle. Aberrancy is important because:

1. It is very common during paroxysmal tachyarrhythmias.
2. It is often overlooked, with the result that supraventricular arrhythmias are misdiagnosed as ventricular arrhythmias and are treated as such.

Almost all physicians are occasionally required to diagnose and treat cardiac arrhythmias and should therefore have the ability to differentiate between supraventricular and ventricular sites of their origin.

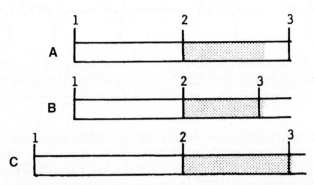

FIGURE 20.1. **A–C.** In the diagrams, 1, 2, and 3 are consecutive beats and the *stippled area* represents the refractory period of some part of the conducting system during the second cycle.

When responsive tissue reacts to a stimulus, the reaction is followed by a dormant interval (the refractory period) during which the tissue cannot respond to another stimulus. This period of rest is necessary for the tissue to recoup and return to a state in which it can again react normally to the stimulus. Characteristics of the refractory period differ for different portions of the conduction system. The His–Purkinje system usually exhibits an "all-or-none" response in contrast to the atrioventricular (AV) node, which exhibits a variable response.

The refractory period of the cardiac conducting pathways is proportional to the length of the preceding cycle (RR interval). Thus, the longer the cycle and slower the rate, the longer the ensuing refractory period, and vice versa. Ventricular aberration can therefore result from a shortened immediate cycle, an extended preceding cycle, or a combination of both (Fig. 20.1). When there are two regular cycles with normal conduction, as shown in Figure 20.1A, the conduction in the third beat (beat 3) is also normal. However, the conduction in the third beat may become aberrant (lower two diagrams) if either the second cycle is shortened (see Fig. 20.1B) or the first cycle is lengthened (see Fig. 20.1C). Shortening of the cycle (see Fig. 20.1B) may bring that beat within the refractory period of part of the conducting system. Lengthening of the preceding cycle (see Fig. 20.1C) prolongs the refractory period so that the next beat, although occurring no earlier than in the previous cycle, falls within the now longer refractory period.

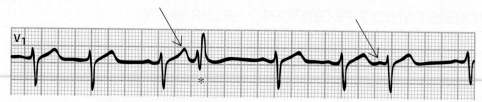

FIGURE 20.2. *Arrows* indicate the premature P waves initiating the fourth and the seventh cycles, and an *asterisk* indicates the right bundle branch aberrancy during the fourth cycle.

Figure 20.2 illustrates right-bundle-branch block (RBBB) aberration of atrial premature beats (APBs). The atrial extrasystole arises after three normally conducted beats, and its impulse arrives at the right bundle branch while the latter is still refractory. The extrasystole is therefore conducted with RBBB aberration. In Figure 20.2, the seventh beat is also an extrasystole, but it is less premature and is therefore conducted normally.

RBBB aberration is much more common (about 80% of all aberration) than is left-bundle-branch block (LBBB) aberration.[1,2] In an individual with cardiac disease, however, LBBB aberration constitutes a greater proportion (about 33%) of the aberrant conduction encountered. In a study by Kulbertus et al,[3] in which investigators were able to produce 116 different aberrant configurations by inducing APBs in 44 patients, RBBB accounted for only 53% of the experimentally produced aberrancies—a smaller than expected proportion.

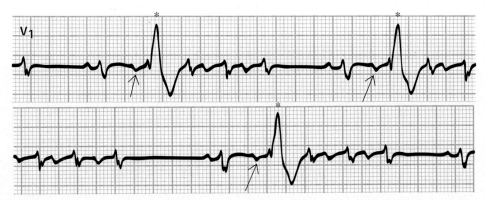

FIGURE 20.3. A continuous lead V1 rhythm strip from a patient with severe chronic obstructive pulmonary disease. *Arrows* indicate the three premature P waves and *asterisks* indicate the aberrantly conducted premature QRS complexes.

Aberrant conduction is a secondary phenomenon, always the result of some primary disturbance, and never requires treatment. At times, the morphology of the aberrant QRS complex is indistinguishable from ventricular ectopy. At other times, however, the morphologies of the QRS complexes provide hints of their having a supraventricular origin.

The first principle in the diagnosis of aberrancy is not to diagnose it unless there is evidence favoring it, because wide QRS complexes are more often produced by beats originating in the ventricular rather than in the supraventricular regions. An axiom in medical diagnosis is: "When you hear hoof beats, think first of a horse rather than a zebra—only consider a zebra if you see its stripes." The six key characteristics of aberration (its "stripes") are presented in Table 20.1.

The first four "stripes" are observable in Figure 20.3, in which the two continuous rhythm strips contain three clusters of rapid beats. Each cluster is initiated by a premature ectopic P wave (stripe 3). The third beat alone has a bizarre appearance (stripe 4). It has a triphasic (rsR′) RBBB pattern (stripe 1), with the initial deflection identical to that of the conducted sinus beats (stripe 2). These points clinch the recognition of aberration.

Table 20.1.
The "Stripes" of Aberration

1. Triphasic morphology
   a. rsR′ variant in V1
   b. qRs variant in V6

2. Initial deflection identical to normal beat (if RBBB)
3. Immediately preceding atrial activity
4. Second-in-the-row phenomenon
5. Alternating BBB patterns separated by single normal beat
6. Identical wide QRS pattern previously diagnosed as aberrancy

Triphasic Lead V1/V6 Morphology of the QRS Complex

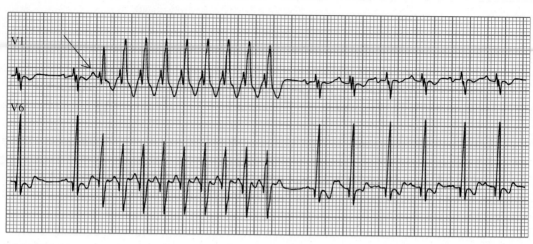

FIGURE 20.4. Simultaneous lead V1 and lead V6 rhythm strips from a woman with severe pulmonary emphysema. An *arrow* indicates the premature P wave.

The shape of the QRS complex is in many cases diagnostic of aberrancy. Triphasic contours (rsR′ in lead V1 and qRs in lead V6) heavily favor the diagnosis of aberration. Figure 20.4 illustrates an atrial tachyarrhythmia with RBBB aberration. The rsR′ pattern in lead V1 and the qRs pattern in lead V6 would each alone be virtually diagnostic of the supraventricular origin of this arrhythmia. Note that the sinus rhythm following termination of the tachyarrhythmia is rapid and irregular, as is typical with severe pulmonary disease (see Chapter 16).

Despite the availability of morphologic clues introduced during the past 40 years[2,4,5] and confirmed more recently,[6-9] many authors persist in ignoring them[10-12] and instead continue to give predominant and undue weight to the presence or absence of independent atrial activity. When independent atrial activity (AV dissociation) is evident, it is a most valuable clue to the diagnosis of ventricular tachycardia (VT). The presence of AV dissociation cannot, however, be relied upon, for three reasons:

1. AV dissociation is present in only a minority of VTs. In one carefully studied series, it was found in only 27 of 100.[13]
2. Even when AV dissociation is present, the independent P waves may be difficult or impossible to recognize in the clinical tracing.
3. Rarely, junctional tachyarrhythmias with bundle-branch block may be dissociated from an independent sinus rhythm (see Fig. 20.4).

Initial Deflection of the Abnormal Beat Is Identical to Normal Beat

There is no reason for a ventricular impulse to produce an initial deflection identical to that of a normally conducted supraventricular impulse. Conversely, because normal ventricular activation begins on the left side, RBBB does not interfere with initial activation unless there is also block in one fascicle of the left bundle. As a result, if a wide QRS complex has a pattern compatible with RBBB and begins with a deflection identical to that of conducted beats, aberration is probably the diagnosis.

Atrial Activity Immediately Preceding the Abnormal Ventricular Beat

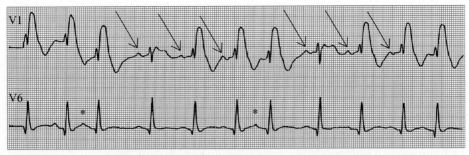

FIGURE 20.5. Simultaneous lead V1 and lead V6 rhythm strips from a woman with chronic angina who presented with severe chest pain. *Arrows* in lead V1 recording indicate sinus P waves preceding the normally and aberrantly conducted QRS complexes, and *asterisks* in lead V6 indicate premature P waves preceding the final (the third in the group of three) aberrantly conducted beats.

Sometimes, the diagnosis of aberration depends on the recognition of P waves preceding the abnormal QRS complex. Figure 20.5 illustrates several paroxysms of wide QRS complexes. A careful inspection reveals, however, that each group of three abnormal ventricular beats is preceded by a premature P wave, thereby confirming the diagnosis of aberrant conduction. The wide QRS complexes should be considered triphasic because there is a downward deflection between the r and K' waves that only sometimes penetrates below the baseline to form an S wave. Note that ventricular conduction becomes aberrant when a short, normal sinus cycle follows a long cycle that follows an APB, and returns to normal only when a long cycle after an APB follows a short cycle preceding the APB. This example also illustrates the value of recording at least two simultaneous ECG leads because the P waves in some cycles are visible only in lead V6, where there is minimal evidence of the aberrantly conducted QRS complexes.

Aberrant Beats Occurring Exclusively as the Second in a Row of Beats

The reason that only the second in a row of beats tends to be aberrant is that it is the only beat that ends a relatively short cycle preceded by a relatively long cycle (see Fig. 20.1). Because the refractory period of the conduction system is proportional to the length of the preceding ventricular cycle, the sequence of a long cycle (lengthening the subsequent refractory period) followed by a short cycle provides conditions for the development of aberration.

Alternating Patterns of Bundle-Branch Block Separated by a Single Normal Beat

When a pattern that could represent either LBBB or RBBB is separated by a single normally conducted beat from a pattern that could represent the other bundle-branch block, it should be strongly presumed that there is bilateral aberration rather than ectopy from alternate ventricles. (See text and Fig. 20.14 later in this chapter.)

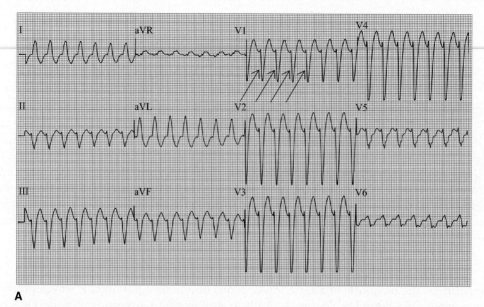

A

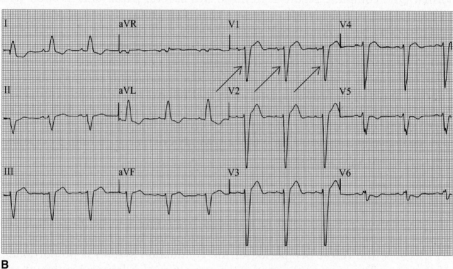

B

FIGURE 20.6. Twelve-lead ECGs from a patient in the postoperative recovery room after coronary artery bypass surgery. *Arrows* indicate the identical QRS complex appearances in the short-axis view in lead V1 during tachycardia **(A)** and preoperative normal sinus rhythm **(B)**.

If one is lucky enough to have available a previous recording that shows the same wide QRS pattern associated with sufficient "stripes" for the diagnosis of aberrancy, the arrhythmia in question is a supraventricular tachyarrhythmia (SVT) with aberrancy. Figure 20.6A shows a tachyarrhythmia that, although the smooth downstroke in lead V1 favors left bundle branch aberrancy, could also represent right-ventricular tachycardia. Figure 20.6B is a recording from the same patient taken 1 year earlier. Because this clearly shows sinus rhythm with LBBB and the QRS complexes of the two recordings are identical, the current tachyarrhythmia can be considered an SVT with left bundle branch aberrancy, most likely atrial flutter with 2:1 AV block.

VENTRICULAR ABERRATION COMPLICATING ATRIAL FLUTTER/FIBRILLATION

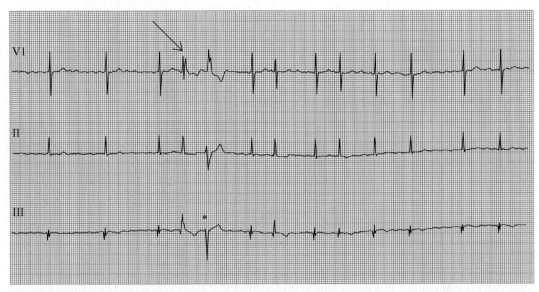

FIGURE 20.7. Simultaneous leads V1, II, and III rhythm strips from an elderly woman with a recent inferior-wall myocardial infarction. An *arrow* indicates the triphasic RsR' in lead V1 for the first wide QRS complex, and an *asterisk* indicates the oppositely directed initial deflection in lead III for the second wide QRS complex.

Ventricular aberration often complicates atrial flutter/fibrillation (see Chapter 17). Interruption of normal intraventricular conduction by wide QRS beats during atrial flutter/fibrillation is more likely to be due to aberration than to a coincidental ventricular premature beat (VPB) or (if there is a series of wide complexes) to VT. Because there is no preceding discrete atrial activity to indicate presence of aberrant conduction, one has to rely more heavily on the morphology of the wide QRS complexes to differentiate aberration from ventricular origin. Accordingly, the rsR' pattern in lead V1 or MCL$_1$ (Fig. 20.7), or the qRs pattern in lead V6, assists in establishing the diagnosis of aberrant conduction. Figure 20.7 provides contrast between an aberrantly conducted beat (the first wide QRS complex) and a VPB (the second wide QRS complex). Note that a short cycle following a long cycle sets the stage for aberrancy.

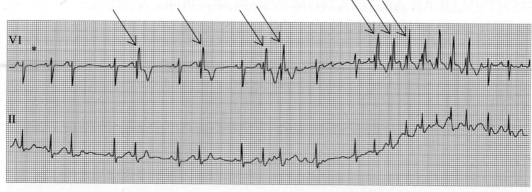

FIGURE 20.8. A lead V1 rhythm strip from an elderly patient with a history of paroxysmal atrial fibrillation. An *asterisk* indicates the normal T wave that allows identification of the subsequent premature P waves. *Arrows* indicate similar triphasic QRS complex morphology (rsR′) for the APBs during sinus rhythm and for the wide beats during atrial flutter/fibrillation.

Gouaux and Ashman[1] first drew attention to the principle that aberrant conduction was likely to complicate atrial flutter/fibrillation when a longer cycle was followed by a shorter cycle (Fig. 20.8). Aberration produced by a long–short sequence is sometimes referred to as the "Ashman phenomenon." It is important to understand that this cycle sequence cannot be used to differentiate aberration from ectopy because, by the *rule of bigeminy*, a lengthened cycle also tends to precipitate a ventricular extrasystole. Therefore, a long–short cycle sequence ending with a wide QRS complex is as likely to represent a VPB as an aberrant beat. Morphologic clues are important in distinguishing these phenomena. Note that in sinus rhythm, a premature P wave is confirmed only by reference to the normal biphasic T wave during the first cycle and that aberrancy occurs only when a long cycle has preceded the short cycle induced by an APB. The fifth premature P wave in Figure 20.8 initiates the atrial flutter/fibrillation.

Several other minor clues help to differentiate aberration from ventricular ectopy in the presence of atrial flutter/fibrillation.[4]

The Presence or Absence of a Longer Returning Cycle

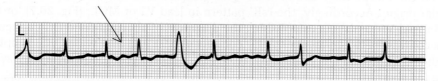

FIGURE 20.9. A lead II rhythm strip from an elderly man with chronic atrial flutter/fibrillation who was being evaluated for elective abdominal surgery. An *arrow* indicates the shorter rather than longer preceding cycle.

Ventricular ectopy tends to be followed by a longer returning cycle. This is because many ectopic ventricular impulses are conducted retrogradely into the AV node. The AV node is therefore made partly refractory by the retrograde invasion, so that the next several atrial impulses cannot penetrate to reach their ventricular destination.

As indicated, a long preceding cycle favors both aberration and ectopy and cannot be used as a point for differentiating the two. On the other hand, the absence of a longer preceding cycle is evidence against aberration and therefore favors ventricular ectopy (Fig. 20.9).

Comparative Cycle Sequences

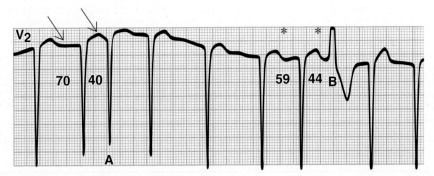

FIGURE 20.10. A lead V2 rhythm strip from a man with severe mitral regurgitation. *Arrows* indicate the even longer and even shorter preceding cycles for another normally conducted beat than for the wide beat (*asterisks*).

If a wide QRS complex ends a longer–shorter cycle sequence, differentiation between aberration and ventricular ectopy may be difficult. If an even longer cycle followed by an even shorter cycle is then followed by a normally conducted beat, the evidence against aberration is strong, and the diagnosis of ventricular ectopy is favored (Fig. 20.10).

Undue Prematurity

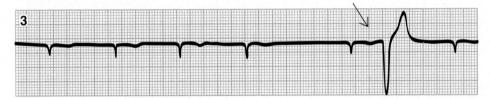

FIGURE 20.11. A lead V1 rhythm strip from a patient with atrial fibrillation following a recent anterior infarction. An *arrow* indicates the immediately preceding cycle, which is remarkably short in comparison with all others.

When so much AV block is present that all conducted cycles are long, the appearance of a wide QRS complex ending a cycle far shorter than any of the normally conducted beats favors the diagnosis of ectopy (Fig. 20.11). It is very unusual for a poorly conducting AV node to suddenly permit extremely early conduction to the ventricular Purkinje system. Note that the atrial flutter/fibrillation in the example shown in Figure 20.11 is so "fine" that, even in lead V1, no atrial activity is visible.

Fixed or Constant Coupling

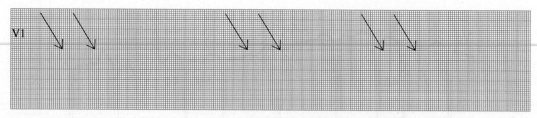

FIGURE 20.12. A lead V1 rhythm strip from an elderly patient with a recent anterior infarction. *Arrows* indicate the fixed intervals coupling all wide beats with their immediately preceding normally conducted beats.

Fixed or constant coupling as a clue to the distinction of aberration from ventricular ectopy is obviously applicable only if several wide QRS beats are available for comparison. If the interval between the normally conducted beat and the ensuing wide QRS beat is constant, ventricular ectopy is favored (Fig. 20.12). In the example, a "coarser" atrial flutter–fibrillation is present, and the absence of conduction with aberrancy is confirmed by variation of the intervals between the onsets of the wide QRS complexes and immediately preceding f waves.

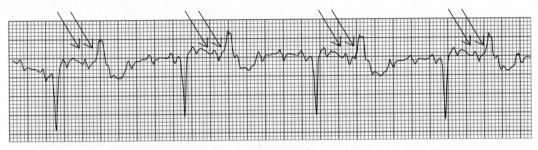

A

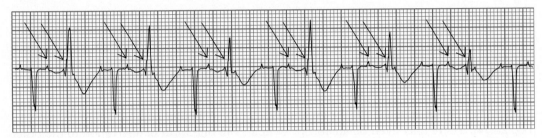

B

FIGURE 20.13. Lead V1 rhythm strips from two patients receiving pharmacologic therapy for atrial flutter complicating chronic heart failure. **A.** Digitalis has been administered to slow the ventricular rate. **B.** Quinidine has been added to the maintenance digitalis to attempt conversion to sinus rhythm. *Arrows* indicate the fixed "F-wave-to-wide-QRS" intervals in both **A** and **B**.

An extremely important form of aberration may complicate the flutter end of the atrial flutter/fibrillation spectrum. Atrial flutter usually manifests an AV conduction ratio of 2:1. If digitalis, propranolol, or verapamil is then administered, the conduction pattern often changes to alternating 2:1 and 4:1. The beats that end the shorter cycles may develop aberrant conduction (Fig. 20.13A), producing the fixed coupling typical of a bigeminal rhythm. If the patient is receiving digitalis, the fixed coupling is likely to evoke a diagnosis of ventricular ectopy and be attributed to digitalis toxicity. The still-needed digitalis is then wrongfully discontinued, when in fact the situation calls for more AV nodal blockade to further reduce conduction to a constant 4:1 with a normal ventricular rate, which is the appropriate goal of therapy. Figure 20.13B presents an example of fixed coupling occurring when slowing of the flutter rate (180 beats per minute) facilitates AV nodal conduction (3:2). In contrast with Figure 20.12, note the constant interval between the onsets of the wide QRS complexes and immediately preceding flutter waves in both Figure 20.13A and B.

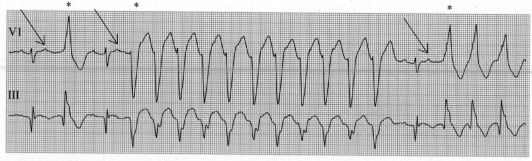

FIGURE 20.14. Simultaneous leads V1 and III rhythm strips from a patient with an acute inferior-wall myocardial infarction. *Arrows* indicate the premature P waves and *asterisks* indicate first the right bundle branch, then the left bundle branch, and then again the right bundle branch aberrancy.

There is a common tendency for an aberrancy of ventricular conduction to be bilateral (Fig. 20.14). There may even be an abrupt switch from one form of aberration to the other (from RBBB to LBBB or vice versa) via a single, intervening, normally conducted beat. This phenomenon is sufficiently characteristic to assist in differentiating bilateral aberrancy from bifocal ventricular ectopy. In Figure 20.14, the initiating premature P waves before each single wide QRS complex or series of wide QRS complexes ensures the supraventricular origin of the ectopy.

CRITICAL RATE

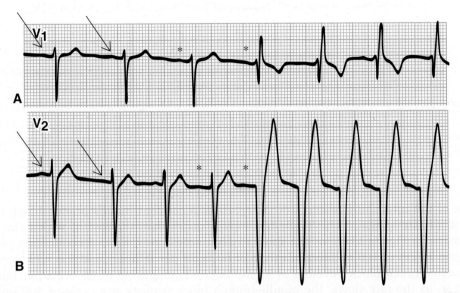

FIGURE 20.15. *Arrows* indicate the baseline atrial rate during normal condition and *asterisks* indicate the accelerated rate that produces the right bundle branch **(A)** and left bundle branch **(B)** aberration.

Most of the examples of aberration presented in the preceding sections occur because an impulse of supraventricular origin traverses the AV node early, suddenly creating a short ventricular cycle. However, aberration also may appear with the gradual acceleration of sinus rhythm. Figure 20.15 presents two examples of slight sinus acceleration in which the cardiac cycle gradually decreases until it becomes shorter than the refractory period of one of the bundle branches and aberrant conduction develops. The persisting refractoriness is encountered in the right bundle branch in the young healthy individual in Figure 20.15A and in an older patient with ischemic cardiomyopathy in Figure 20.15B. The wide QRS complexes will persist until the cycle lengthens sufficiently for normal conduction to occur.

The rate at which the bundle-branch block develops is known as the *critical rate*, and when such block comes and goes with changes in the heart rate, the condition is known as *rate-dependent bundle-branch block* (in this instance, *tachycardia-dependent bundle-branch block*). The tachycardia may be either true (>100 beats per minute) or relative (faster than the preexisting rate).

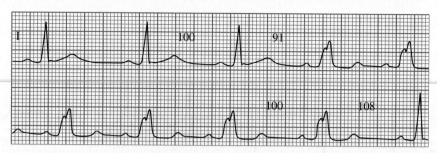

FIGURE 20.16. A continuous lead I rhythm strip from an elderly woman with chronic hypertension and cardiac failure. Numbers indicate the intervals between both normally and abnormally conducted beats (100 milliseconds), preceding the onset of left bundle branch branch aberrancy (91 milliseconds), and preceding the return to normal conduction (108 milliseconds).

One of the interesting features of tachycardia-dependent bundle-branch block is that the critical rate at which the block develops is faster than the rate at which the block disappears. In Figure 20.16, as the sinus rhythm accelerates, normal conduction prevails at a cycle length of 100 milliseconds (rate of 60 beats per minute), and the cycle at which the bundle-branch block develops is 91 milliseconds long (rate of 66 beats per minute). However, as the rate slows, the bundle-branch block persists at a cycle of 100 milliseconds (rate of 60 beats per minute), and for normal conduction to resume, the cycle must lengthen further to 108 milliseconds (rate of 56 beats per minute).

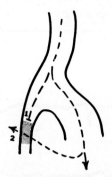

FIGURE 20.17. Diagram of the two mechanisms responsible for the difference in the critical rate during acceleration and deceleration. 1 indicates the inability of the supraventricular impulse to initially penetrate the right bundle branch, and 2 indicates subsequent penetration of the right bundle branch via the transseptal "detour."

There are two reasons for this difference in rate requirement for the development of bundle-branch block during acceleration and deceleration:

1. Because the refractory period of the ventricular conduction system is proportional to the length of the preceding ventricular cycle, it follows that as the ventricular rate accelerates, the refractory periods become progressively shorter (i.e., the potential for conduction progressively improves, and there is therefore a tendency to preserve normal conduction). The converse is true as the ventricular rate slows: Refractory periods become longer, and the potential for conduction diminishes, making aberration more likely.

2. More important, however, is the factor that is diagrammed in Figure 20.17. The shaded area in the right bundle branch indicates the refractory segment that fails to conduct when the impulse first arrives, causing RBBB aberration. An instant later, the refractory segment in the right bundle branch has recovered and is receptive for conduction of the impulse, which has meanwhile negotiated the left bundle branch. For the impulse to travel down the left bundle branch and through the interventricular septum to the distal right bundle branch requires about 0.06 second. Thus, the previously refractory right bundle branch is depolarized about 0.06 second after the beginning of the QRS complex. The conventional measurement of cycle length from the beginning of the final normal QRS complex to the beginning of ensuing wide QRS complex does not provide an indication of the time required for right bundle branch recovery; the cycle of the right bundle branch did not begin until halfway through the wide QRS complex. It follows that for normal conduction to resume, the critical cycle during deceleration must be longer than the critical cycle during acceleration by about 0.06 second. This calculation fits with the observed condition in Figure 20.16.

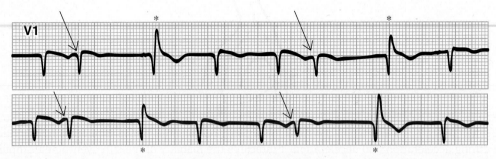

FIGURE 20.18. Lead V1 rhythm strip from a patient with acute anterior infarction. *Arrows* indicate the normally conducted APBs and *asterisks* indicate the right bundle branch aberration following the pauses.

Abnormal intraventricular conduction sometimes occurs only at the end of a lengthened ventricular cycle. Because one would expect conduction to be better after an extremely long ventricular cycle (because there is ample time for even the prolonged refractory period to be completed), the occurrence of this type of aberration seems paradoxical. It is referred to as *bradycardia-dependent bundle-branch block* and the bradycardia can be either true (<60 beats per minute) or relative (slower than the preexisting rate). The rate at which the bundle-branch block develops is known as the *paradoxical critical rate*. In Figure 20.18, normal conduction is present at a rate of 82 beats per minute, and the bundle-branch block develops only if the cycle length increases to a point equaling a rate of 68 beats per minute. The sinus rhythm is repeatedly interrupted by atrial extrasystoles. All of the conducted beats ending the lengthened cycles following extrasystolic beats show RBBB, but the shorter sinus cycles and the even shorter extrasystolic cycles show more normal intraventricular conduction. As with tachycardia-dependent bundle-branch block, the rate at which bradycardia-dependent bundle-branch block develops is known as the critical rate.

The cause of bradycardia-dependent bundle-branch block is the spontaneous depolarization of pacemaking cells in the bundle branches in an attempt to terminate the prolonged delay in the ventricular cycle. However, a supraventricular impulse arrives before these ventricular Purkinje cells achieve the threshold required for pacemaking or "capturing" the ventricular rhythm. The supraventricular impulse is conducted slowly through these bundle-branch cells because they are no longer in their fully repolarized state. The impulse is therefore conducted more rapidly through the uninvolved bundle branch, creating aberrancy.[17,18]

Ashman phenomenon: an aberration in the intraventricular conduction of an impulse that completes a short cardiac cycle following a long cycle because the long cycle results in delay of repolarization.

Bradycardia-dependent bundle-branch block: an aberration in conduction that develops because of a gradual deceleration of the sinus rhythm.

Critical rate: a cycle length so short that part of the ventricular Purkinje system has not yet recovered from its previous activation, resulting in aberrant conduction of a supraventricular impulse.

Ectopy: any number of beats, ranging from a single PB to a sustained tachyarrhythmia, arising from outside the sinus node.

Paradoxical critical rate: a cycle length so long that part of the ventricular Purkinje system has already begun the process of impulse formation and therefore conducts the supraventricular impulse so slowly that aberrancy occurs.

Rate-dependent bundle-branch block: an aberration that develops as the result of a gradual change in sinus rhythm.

Rule of bigeminy: the likelihood that a VPB will occur after a long cycle because the long cycle results in delay of repolarization, facilitating reentry of the impulse causing the VPB.

Tachycardia-dependent bundle-branch block: an aberration that develops because of a gradual acceleration of sinus rhythm.

REFERENCES

1. Gouaux JL, Ashman R. Auricular fibrillation with aberration simulating ventricular paroxysmal tachycardia. *Am Heart J.* 1947;34:366.

2. Sandler IA, Marriott HJL. The differential morphology of anomalous ventricular complexes of RBBB-type in lead V1; ventricular ectopy versus aberration. *Circulation.* 1965;31:551.

3. Kulbertus HE, de Laval-Rutten F, Casters P. Vectorcardiographic study of aberrant conduction; anterior displacement of QRS, another form of intraventricular block. *Br Heart J.* 1976;38:549–557.

4. Marriott HJL, Sandler IA. Criteria, old and new, for differentiating between ectopic ventricular beats and aberrant ventricular conduction in the presence of atrial fibrillation. *Prog Cardiovasc Dis.* 1966;9:18.

5. Marriott HJL. Differential diagnosis of supraventricular and ventricular tachycardia. *Geriatrics.* 1970;25:91–101.

6. Gulamhusein S, Yee R, Ko PT, et al. Electrocardiographic criteria for differentiating aberrancy and ventricular extrasystole in chronic atrial fibrillation: validation by intracardiac recordings. *J Electrocardiol.* 1985;18:41–50.

7. Vera Z, Cheng TO, Ertem G, et al. His bundle electrography for evaluation of criteria in differentiating ventricular ectopy from aberrancy in atrial fibrillation. *Circulation.* 1972;45[Suppl II]:355.

8. Wellens HJJ, Bar FW, Lie KI. The value of the electrocardiogram in the differential diagnosis of a tachycardia with a widened QRS complex. *Am J Med.* 1978;64:27–33.

9. Wellens HJJ, Bar FW, Vanagt EJ, et al. Medical treatment of ventricular tachycardia; considerations in the selection of patients for surgical treatment. *Am J Cardiol.* 1982;49:186–193.

10. Bailey JC. The electrocardiographic differential diagnosis of supraventricular tachycardia with aberrancy versus ventricular tachycardia. *Pract Cardiol.* 1980;6:118.

11. Pietras RJ, Mautner R, Denes P, et al. Chronic recurrent right and left ventricular tachycardia: comparison of clinical, hemodynamic and angiographic findings. *Am J Cardiol.* 1977;40:32–37.

12. Zipes DP. Diagnosis of ventricular tachycardia. *Drag Ther.* 1979;9:83.

13. Niazi I, McKinney J, Caceres J, et al. Reevaluation of surface ECG criteria for the diagnosis of wide QRS tachycardia. *Circulation.* 1987;76(suppl IV):412.

14. Marriott HJL, Bieza CF. Alarming ventricular acceleration after lidocaine administration. *Chest.* 1972;61:682–683.

15. Sherf L, James TN. A new electrocardiographic concept: synchronized sinoventricular conduction. *Dis Chest*. 1969;55:127–140.

16. Kistin AD. Problems in the differentiation of ventricular arrhythmia from supraventricular arrhythmia with abnormal QRS. *Prog Cardiovasc Dis*. 1966;9:1.

17. Gambetta M, Childers RW. Reverse rate related bundle branch block. *J Electrocardiol*. 1973;6:153–157.

18. Massumi RA. Bradycardia-dependent bundle branch block. A critique and proposed criteria. *Circulation*. 1968;38: 1066–1073.

21

Decreased Automaticity

GALEN S. WAGNER

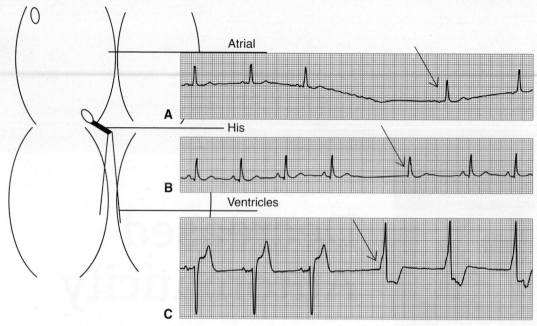

FIGURE 21.1. The *small ovals* in the schematic diagram indicate the SA and AV nodes, and the common bundle (*His*) and bundle branches are shown to lead toward the ventricles from the AV node. *Arrows* indicate the atrial **(A)**, His-bundle **(B)**, and ventricular escape **(C)** beats that terminate the pauses after the sinus node has failed to maintain its dominant rhythmicity. (From Wagner GS, Waugh RA, Ramo BW. *Cardiac Arrhythmias*. New York, NY: Churchill Livingstone; 1983:4, with permission.)

When the automaticity of the sinus node is decreased, the result is a bradyarrhythmia originating either from the sinus node itself or from a "lower" site in the pacemaking and conduction system that spontaneously depolarizes to maintain a cardiac rhythm (see Fig. 1.7). When the decelerated rhythm originates from the sinus node, the term *sinus bradycardia* is used; when it originates from a lower site, the terms *atrial rhythm, junctional rhythm*, or *ventricular rhythm* are used. These are not truly arrhythmias but rather *escape rhythms* that attempt to compensate for the problem of decreased sinus node automaticity. Figure 21.1 illustrates the various consequences of the slowing of sinus automaticity to <60 beats per minute. The automaticity of the distal sites is suppressed if the sinus node is pace-making normally, but their automaticity returns (escapes) at its own, slower rate when the sinus node fails. Escape beats emerge from an atrial (see Fig. 21.1A), His bundle (see Fig. 21.1B), or ventricular Purkinje (see Fig. 21.1C) site after the sinus impulses fail to appear.

There are three causes of decreased automaticity:

1. Physiologic slowing of the sinus rate.
2. Physiologic or pathologic enhancement of parasympathetic nervous activity.
3. Pathologic pacemaker failure

MECHANISMS OF BRADYARRHYTHMIAS OF DECREASED AUTOMATICITY

Physiologic Slowing of the Sinus Rate

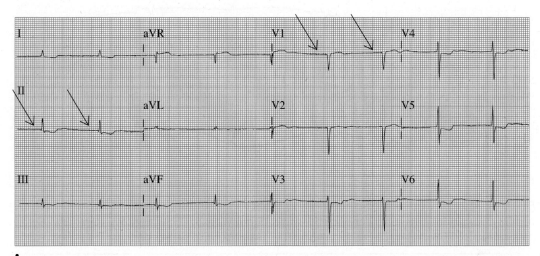

A

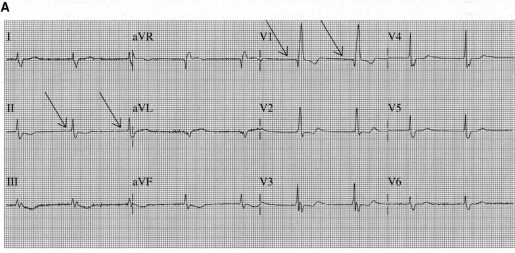

B

FIGURE 21.2. Twelve-lead ECGs from **(A)** a woman receiving β-adrenergic–blocking therapy for ischemic heart disease and **(B)** an otherwise healthy man on the day after prostate surgery. *Arrows* indicate complete absence of P waves preceding the normal **(A)** and abnormally wide QRS complexes **(B)**.

Although a rate of <60 beats per minute is technically termed a "bradyarrhythmia," it is often a normal variation of cardiac rhythm (especially in trained athletes, whose heart rates may be as low as in the 30s of beats per minute at rest). The rhythm may be either sinus bradycardia or, as shown in Figure 21.2, a junctional (see Fig. 21.2A) or ventricular (see Fig. 21.2B) escape rhythm. Bradycardia is a physiologic reaction to relaxation or sleep, when the parasympathetic effect on cardiac automaticity dominates over the sympathetic effect. Even during the expiratory phase of the respiratory cycle, there is slowing of the sinus rate, often into the bradycardic range (see Fig. 3.15). The lead V1–positive QRS complexes in Figure 21.2B indicate that the escape site is in the left bundle.

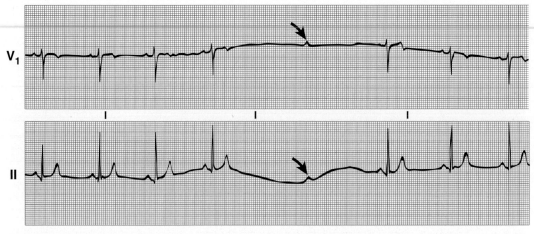

FIGURE 21.3. Simultaneous recording of leads V1 and II from a patient soon after cholecystectomy. *Arrows* indicate a nonconducted P wave. (From Wagner GS, Waugh RA, Ramo BW. *Cardiac Arrhythmias.* New York, NY: Churchill Livingstone; 1983:208, with permission.)

All cells with pacemaking capability are under some influence of the sympathetic and parasympathetic divisions of the autonomic nervous system. This influence is greatest in the sinus node and diminishes in the lower sites with pacemaking capacity. Usually, the changing autonomic balance causes a gradual increase or decrease in the pacing rate. However, many factors can induce a sudden increase in parasympathetic activity and decrease in sympathetic activity. These factors include:

1. Carotid sinus massage.
2. Hypersensitivity of the carotid sinus.
3. Straining (i.e., a Valsalva maneuver).
4. Ocular pressure.
5. Increased intracranial pressure.
6. Sudden movement from a recumbent to an upright position.
7. Drugs that cause pooling of blood by dilating the veins.

This increase in parasympathetic activity is termed a *vasovagal reaction* (*vasovagal reflex*) because it has a prominent component of vascular relaxation in addition to cardiac slowing and because it is mediated by the vagus nerve. Typical bradyarrhythmias that occur suddenly during a vasovagal reaction are presented in Figure 21.3. A sudden increase in parasympathetic activity is manifested by both slowing of the sinus rate and failure of atrioventricular (AV) conduction (note the nonconducted P wave in the electrocardiogram [ECG] shown in Fig. 21.3). The increase in parasympathetic activity also suppresses escape pacemakers, and the resulting pause is interrupted only by the return of sinus rhythm. The combination of vascular relaxation and cardiac slowing results in a reduction in cardiac output so severe that it may cause dizziness or even loss of consciousness. This is termed *vasovagal syncope* or fainting. It is typically reversed when the individual falls into a recumbent position, thereby increasing venous return to the heart. When a person who has fainted is encountered, consciousness can usually be restored by lowering the head and chest and elevating the legs.

A single physiologic vasovagal reaction can have severe pathologic consequences if the individual is injured during a consequent fall or if the change in body position required to restore venous return to the heart is not possible. Indeed, the autonomic reflex itself may become pathologic, resulting in *neurocardiogenic syncope*.[1-3] Repeated, severe, and sudden episodes of bradyarrhythmia with vasodilation require medical intervention to prevent serious injury or death.

Pathologic Pacemaker Failure

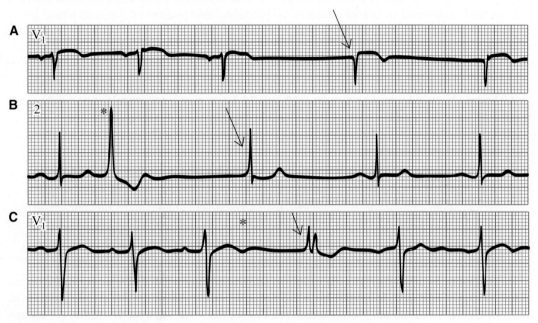

FIGURE 21.4. Rhythm strips from three individuals during postoperative monitoring: lead V1 **(A and C)** and lead II **(B)**. *Arrows* indicate junctional escape beats in **A** and **B** and the ventricular escape beat in **C**. *Asterisks* indicate the ventricular premature beat in **B** and nonconducted APB in **C**. (From Marriott HJL. *ECG/PDQ*. Baltimore, MD: Williams & Wilkins; 1987:171, with permission.)

When a sudden period of complete absence of P waves appears in the ECG, the term *asystole* is used. The term *sick sinus syndrome* is often applied to this situation; it is tempting to attribute the problem solely to the sinus node and pathologic pacemaker failure. However, if the problem was indeed limited to the sinus node, it would not produce any serious bradyarrhythmia because a 1- to 2-second pause in sinus rhythm would be interrupted by escape from a lower site with the capacity for impulse formation (Fig. 21.4). After three sinus beats (see Fig. 21.4A), there is no further evidence of atrial activity, but then two junctional escape beats result. The pause following a ventricular premature beat (see Fig. 21.4B) ends with a junctional escape beat. After three sinus beats (see Fig. 21.4C), a nonconducted atrial premature beat (APB) provides a cycle long enough for the ventricular Purkinje system to provide an escape beat. Therefore, a prolonged atrial pause is caused by either:

1. Enhanced parasympathetic activity or
2. Impairment of all cells with impulse formation capability.

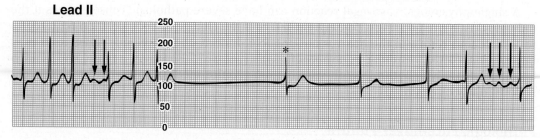

Lead II

FIGURE 21.5. A lead II rhythm strip from a patient with paroxysmal atrial fibrillation. *Arrows* indicate the F waves and an *asterisk* indicates the junctional escape after a 2.5-second pause. (From Wagner GS, Waugh RA, Ramo BW. *Cardiac Arrhythmias.* New York, NY: Churchill Livingstone; 1983:210, with permission.)

Although "sick pacemaker syndrome" would be a more accurate term, "sick sinus syndrome" is used here because of its general acceptance. Its characteristics are:

1. Bradyarrhythmia at rest.
2. Incapability to appropriately increase the pacemaking rate with increased sympathetic nervous activity.
3. Absence of escape rhythms when the sinus rate slows.
4. Sensitivity to suppression of impulse formation by various drugs.
5. Sensitivity to suppression of impulse formation during a reentrant tachyarrhythmia[4,5] (Fig. 21.5).

In the example of atrial flutter/fibrillation shown in Figure 21.5, the arrhythmia terminated abruptly and was followed by a 2.5-second pause. All potential atrial, junctional, and ventricular pacemakers were suppressed during the atrial tachyarrhythmia. An escape junctional pacemaker eventually emerged. After three beats, atrial reentry recurred and atrial flutter/fibrillation reappeared.

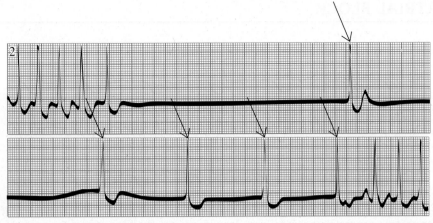

FIGURE 21.6.   A lead II rhythm strip from a patient with history of recurrent syncopal episodes. *Arrows* indicate the junctional escape rhythm following the initial failure of emergence of an adequate escape rhythm.

Sick sinus syndrome is a part of the *tachycardia–bradycardia syndrome*[6,7] in which bursts of an atrial tachyarrhythmia, often atrial fibrillation, alternate with prolonged pauses. In Figure 21.6, an irregular atrial tachyarrhythmia (probably atrial fibrillation) stops abruptly and is followed by a 4-second pause. Because the sinus node fails to establish a rhythm, there is only slow junctional escape and then the return of an atrial tachyarrhythmia.

Although sick sinus syndrome predominantly affects the elderly, it has been recognized as early as the first day of life.[8] Temporary and reversible manifestations of the syndrome can be caused by digitalis, quinidine, β-blockers, or aerosol propellants. The chronically progressive sick sinus syndrome was formerly believed to be due to ischemia, but a postmortem angiographic study of the sinus nodal artery confirmed vascular involvement in fewer than one third of 25 subjects with the chronic syndrome.[9] Sick sinus syndrome may result from inflammatory diseases, cardiomyopathy, amyloidosis,[10] collagen disease, metastatic disease, or surgical injury. In many patients, no cause is evident, and the syndrome is therefore classified as idiopathic. In these patients, it may be part of a sclerodegenerative process also affecting the lower parts of the cardiac pacemaking and conduction systems. Two complications that affect the prognosis of patients with sick sinus syndrome are atrial fibrillation and AV block. During a 3-year follow-up study, atrial fibrillation developed in 16% and AV block developed in 8% of patients.[11]

The diagnosis of sick sinus syndrome can usually be made from the standard ECG or from a 24-hour Holter recording carefully correlated with the patient's clinical history. Pauses of ≥3 seconds in sinus rhythm, although uncommon, do not necessarily indicate a poor prognosis, cause symptoms, or require artificial pacemaker implantation if the patient is asymptomatic.[12] In some patients, definitive tests may be required. One of the best of these is measurement of the sinus node recovery time after rapid atrial pacing, which is useful in recognizing sinoatrial (SA) block as the underlying mechanism for sick sinus syndrome.[13-15] Disorders of cardiac impulse formation probably account for half of all implantations of permanent pacemakers.[16]

SINOATRIAL BLOCK

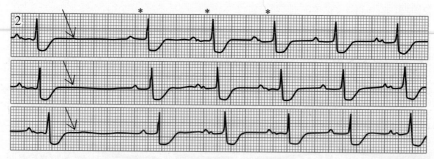

FIGURE 21.7. A continuous lead II rhythm strip from an elderly patient receiving digitalis therapy for chronic congestive heart failure. *Arrows* indicate the times when P waves should have emerged from the sinus node pacemaker, and *asterisks* indicate the accompanying first-degree AV block (PR interval = 0.28 second).

Although SA block is caused by failure of an impulse to emerge from the sinus node, it is often impossible to determine whether this or some other mechanism is responsible for an absent P wave. SA block should be diagnosed only when a mathematical relationship between the longer and shorter sinus cycles can be demonstrated or when the sinus cycles show the characteristic classical Wenckebach sequence of Mobitz type I block (see Chapter 22).

SA block is characterized by the intermittent failure of an impulse to emerge from the SA node, resulting in the occasional complete absence of beats (Fig. 21.7). The long cycle at the beginning of each strip is due to an absent sinus beat, in which an entire P–QRS–T sequence is missing. Note that the pauses are approximately equal to twice the observed sinus cycle length. When no such pattern can be established, "sinus pause" is a useful and appropriate term for the abnormally long cycle, accompanied by indication of its duration (e.g., a 4.5-second sinus pause).

PERSPECTIVE ON SINUS PAUSES

Although sudden pauses in sinus rhythm are common and important arrhythmias, it is often impossible to determine their etiology with the standard ECG or any other clinical test. When the sinus pauses are brief, the differential diagnosis includes sinus node failure, SA block, and an APB that fails to conduct to the ventricles (see Chapter 15). It is often impossible to reach a conclusion about the etiology of a sudden sinus pause because underlying sinus arrhythmia makes it difficult to determine whether the pause is a precise multiple of the PP interval (see Fig. 21.7). Also, when a nonconducted APB is present, the premature P wave is often obscured by a T wave (see Figs. 15.7 and 15.8).

When sudden pauses in sinus rhythm are prolonged, nonconducted APBs are not a consideration, and failure of all pacemaking cells, rather than only of the sinus node, must be considered. The differentiation of abnormal control of these pacemakers by the autonomic nervous system from abnormality within the pacemaking cells is often difficult to make.

When pauses in sinus rhythm are brief, no clinical intervention is required, and the patient may not be at future risk for either the generalized pacemaker failure or autonomic abnormality that produces prolonged pauses. When sinus pauses are prolonged, it may be necessary to proceed with treatment without differentiating between a neurologic and cardiologic etiology.

GLOSSARY

Asystole: a pause in the cardiac electrical activity with neither atrial nor ventricular waveforms present on the ECG.

Atrial rhythm: a rhythm with a rate of <100 beats per minute and with abnormally directed P waves (indicating origination from a site in the atria other than the sinus node) preceding each QRS complex.

Escape rhythms: rhythms that originate from sites in the pacemaking and conduction system other than the sinus node after a pause created by the failure of either normal sinus impulse formation or AV impulse conduction.

Junctional rhythm: a rhythm with a rate of <100 beats per minute with an inverted P-wave direction visible in the frontal plane leads and normally appearing QRS complexes. The P waves may precede or follow the QRS complexes or may be obscured because they occur during the QRS complexes.

Neurocardiogenic syncope: a condition that occurs when an individual experiences a vasovagal reaction that causes loss of consciousness. It may be diagnosed by using a head-up tilt test.

Sick sinus syndrome: inadequate function of cardiac cells with pacemaking capability, resulting in continuous or intermittent slowing of the heart rate at rest and an inability to appropriately increase the rate with exercise.

Tachycardia–bradycardia syndrome: a condition in which both rapid and slow cardiac rhythms are present. The rapid rhythms tend to appear when the rate slows abnormally, whereas the slow rhythms are prominent immediately after the sudden cessation of a rapid rhythm.

Vasovagal reaction (vasovagal reflex): sudden slowing of the heart rate either from decreased impulse formation (sinus pause) or decreased impulse conduction (AV block) resulting from increased activity of the parasympathetic or decreased activity of the sympathetic nervous system. The slowing of the cardiac rhythm is accompanied by peripheral vascular dilation.

Vasovagal syncope: loss of consciousness caused by a vasovagal reaction. Consciousness is almost always regained when the individual falls into a recumbent position because this results in increased venous return to the heart.

Ventricular rhythm: a rhythm with a rate of <100 beats per minute with abnormally wide QRS complexes. There may be either retrograde association or AV dissociation.

REFERENCES

1. Abboud FM. Neurocardiogenic syncope. *N Engl J Med.* 1993;328:1117–1120.
2. Fouad FM, Siitthisook S, Vanerio G, et al. Sensitivity and specificity of the tilt table test in young patients with unexplained syncope. *Pace.* 1993;16:394–400.
3. Thilenius OG, Ryd KJ, Husayni J. Variations in expression and treatment of transient neurocardiogenic instability. *Am J Cardiol.* 1992;69:1193–1195.
4. Lown B. Electrical reversion of atrial fibrillation. *Br Heart J.* 1967;29:469–489.
5. Ferrer MI. *The Sick Sinus Syndrome.* Mt. Kisco, NY: Futura Publishing; 1974.
6. Kaplan BM, Langendorf R, Lev M, et al. Tachycardia-bradycardia syndrome (so-called "sick sinus syndrome"). *Am J Cardiol.* 1973;31:497–508.
7. Moss AJ, Davis RJ. Brady-Tachy syndrome. *Prog Cardiovasc Dis.* 1974;16:439–454.
8. Ector H, Van der Hauwaert LG. Sick sinus syndrome in childhood. *Br Heart J.* 1980;44:684–691.
9. Shaw DB, Linker NJ, Heaver PA, et al. Chronic sinoatrial disorder (sick sinus syndrome): a possible result of cardiac ischemia. *Br Heart J.* 1987;58:598–607.
10. Evans R, Shaw DB. Pathological studies in sinoatrial disorder (sick sinus syndrome). *Br Heart J.* 1977;39:778–786.

11. Sutton R, Kenny RA. The natural history of sick sinus syndrome. *Pacing Clin Electrophysiol.* 1986;9:1110–1114.

12. Hilgard J, Ezri MD, Denes P. Significance of ventricular pauses of three seconds or more detected on twenty-four-hour Holter recordings. *Am J Cardiol.* 1984;55:1005.

13. Chung EK. Sick sinus syndrome: current views. Part II. *Mod Concepts Cardiovasc Dis.* 1980;49:67–70.

14. Gann D, Tolentino A, Samet P. Electrophysiologic evaluation of elderly patients with sinus bradycardia. *Ann Intern Med.* 1979;90:24–29.

15. Yeh SJ, Lin FC, Wu D. Complete sinoatrial block in two patients with bradycardia-tachycardia syndrome. *J Am Coll Cardiol.* 1987;9:1184–1188.

16. Kaplan BM. Sick sinus syndrome. *Arch Intern Med.* 1978;138:28.

22

Atrioventricular Block

GALEN S. WAGNER

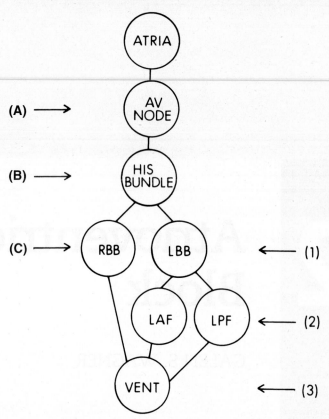

FIGURE 22.1. Figure 6.1 is reproduced here to schematically illustrate the anatomic layers of AV-junctional (AV node [A] and His bundle [B]) and ventricular (RBB and LBB [C]) structures potentially capable of causing AV block. The numbers 1, 2, and 3 are anatomic structures in the ventricles incapable of initiating a narrow (<0.12 second) QRS complex.

Atrioventricular (AV) block refers to an abnormality in electrical conduction between the atria and ventricles. The term *heart block* has also been used to describe this abnormality. Normal AV conduction was discussed in Chapter 3, and the parts of the cardiac pacemaking and conduction system that electrically connect the atrial and ventricular myocardia are illustrated in Figure 22.1. The term *degree* is used to indicate the severity of AV block. This severity varies from minor (first degree), in which all impulses are conducted with delay; through moderate (second degree), in which some impulses are not conducted; to complete (third degree), in which no impulses are conducted. Any of these three levels of severity of AV block can be caused by conduction abnormality in the AV node (level A in Fig. 22.1), His bundle (level B in Fig. 22.1), or both the right bundle branch (RBB) and left bundle branch (LBB) (level C in Fig. 22.1).

SEVERITY OF ATRIOVENTRICULAR BLOCK

First-Degree Atrioventricular Block

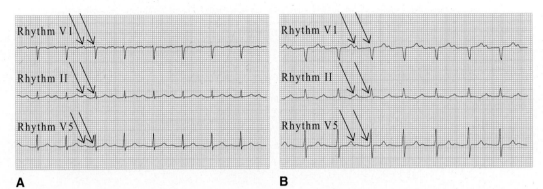

FIGURE 22.2. Simultaneous three-lead (V1, II, and V5) rhythm strips showing examples of first-degree AV block from healthy patient **(A)** and a **(B)** woman receiving no medications. *Arrows* indicate PR intervals of 0.25 **(A)** and 0.35 second **(B)**.

The "normal" PR interval has a duration of 0.12 to 0.20 second. *First-degree* AV *block* is generally defined as a prolongation of AV conduction time (PR interval) to >0.20 second. In analyses of records from normal young persons, the incidence of first-degree block by this definition ranged from 0.5%[1] to 2%.[2] In healthy middle-aged men, a prolonged PR interval in the presence of a normal QRS complex was found not to affect prognosis and to be unrelated to ischemic heart disease.[3] Figure 22.2 illustrates two examples of first-degree AV block. The first of these (see Fig. 22.2A) is minor, with a PR interval of 0.24 second, and the second (see Fig. 22.2B) shows extreme PR lengthening. Note that in Figure 22.2B, the P wave is superimposed on the T wave of the preceding cycle.

Second-Degree Atrioventricular Block

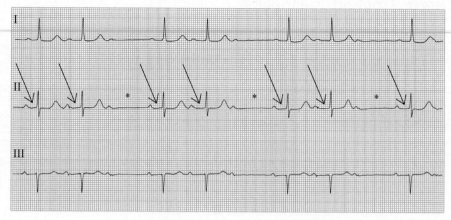

FIGURE 22.3.   Leads I, II, and III rhythm strips from an elderly patient receiving digitalis therapy for chronic heart failure. *Arrows* indicate first-degree AV block and *asterisks* indicate second-degree AV block.

By definition, *second-degree AV block* is present when one or more, but not all, atrial impulses fail to reach the ventricles. Examples of atrial premature beats that are not conducted because they occur early were presented in Chapter 15 (see Figs. 15.7 and 15.8). This situation is not considered AV block because it is normal. Figure 22.3 presents an example of both first- and second-degree AV block in which on-time P waves either have delayed AV conduction (first and second cycles of the series) or no AV conduction (third cycle).

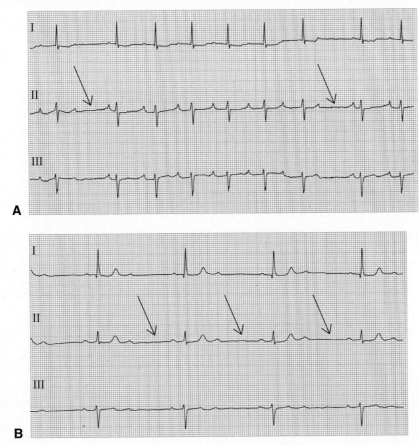

FIGURE 22.4. Leads I, II, and III rhythm strips from a patient with chronic pulmonary disease and receiving digitalis therapy **(A)** and a woman with hypertension and receiving both β-adrenergic and calcium antagonist therapy **(B)**. *Arrows* indicate failure of AV conduction and therefore the presence of second-degree AV block.

A second-degree AV block may be intermittent (Fig. 22.4A) or continuous (see Fig. 22.4B). Note that in Figure 22.4A, the second-degree block occurs only after a sequence of six conducted beats, of which the first shows no AV block and the latter five show first-degree block (7:6 block). In Figure 22.4B, there is continually alternating first- and second-degree AV block with a 2:1 AV ratio. This is termed 2:1 (AV) block.

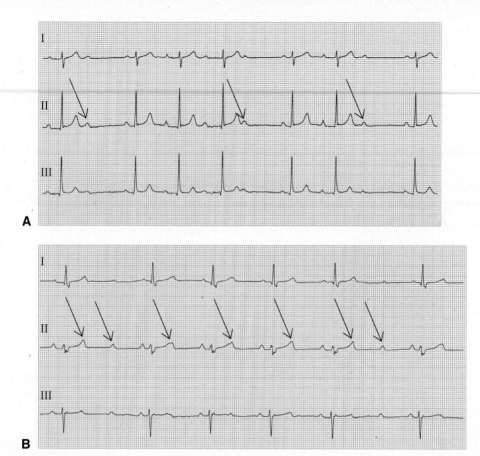

FIGURE 22.5. Leads I, II, and III rhythm strips from a patient with chronic bronchitis and cor pulmonale **(A)** and a 79-year-old woman with acute pulmonary edema **(B)**, both of whom were receiving long-term digitalis therapy for heart failure. *Arrows* indicate P waves that completely fail to conduct to the ventricles.

Second-degree AV block may have any ratio of P waves to QRS complexes (Fig. 22.5). In Figure 22.5A, there are the commonly appearing 3:2 and 4:3 AV conduction ratios. However, in Figure 22.5B the sinus rate is in the tachycardia range, and the more rapid "bombardment" of the AV node causes the 2:1 ratio to be intermittently increased to 3:1.

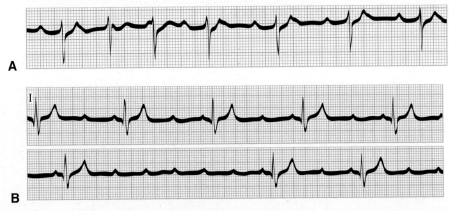

FIGURE 22.6. Lead II rhythm strips from elderly patients receiving digitalis therapy. The ventricular rates are in the normal (60 to 100 beats per minute) **(A)** and bradycardic (15 to 40 beats per minute) **(B)** ranges. Note the prolonged pause in the ventricular rhythm (3.5 seconds) in **B**.

When determining the clinical significance of second-degree AV block, the atrial rate should be considered. As discussed in Chapter 17, conduction of some, but not all, atrial impulses is essential for clinical stability in the presence of atrial flutter/fibrillation. Chapter 16 (see Fig. 16.6) indicates that second-degree AV block commonly occurs along with atrial tachycardia, particularly when there is digitalis toxicity. When "AV block" occurs in the presence of an atrial tachyarrhythmia, the block itself is considered a normal occurrence and not an additional arrhythmia (Fig. 22.6A) unless the ventricular rate is reduced into the bradycardic range (see Fig. 22.6B).

When both second-degree AV block and sinus pauses are present (see Chapter 21), the cause is most likely not within the heart itself but rather in its autonomic nervous control. Second-degree AV block usually occurs in the AV node[4,5] and is associated with reversible conditions such as the acute phase of an inferior myocardial infarction or treatment with digitalis, a β-adrenergic blocker, or a calcium channel–blocking drug. Because second-degree AV block is generally a transient disturbance in rhythm, it seldom progresses to complete AV block. However, in one study of 16 children manifesting second-degree AV block, 7 developed complete block.[6] Chronic second-degree AV block may occasionally occur in many conditions, including aortic valve disease, atrial septal defect, amyloidosis, Reiter syndrome, and mesothelioma of the AV node.

Third-Degree Atrioventricular Block

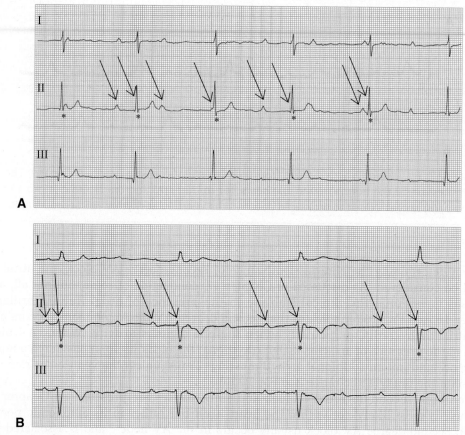

FIGURE 22.7. Leads I, II, and III rhythm strips from two patients presenting with complaints of dyspnea on exertion. *Arrows* indicate the varying PR-interval relationships and *asterisks* indicate the regular junctional **(A)** and ventricular **(B)** escape rates.

When no atrial impulses are conducted to the ventricles, the cardiac rhythm is termed "third-degree AV block," and the clinical condition is determined by the escape capability of the more distal Purkinje cells. The junctional or ventricular escape rhythm in the presence of third-degree AV block is almost always precisely regular because these sites are not as influenced by the sympathetic/parasympathetic balance as is the sinus node. Figure 22.7A shows junctional escape in a case of third-degree AV block, but Figure 22.7B shows ventricular escape, which occurs at a slower rate.

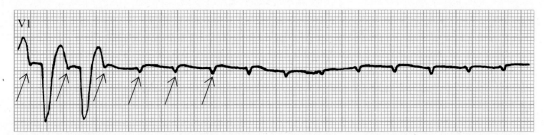

FIGURE 22.8. A lead V1 rhythm strip from elderly patient on telemetry monitoring during hospitalization following an episode of syncope. *Arrows* indicate the continuing sinus tachycardia before and after the onset of complete AV block.

In most clinical instances, complete AV block is at least partly compensated by an escape rhythm originating from an area distal to the site of the block. However, complete AV block of sudden onset may cause syncope with catastrophic results, or even sudden death, when there is no escape rhythm (Fig. 22.8). As seen in the figure, P waves occur immediately after the T waves, and the first two P waves are conducted without even first-degree block, but the third and all subsequent P waves are not conducted at all. Thus, third-degree AV block need not be preceded by first- or second-degree AV block.

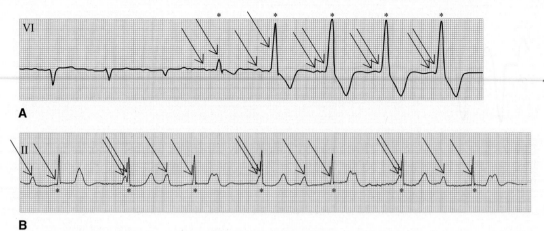

A

B

FIGURE 22.9. Rhythm strips from two patients receiving digitalis therapy for congestive heart failure. **A.** Lead V1. **B.** Lead II. Note in **A** that the initial independent ventricular beat is a "fusion beat" produced partly by conduction from the atria and partly from the ventricular pacing site. *Arrows* indicate the varying relationships between adjacent P waves and QRS complexes, and *asterisks* indicate the regular ventricular rates. Note that the P waves are unusually small in **A** and unusually large in **B**.

Third-degree AV block always produces AV dissociation with its independent atrial and ventricular rhythms; however, AV dissociation may result from other sources than third-degree AV block. Decreased sinus automaticity (see Chapter 21), increased junctional and ventricular automaticity (see Chapter 16), and reentrant ventricular tachycardia (see Chapter 19) can all produce AV dissociation by creating the condition in which anterograde impulses fail to traverse the AV node. They encounter the refractoriness that follows AV nodal activation by retrograde impulses. Therefore, AV dissociation caused solely by impaired function of the AV conduction system should actually be termed "AV dissociation due to AV block" (see Fig. 22.7A, B) and AV dissociation caused solely by an accelerated distal pacing site should be termed "AV dissociation due to refractoriness" (Fig. 22.9A). Both causes can coexist, producing "AV dissociation due to a combination of AV block and refractoriness," when there are P waves that are obviously not conducted to the ventricles but the ventricular rate is slightly above the upper limit of the bradycardic range of 60 beats per minute (see Fig. 22.9B). The term "interference" is often used to describe the condition of refractoriness that either causes or contributes to the two types of AV dissociation described here.

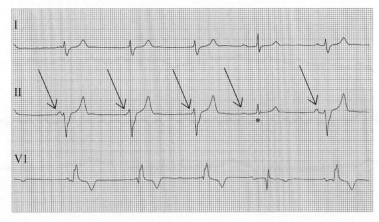

FIGURE 22.10. Leads I, II, and V1 rhythm strips from a patient receiving digitalis therapy for congestive heart failure. *Arrows* indicate P-wave locations (the irregularity is due to sinus arrhythmia) and an *asterisk* indicates a QRS complex produced by atrial capture.

Often, the AV dissociation produced by third-degree AV block is "isoarrhythmic," with similar atrial and ventricular rates and with P waves and QRS complexes occurring almost simultaneously. Insight into the presence or absence of AV block can be attained only when a P wave appears at a time sufficiently remote from a QRS complex that the ventricular refractory period would be expected to have been completed. In Figure 22.10, there is AV dissociation during the first three cycles, in which the independent sinus and ventricular rhythms are similar. Then, when variation in rate caused by respiration (sinus arrhythmia) accelerates the sinus rate but does not affect the ventricular escape focus during the fourth cycle, atrial capture occurs. This event proves AV conduction to be possible and eliminates complete AV block as a contributor to the AV dissociation.

Block in both the RBB and LBB (level C in Fig. 22.1), rather than block at the AV node or in the His bundle, is usually the cause of chronic complete AV block.[7-10] Idiopathic fibrosis, called either Lev disease or Lenègre disease, is the most common cause of chronic complete AV block.[7,11] Acute complete AV block within the AV node results from inferior myocardial infarction, digitalis intoxication, and rheumatic fever.[12] Acute complete AV block within the bundle branches results from extensive septal myocardial infarction.[13,14] Complete AV block may also be congenital, as when it results from maternal anti-Ro antibodies affecting the AV node.[15]

In the presence of chronic LBB or RBB block, the individual is at some risk of suddenly developing complete AV block. After this occurs, the ventricles either remain inactive (ventricular asystole; see Fig. 22.8) and the patient experiences syncope or even sudden death, or a more distal pacing site takes over (see Fig. 22.7B) and controls the ventricles (ventricular escape). In this event, the atria continue to beat at their own rate and the ventricles beat at a slower rhythm. This independence (AV dissociation due to AV block) is readily recognized in the ECG recording from the lack of relationship between the infrequent QRS complexes and the more frequent P waves. Each maintains its own rhythm.

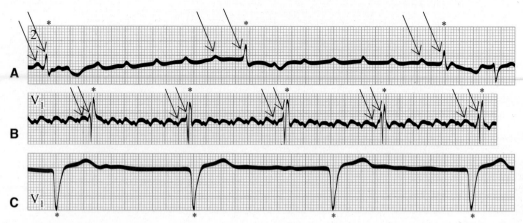

FIGURE 22.11. Three examples of atrial tachyarrhythmias with third-degree AV block and lower escape rhythms. In **A** and **B**, the QRS duration of <0.12 second indicates escape from the common bundle, but in **C**, the QRS duration of 0.16 second indicates either escape from the common bundle accompanied by LBB block or escape from the RBB. *Arrows* indicate the varying P-QRS **(A)** and F-QRS **(B)** intervals, and *asterisks* indicate the constant ventricular rates in all three examples.

Differentiation between second- and third-degree AV block is accomplished by considering the relationship among the ventricular waveforms in a series of cycles (RR intervals) and the relationship between the atrial and ventricular waveforms in each of these cycles (PR or flutter-R intervals). If the RR interval is irregular, some AV conduction can be assumed, and second-degree block is present. If the RR interval is regular, a constant PR or flutter-R interval indicates second-degree AV block, whereas a varying PR or flutter-R interval indicates third-degree block, with an escape rhythm generated by a lower site. Figure 22.11 presents examples of AV block occurring in the presence of three different atrial tachyarrhythmias: sinus tachycardia (see Fig. 22.11A), atrial flutter (see Fig. 22.11B), and atrial fibrillation (see Fig. 22.11C). Consecutive RR intervals are constant in all of the examples, at 2.84, 1.40, and 1.96 seconds, respectively. In Figure 22.11A and B, it is obvious that there is third-degree AV block because the adjacent PR relationships in Figure 22.11A and flutter wave-R relationships in Figure 22.11B are quite variable. In Figure 22.11C, third-degree AV block can be assumed because the absence of regular atrial activity in atrial fibrillation prohibits any constancy in AV conduction relationships.

LOCATION OF ATRIOVENTRICULAR BLOCK

As discussed in Chapter 6 and presented schematically in Figure 22.1, AV block can be located in the AV node, the common bundle, or the bundle branches. This distinction is important because both the etiology and prognosis are quite different with proximal (AV nodal) versus distal (infranodal) block. Fortunately, block within the common bundle is so rare that the clinical decision about the location of an AV block is essentially limited to the AV node versus the bundle branches.

Two aspects of the electrocardiographic appearance of rhythm may help in differentiating AV block at the AV node versus AV block in a bundle branch: (a) the consistency of the PR intervals of conducted impulses and (b) the width of the QRS complexes of either conducted or escape impulses. Because only the AV node has the ability to vary its conduction time, the Purkinje cells of the common bundle and bundle branches must conduct at a particular speed or not at all. Therefore, when a varying PR interval is present, the AV block is most likely within the AV node.

A QRS complex of normal duration (<0.12 second) can occur only when the impulse producing the complex has equal access to both the RBB and LBB. Therefore, when an AV block is located at the bundle-branch level, the conducted or escape QRS complexes must be ≥0.12 second. The diagnosis is complicated by the possibility of either a fixed bundle-branch block accompanying AV nodal block or an aberrancy of intraventricular conduction (Chapter 20). Consequently, a QRS complex of normal duration confirms that a block has an AV nodal location, whereas a QRS complex of prolonged duration is not helpful in locating the site of an AV block.

The AV node has this ability to vary its conduction time, because its cells have uniquely prolonged periods of partial refractoriness as they return from their depolarized to their repolarized states. Therefore, in less than complete AV block, a nodal versus an infranodal (bilateral bundle) location can be determined by observing whether the PR interval is variable, as in the first case, or constant, as in the second.

AV conduction patterns can be considered only when some conduction is present (first- or second-degree AV block). No differentiation between an AV nodal and an infranodal location is possible in *complete (third-degree) block* with wide escape QRS complexes (see Fig. 22.7B).

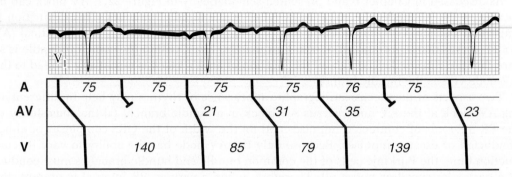

FIGURE 22.12. A lead V1 rhythm strip accompanied by a ladder diagram with atrial (A), AV nodal (AV), and ventricular (V) levels. The various intervals are indicated in hundredths of a second.

The classic form of AV nodal block is reflected by the *Wenckebach sequence*, in which the PR interval may begin within normal limits but is usually somewhat prolonged. With each successive beat, the PR interval gradually lengthens until there is failure to conduct an impulse to the ventricles. Examples are presented in Figures 22.3, 22.4A, and 22.5A. Following the nonconducted P wave, the PR interval reverts to normal (or near normal) and the sequence is repeated. At times, the PR interval may increase to surprising lengths.

Progressive lengthening of the PR interval occurs in the Wenckebach sequence because each successive atrial impulse arrives progressively earlier in the relative refractory period of the AV node and therefore takes progressively longer to penetrate the node and reach the ventricles. This is a physiologic mechanism during atrial flutter/fibrillation, but its occurrence at normal heart rates implies impairment of AV conduction.[16] The progressive lengthening of the PR interval usually follows a predictable pattern: The maximal increase in the PR interval occurs between the first and second cardiac cycles, and the increase between subsequent cycles then becomes progressively smaller. Three characteristic features of the cardiac cycle, which can be figuratively referred to as the *footprints of the Wenckebach sequence*, occur with AV nodal block: (a) the beats tend to cluster in small groups, particularly in pairs, because 3:2 P-to-QRS ratios are more common than 4:3 ratios, which are more common than 5:4 ratios, and so forth; (b) in each group of ventricular beats, the first cycle is longer than the second cycle, and there is a tendency for progressive shortening to occur in successive cycles; and (c) the longest cycle (the one containing the dropped ventricular beat) is less than twice the length of the shortest cycle (Fig. 22.12).

This phenomenon influences the rhythm of the ventricles. After the pause produced by complete failure of AV conduction, the RR intervals in the ECG tend to decrease progressively, and the long cycle (the one containing the nonconducted beat) is of shorter duration than two of the shorter cycles because it contains the shortest PR interval. This pattern of progressively decreasing RR intervals preceding a pause in AV conduction that lasts for less than twice the duration of the shortest RR interval is of only academic interest in the presence of AV nodal block, but a similar pattern of PP intervals may provide the only clue to the presence of sinus nodal exit block (see Chapter 21).

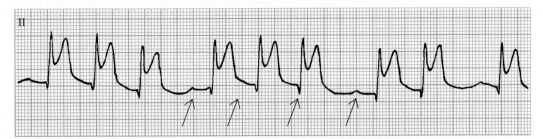

FIGURE 22.13. A continuous recording of lead II from a patient with acute inferior myocardial infarction. *Arrows* indicate both the obvious and the assumed locations of sinus-originated P waves.

When second-degree AV block appears during an acute inferior myocardial infarction, the elevation of the ST segment in the ECG may obscure many of the P waves, as seen in Figure 22.13. The visible P waves with prolonged PR intervals during the pauses allow diagnosis of first-degree block, but only the typical RR-interval pattern allows a diagnosis of second-degree AV nodal block.

The features described are typical of a classic Wenckebach period, but AV nodal block rarely fits this pattern, because both the sinus rate and the AV conduction are under the constant influence of the autonomic nervous system.[17,18] Among common variations from the classic pattern are (a) the first incremental increase in PR interval may not be the greatest, (b) the PR intervals may not lengthen progressively, (c) the last PR increment may be the longest of all, and (d) a nonconducted atrial beat may not occur.[17] The only criterion needed to identify the form of AV block that typically occurs in the AV node is a variation in the PR intervals. The term *Mobitz type I* or simply *type I* AV block is used when variation of the PR intervals is virtually diagnostic of block in the AV node.

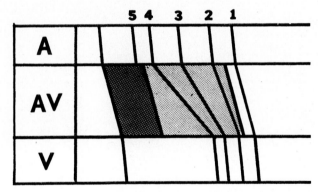

FIGURE 22.14. A ladder diagram illustrating the effect of progressively earlier entry of atrial impulses 1 to 5 into the AV node (AV). The *light stippled area* indicates the AV node's relative refractory period, during which impulses 2, 3, and 4 encounter progressively slower conduction. The *dark stippled area* indicates the node's absolute refractory period, during which impulse 5 cannot be conducted to the ventricles.

The earlier an impulse arrives during the prolonged partial refractory period of the AV node, the longer the time required for conduction of the impulse through to the ventricles. Therefore, when the AV node remains in its refractory period, the shorter the interval between a conducted QRS complex and the next conducted P wave (*RP interval*), the longer is the following conduction time (PR interval). This inverse or reciprocal relationship between RP and PR intervals is illustrated schematically in Figure 22.14.

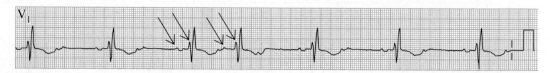

FIGURE 22.15. A lead V1 rhythm strip from an elderly patient on digitalis therapy for congestive heart failure. *Arrows* indicate the varying PR intervals during the third and fourth cycles that prove the capacity for variable conduction times.

The need to consider the variability in AV conduction times to determine the location of an AV block is illustrated in Figure 22.15. There is normal sinus rhythm with second-degree AV block and RBB block. For the initial complete cardiac cycles, the RP intervals are constant (1.36 seconds) and the PR intervals are also constant (0.24 second). It is tempting to locate the AV block below the AV node because the PR intervals do not vary and there is an obvious intraventricular conduction problem. However, the possibility of AV nodal block has not been eliminated because, with a constant RP interval, the AV node would be expected to conduct with a constant PR interval. Only when the conduction ratio changes from 2:1 (P waves 1 to 4) to 3:2 (P waves 5 to 7) is a change produced in the RP interval (from 1.36 to 0.56 seconds). This shorter RP interval is accompanied by a reciprocally greater PR interval (from 0.24 to 0.36 second), identifying the AV node rather than the ventricular Purkinje system as the location of the AV block.

INFRANODAL (PURKINJE) BLOCK

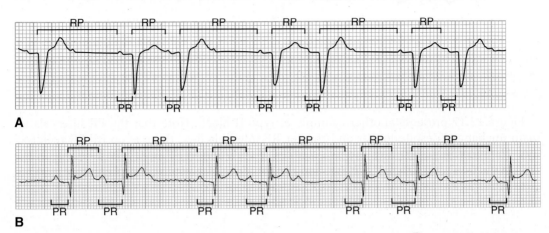

FIGURE 22.16. Lead II rhythm strips from a woman with recurrent presyncopal episodes **(A)** and another patient with an acute inferior myocardial infarction **(B)**. *Brackets* indicate the variable RP/constant PR pattern typical of type II AV block in **A** and the variable RP/variable PR pattern typical of type I AV block in **B**.

Although infranodal (i.e., occurring in the Purkinje system) block is much less common than AV nodal block, it is a much more serious condition. It is almost always preceded by a bundle-branch block pattern for the conducted beats, with the nonconducted beats resulting from intermittent block in the other bundle branch.[4,5] Continuous block in the other bundle branch results in syncope or heart failure if ventricular escape occurs and sudden death if there is no ventricular escape. *Infranodal block* is almost always due to bilateral bundle-branch block (level C in Fig. 22.1) rather than His-bundle block (level B in Fig. 22.1). First-degree AV block may or may not accompany the bundle-branch block, but there is usually no stable period of second-degree AV block. Infranodal block is typically characterized by a sudden progression from no AV block to third-degree (complete) AV block. Because it occurs in the distal part of the pacemaking and conduction system, the escape rhythm may be too slow or too unreliable to support adequate circulation of blood, thereby causing serious and even fatal clinical events.

Unlike the cells in the AV node, those in the Purkinje system have an extremely short relative refractory period. Therefore, they either conduct at a particular speed or not at all. Infranodal block is characterized by a lack of lengthening of the PR interval preceding the nonconducted P wave and a lack of shortening of the PR interval in the following cycle. This is termed *Mobitz type II* or simply *type II* AV block. It should be diagnosed whenever there is second-degree AV block with a constant PR interval despite a change in the RP interval. Indeed, the distinction between type I and type II blocks does not require the presence of a nonconducted P wave and can therefore be made in the presence of first-degree AV block alone.

The cardiac rhythm shown in Figure 22.16A should be compared with that in Figure 22.16B. The consistent 3:2 AV ratio provides varying RP intervals. However, in Figure 22.16A, the PR intervals remain constant at 0.20 second, in contrast with Figure 22.16B in which the varying PP intervals result in varying PR intervals. Therefore, the AV block producing the rhythm shown in Figure 22.16A is in a location that is incapable of varying its conduction time even when it receives impulses at varying intervals. The PR intervals are independent of, rather than reciprocal to, their associated RP intervals. This type II block in Figure 22.16A is indicative of an infranodal (Purkinje) site of failure of AV conduction, in contrast to type I block in Figure 22.16B, which is indicative of an AV nodal site.

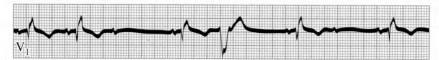

FIGURE 22.17. A lead V1 rhythm strip from a patient with chronic congestive heart failure. There is a lack of increase in the PR interval when a decrease occurs in the RP interval.

Figure 22.17 presents another example of type II block. Note that the PR intervals remain unchanged despite longer and shorter RP intervals (i.e., there is no RP/PR reciprocity). The recording illustrates the two sources of variation in RP intervals: a change in the AV conduction ratio (from 1:1 to 2:1) and the presence of a ventricular premature beat.

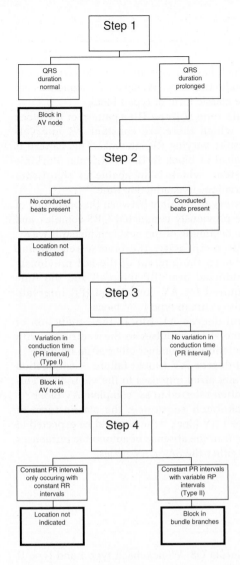

Step 1

QRS duration normal

QRS duration prolonged

Block in AV node

Step 2

No conducted beats present

Conducted beats present

Location not indicated

Step 3

Variation in conduction time (PR interval) (Type I)

No variation in conduction time (PR interval)

Block in AV node

Step 4

Constant PR intervals only occuring with constant RR intervals

Constant PR intervals with variable RP intervals (Type II)

Location not indicated

Block in bundle branches

FIGURE 22.18. The four-step algorithm for identifying the location of AV block from an ECG recording. Step 1: Consider the duration of the QRS complex. Step 2: Consider whether conducted beats are present. Step 3: Consider whether there is variation in the conduction times. Step 4: Consider whether there are constant PR intervals with changing RP intervals. Situations that indicate an end point in the algorithm are indicated by boxes *with accentuated borders.*

A stepwise method for determining the location of AV block is illustrated in Figure 22.18. This algorithm does not consider the localization of AV block within the common bundle because of the rarity of AV block in this location. (Such a location should be considered only when a QRS complex of normal duration [step 1] is accompanied by a pattern characteristic of type II block [step 4].) Note that both steps 2 and 4 may lead to situations in which it is impossible to determine the location of a block from a particular ECG recording. In this case, additional recordings should be obtained. If these are also nondiagnostic, the patient should be managed as though the block were located in the bundle branches because such a location has the most serious clinical consequences. This usually requires insertion of a temporary pacemaker, which provides time for further studies to determine the location of the AV block. *His-bundle electrograms* can be obtained via intracardiac recordings. A prolonged atrial-to-His interval (from the onset of the atrial signal to the time of the His-bundle signal), or the absence of a signal from the His bundle, indicates block in an AV nodal location, whereas a prolonged His-to-ventricle interval (from the His-bundle signal to the onset of the ventricular signal), or absence of a signal from the ventricles after a His signal, indicates block in a bilateral bundle branch location (see Fig. 14.11).

Atrioventricular (AV) block: a conduction abnormality located between the atria and the ventricles. Both the severity and the location of the abnormality should be considered.

Degree: a measure of the severity of AV block.

First-degree AV block: conduction of atrial impulses to the ventricles with PR intervals of >0.21 second.

Footprints of the Wenckebach sequence: the pattern of clusters of beats in small groups, with gradually decreasing intervals between beats, preceding a pause that is less than twice the duration of the shortest interval.

Heart block: another term used for AV block.

His-bundle electrograms: intracardiac recordings obtained via a catheter positioned across the tricuspid valve adjacent to the common or His bundle. These recordings are used clinically to determine the location of AV block when this is not apparent from the surface ECG recordings.

Infranodal block: AV block that occurs distal to or below the AV node and therefore within either the common bundle or in both the RBB and LBB.

Mobitz type I (type I): a pattern of AV block in which there are varying PR intervals. This pattern is typical of block within the AV node, which has the capacity for wide variations in conduction time. Wenckebach sequences are the classic form of type I block.

Mobitz type II (type II): a pattern of AV block in which there are constant PR intervals despite varying RP intervals. This pattern is typical of block in the ventricular Purkinje system, which is incapable of significant variations in conduction time.

RP interval: the time between the beginning of the previously conducted QRS complex and the beginning of the next conducted P wave.

RP/PR reciprocity: the inverse relationship between the interval of the last previously conducted beat (RP interval) and the time required for AV conduction (PR interval). This occurs in type I AV block.

Second-degree AV block: the conduction of some atrial impulses to the ventricles, with the failure to conduct other atrial impulses.

Third-degree AV block: failure of conduction of any atrial impulses to the ventricles. This is often referred to as "complete AV block."

Wenckebach sequence: the classic form of type I AV block, which would be expected to occur in the absence of autonomic influences on either the SA or AV nodes.

REFERENCES

1. Johnson RL, Averill KH, Lamb LE. Electrocardiographic findings in 67,375 asymptomatic individuals. VII. A-V block. *Am J Cardiol.* 1960;6:153.

2. Van Hemelen NM, Robles de Medina EO. Electrocardiographic findings in 791 young men between the ages of 15 and 23 years; I. Arrhythmias and conduction disorders. (Dutch). *Ned Tijdschr Geneeskd.* 1975;119: 45–52.

3. Erikssen J, Otterstad JE. Natural course of a prolonged PR interval and the relation between PR and incidence of coronary heart disease. A 7-year follow-up study of 1832 apparently healthy men aged 40–59 years. *Clin Cardiol.* 1984;7:6–13.

4. Damato AN, Lau SH. Clinical value of the electrogram of the conduction system. *Prog Cardiovasc Dis.* 13:119–140.

5. Narula OS. Wenckebach type I and type II atrioventricular block (revisited). *Cardiovasc Clin.* 1974;6:137–167.

6. Young D, Eisenberg R, Fish B, et al. Wenckebach atrioventricular block (Mobitz type I) in children and adolescents. *Am J Cardiol.* 1977;40:393–393.

7. Lenegre J. Etiology and pathology of bilateral bundle branch block in relation to complete heart block. *Prog Cardiovasc Dis.* 1964;6:409.

8. Lepeschkin E. The electrocardiographic diagnosis of bilateral bundle branch block in relation to heart block. *Prog Cardiovasc Dis.* 1964;6:445.

9. Rosenbaum MB, Elizari MV, Kretz A, et al. Anatomical basis of AV conduction disturbances. *Geriatrics.* 1970;25:132–144.

10. Steiner C, Lau SH, Stein E, et al. Electrophysiological documentation of trifascicular block

as the common cause of complete heart block. *Am J Cardiol.* 1971;28:436–441.

11. Louie EK, Maron BJ. Familial spontaneous complete heart block in hypertrophic cardiomyopathy. *Br Heart J.* 1986;55:469–474.

12. Rotman M, Wagner GS, Waugh RA. Significance of high degree atrioventricular block in acute posterior myocardial infarction. The importance of clinical setting and mechanism of block. *Circulation.* 1973;47:257–262.

13. Hindman MC, Wagner GS, JaRo M, et al. The clinical significance of bundle branch block complicating acute myocardial infarction. I. Clinical characteristics, hospital mortality, and one year follow-up. *Circulation.* 1978;58:679–688.

14. Hindman MC, Wagner GS, JaRo M, et al. The clinical significance of bundle branch block complicating acute myocardial infarc-

tion. II. Indications for temporary and permanent pacemaker insertion. *Circulation.* 1978;58:689–699.

15. Ho SY, Esscher E, Anderson RH, et al. Anatomy of congenital complete heart block and relation to maternal anti-Ro antibodies. *Am J Cardiol.* 1986;58:291–294.

16. Brodsky M, Wu D, Denes P, et al. Arrhythmias documented by 24 hour continuous electrocardiographic monitoring in fifty male medical students without apparent heart disease. *Am J Cardiol.* 1977;39:390–395.

17. Denes P, Levy L, Pick A, et al. The incidence of typical and atypical atrioventricular Wenckebach periodicity. *Am Heart J.* 1975;89:26–31.

18. Narula OS. *His Bundle Electrocardiography and Clinical Electrophysiology.* Philadelphia, PA: FA Davis; 1975:146–160.

23

Artificial Cardiac Pacemakers

WESLEY K. HAISTY, JR., TOBIN H. LIM,
AND GALEN S. WAGNER

BASIC CONCEPTS OF THE ARTIFICIAL PACEMAKER

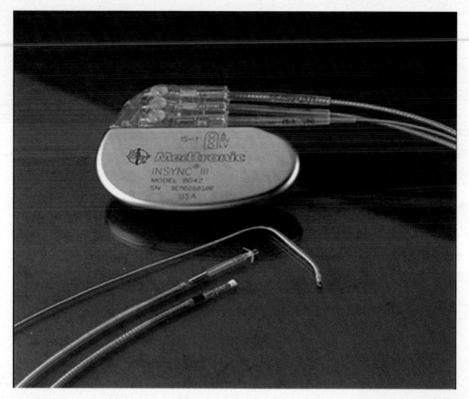

FIGURE 23.1. Biventricular pacemaker with three leads. Top lead: coronary sinus (LV) pacing lead. Middle lead: Right ventricular pacing lead. Bottom lead: Active fixation pacing lead for the right atrium.

Artificial cardiac pacemakers are used for a wide range of cardiac arrhythmias and conduction disorders. Pacemakers are used for treatment of symptomatic bradyarrhythmias caused by abnormal cardiac impulse formation or conduction.[1] Pacemakers are used in patients with tachyarrhythmias when (a) pharmacologic therapy carries a risk of bradyarrhythmias or more serious arrhythmias or (b) when electrical stimuli are required to stop the tachyarrhythmia. Pacemakers are combined with the capability of cardiac *defibrillation* in implanted devices for treatment of prior or potential life-threatening ventricular arrhythmias.[2] Pacemakers that pace both cardiac ventricles are used for treatment of heart failure in patients with reduced and poorly coordinated left-ventricular (LV) contraction associated with severe slowing of intraventricular conduction.[3]

Figure 23.1 shows the components of an implantable artificial pacemaker system designed to pace the right atrium and both cardiac ventricles (biventricular pacing). Electronic impulses originate from a *pulse generator* surgically placed subcutaneously in the pectoral area that is connected to transvenous leads with small electrodes mounted at their distal ends. These electrodes are positioned adjacent to the endocardial surfaces of the right atrium and right ventricle. The third lead is placed in an epicardial vein to pace the left ventricle. Temporary pacing can be achieved with an external pulse generator connected either to transvenous leads positioned like those for permanent pacing or to large precordial electrodes (Zoll device). With open-heart surgery, temporary or permanent epicardial electrodes may be placed on the atria or ventricles.

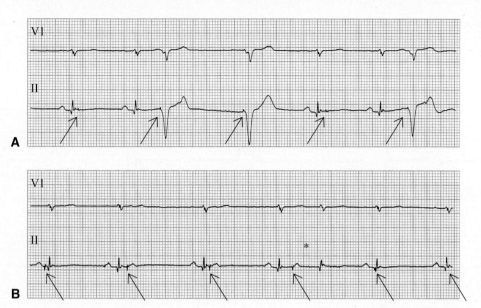

FIGURE 23.2. **A and B.** Fixed-rate ventricular and atrial pacing systems, respectively. *Arrow,* small pacing artifacts at a rate of 50 beats per minute; *asterisk,* prolonged PR interval.

When the cardiac rhythm is initiated by the impulses from an artificial pacemaker, *pacemaker artifacts* can usually be detected on an electrocardiogram (ECG) recording as positively or negatively directed vertical lines (Fig. 23.2). *Fixed-rate pacing* of the ventricles (see Fig. 23.2A) and the atria (see Fig. 23.2B) are illustrated. Note that this pacing system has no capability of "sensing" the patient's intrinsic rhythms and continues to generate impulses despite the resumption of sinus rhythm. In Figure 23.2A, the second, third, and fifth pacemaker impulses capture the ventricles. Thus, the patient's sinus rhythm is competing with a fixed-rate ventricular pacemaker. The regular rhythm of the pacemaker spikes is not disturbed by the intrinsic beats of the heart. The atrial pacemaker (see Fig. 23.2B) competes with sinus rhythm and initiates atrial premature beats (APBs) in the second, third, and fourth that fail to conduct until the fourth APB impulse conducts with a long PR interval. Modern pacemakers contain sophisticated sensing capabilities, and "fixed-rate" systems such as those described are no longer used.

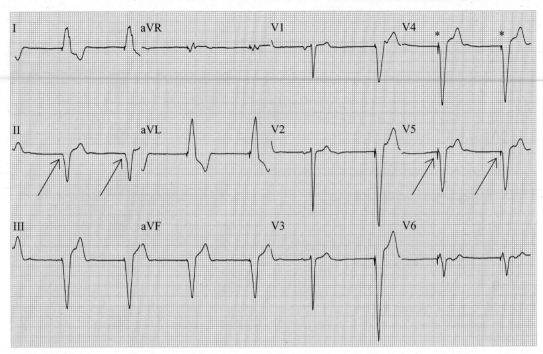

FIGURE 23.3. *Arrows,* prominent (lead V5) and absent (lead II) pacing artifacts in different leads; *asterisks,* varying artifact amplitudes (V4) characteristic of digital ECG recordings.

As illustrated in Figure 23.3, the amplitude of pacemaker artifacts in the ECG varies among leads, and the artifacts may not be apparent at all in a single-lead recording. The pacing artifacts are prominent in many leads (V2 to V6) but minimal in others and entirely absent in lead II. If only lead II were observed, there would be no evidence that the cardiac rhythm was artificially generated. The amplitude of the pacing spike also depends on the programmed output and configuration of the pacing system. This pacing spike amplitude is increased when unipolar pacing is used and may vary from beat to beat when digital ECG recording systems are used (see Fig. 23.3).

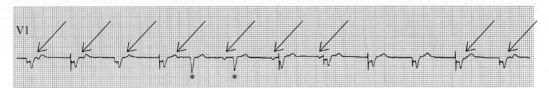

FIGURE 23.4. *Arrows*, patient's intrinsic sinus P waves; *asterisks*, QRS complexes of intrinsic ventricular activation that inhibit impulse generation from the demand pacemaker.

All current artificial pacemakers have a built-in standby or *demand mode* because the rhythm disturbances that require their use may occur intermittently.[2] Figure 23.4 provides an example of a normally functioning atrial demand pacemaker. In this mode, the device senses the heart's intrinsic impulses and does not generate artificial impulses while the intrinsic rate exceeds the rate set for the pulse generator. If the intrinsic pacing rate falls below the set artificial pacing rate, all cardiac cycles are initiated by the artificial pacemaker, and no evaluation of its sensing function is possible. In this example, the pacemaker cycle length is 840 milliseconds (0.84 second). Intrinsic beats occur in the lead V1 rhythm strip and are appropriately sensed by the demand pacemaker. Note the prolonged PR interval (0.32 second) required for the first intrinsic ventricular activation.

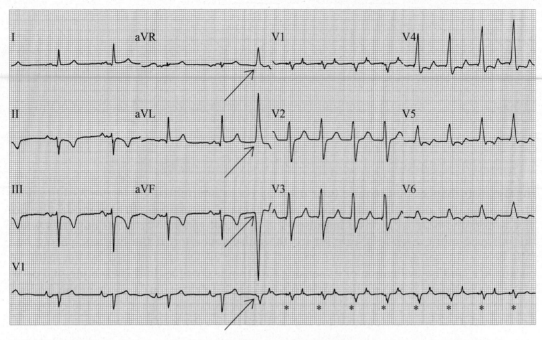

FIGURE 23.5. *Arrows*, magnet application; *asterisks*, rapid magnet-induced pacing rate.

If the intrinsic rate is greater than that of the artificial pacemaker, the pacing capability of the demand device may not be detectable on an ECG recording. The activity of the device can only be observed when a bradyarrhythmia occurs (Fig. 23.5) or when a magnet is applied. The magnet converts the pacemaker to fixed-rate pacing. Most current pacemakers also increase their pacing rate during magnet application to minimize competition with the patient's intrinsic rhythm. In the example shown in Figure 23.5, the patient's sinus bradycardia is interrupted by magnet application, causing an increase in the pacemaker rate to 100 beats per minute. Note the P waves following the pacemaker-induced QRS complexes, indicating 1:1 ventriculoatrial conduction.

PACEMAKER MODES AND DUAL-CHAMBER PACING

Table 23.1.

The NASPE/BPEG Generic (NBG) Pacemaker Code

Position	I	II	III	IV	V
Category	Chamber(s) paced 0 = None A = Atrium	Chamber(s) sensed 0 = None A = Atrium	Response to sensing 0 = None T = Triggered	Programmability, rate modulation 0= None P = Simple	Antitachyarrhythmia function(s) 0 = None P = Pacing
Programmable (antitachyarrhythmia)	V = Ventricle D = Dual (A + V)	V = Ventricle D = Dual (A + V)	I = Inhibited D= Dual (T + I)	M = Multiprogrammable C = Communicating R = Rate modulation	S = Shock D = Dual (P + S)

Note: Positions I through III are used exclusively for antibradyarrhythmia function.

The North American Society of Pacing and Electrophysiology Mode Code Committee and the British Pacing and Electrophysiology Group jointly developed the NASPE/BPEG Generic (NBG) code for artificial pacemakers.[4] This code, presented in Table 23.1 and described below, includes three letters to designate the bradycardia functions of a pacemaker; a fourth letter to indicate the pacemaker's programmability and rate modulation; and a fifth letter to indicate the presence of one or more antitachyarrhythmia functions.

The first three letters of the NBG code can be easily remembered by ranking pacemaker functions from most to least important. Pacing is the most important function of such an instrument, followed by sensing, and then by the response of the pacemaker to a sensed event. The first letter designates the cardiac chamber(s) that the instrument paces. The second letter designates the chamber(s) that the pacemaker senses. Entries for pacing and sensing include "A" for atrium, "V" for ventricle, "D" for dual (atrium and ventricle), and "O" for none. The third letter in the NBG code designates the response to sensed events. Entries for this third letter include "I" for inhibited, "D" for both triggered and inhibited, and "O" for none. The fourth letter describes two different functions: (a) the degree of programmability of the pacemaker ("M" for multiprogrammability, "P" for simple programmability, and "O" for no programmability) and (b) the presence of rate responsiveness ("R" for the presence, and omission of a fourth letter for the absence of rate responsiveness). The fifth letter of the NBG code is seldom used.

Commonly used pacemakers include those with the VVI, AAI, and DDD modes, with VVIR, AAIR, and DDDR designating the rate-modulated modes.[5,6] VVI pacemakers (see Figs. 23.3 to 23.5) pace the ventricle, sense the ventricle, and are inhibited by sensed intrinsic events. These instruments represent the classic ventricular demand pacemaker that paces at the programmed rate unless the instrument senses intrinsic ventricular activity at a faster rate. The VVI pacemaker has only a single rate (usually called the "minimum rate") to be programmed. By analogy with VVI pacemakers, AAI pacemakers pace the atrium, sense the atrium, and are inhibited by sensed atrial beats. AAI pacemakers also have only a single programmable rate. Both VVI and AAI pacemakers are *"single-chamber"* pacemakers; they both have only one lead pacing and sensing one cardiac chamber.

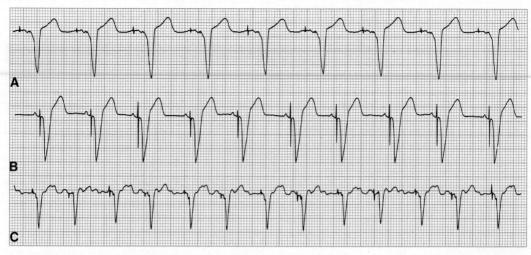

FIGURE 23.6. **A.** Atrial and ventricular minimum-rate-behavior pacing. **B.** Ventricular pacing at the atrially tracked rate with the programmed AV interval. **C.** Ventricular pacing at varying intervals following sensed atrial flutter waves exhibiting maximum-rate behavior.

DDD pacemakers are typically *"dual-chamber"* pacemakers; they pace both the right atrium and right ventricle or both ventricles and sense atrial and ventricular impulses. They are triggered by P waves to pace the ventricle at the programmed atrioventricular (AV) interval and are inhibited by ventricular sensing to not compete with the patient's underlying rhythm. DDD pacing varies according to the patient's underlying atrial rate. If the patient's atrial rate is below the minimum tracking rate in the DDD mode, the pacemaker shows "minimum rate behavior," pacing both the atrium and the ventricle (Fig. 23.6A). If the sinus rate is above the minimum rate in the DDD mode, the pacemaker tracks atrial activity and paces the ventricle at the programmed AV interval (see Fig. 23.6B). To prevent tracking of rapid atrial rhythms, the DDD pacemaker requires a programmed maximum tracking rate. More rapid atrial rates are sensed, but ventricular pacing is limited to the programmed upper tracking rate ("maximum-rate behavior"; see Fig.23.6C). If the pacemaker is programmed appropriately, AV intervals following the sensed atrial activity vary and resemble those in AV nodal block.

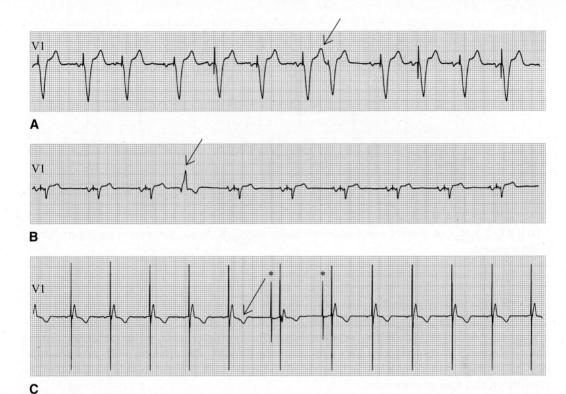

A

B

C

FIGURE 23.7. **A.** *Arrow*, sensed APB. **B.** *Arrow*, sensed VPB. **C.** *Arrow*, unsensed APB; *asterisks*, minimum-rate AV pacing following the APB-induced pause and continuing until intrinsic sinus rhythm exceeds this minimum pacing rate.

Figure 23.7 shows lead V1 rhythm strips from three patients with syncope owing to intermittent AV block. Displayed are the normal functions of three DDD pacemakers when the atrial rate is above the programmed minimum rate and below the programmed maximal tracking rate of the pacemaker. The DDD pacemaker is best understood by knowing that it approximates normal AV function and conduction and that its function closely approximates normal cardiac physiology. The AV intervals provided by DDD pacemakers may shorten with an increased pacing rate. The DDD pacemaker tracks both sinus arrhythmia and APBs (occurring at the peak of a T wave, triggering ventricular pacing; see Fig. 23.7A) and senses and is reset by ventricular premature beats (VPBs; see Fig. 23.7B). The pacemaker may lengthen the AV interval for closely coupled APBs but may not sense very closely coupled APBs when they occur in its atrial refractory period (see Fig. 23.7C). Note the minimum-rate AV pacing following the APB-induced pause and continuing until intrinsic sinus rhythm exceeds this minimum pacing rate in Figure 23.7C.

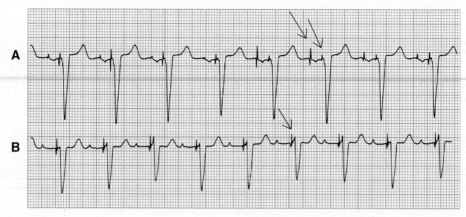

FIGURE 23.8. **A.** *Arrows*, atrial and ventricular pacing. **B.** *Arrow*, ventricular pacing tracking a rapid sinus rate.

VVIR and DDDR pacemakers have the capacity for rate modulation by having their minimum rate automatically increased through an activity sensor. Common sensors include a piezoelectric crystal (activity), accelerometer (body movement), or impedance sensing device (sensing of respiratory rate or minute ventilation). Pacemakers with rate modulation have programmed maximal sensor rates and may have programmable parameters for sensitivity and rate of response.

DDDR pacing and modulation of the minimum rate through sensor activity is shown in Figure 23.8A. Consecutive beats with both atrial and ventricular pacing confirm minimum-rate pacing. The minimum rate has been "modulated" and increased to 84 beats per minute as a result of sensor activity (see Fig. 23.8A). Figure 23.8B displays the same pacemaker tracking the same patient's sinus rhythm at a rate faster than that with the sensor-driven pacing shown in Figure 23.8A. Note the sensor has not increased the pacemaker's minimum rate while tracking a rapid sinus rate. Thus, the DDDR pacemaker can increase the rate of ventricular pacing either through an increased rate of atrial pacing driven by the sensor or through sensing of an increased intrinsic sinus rate. Maximal sensor rate and maximal tracking rate may be independently programmed in dual-chamber pacemakers.

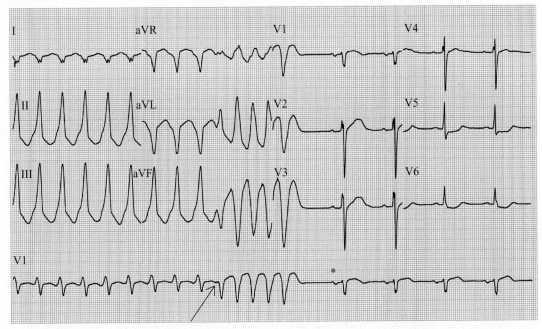

FIGURE 23.9 *Arrow*, beginning of a five-beat train that terminates the tachycardia; *asterisk*, return of sinus rhythm.

Pacemaker systems may include antitachycardia pacing (ATP), but current practice usually limits ATP to supraventricular tachyarrhythmias. However, Figure 23.9 presents an example using ATP to terminate a monomorphic ventricular tachycardia in a patient with palpitations and dizziness before pacemaker implantation. Note the very small pacing artifacts visible in lead aVF.

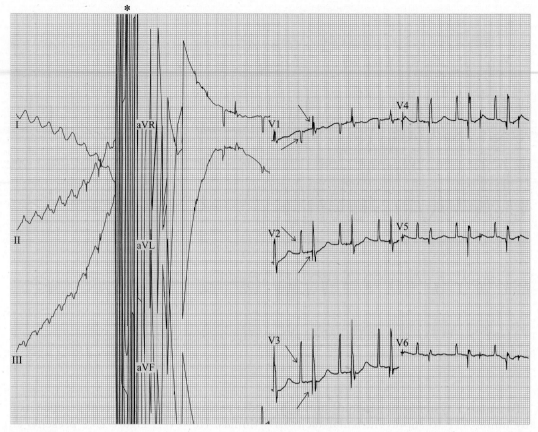

FIGURE 23.10. *Asterisk,* high-energy ICD artifact terminating the tachycardia; *arrows,* return of dual-chamber pacing.

ATP for ventricular tachycardia is usually included in an implantable cardioverter defibrillator (ICD). This complex device protects the patient from acceleration of a tachyarrhythmia or even induction of ventricular fibrillation as a complication of ATP (Fig. 2.10). As seen in Figure 23.10, a polymorphic ventricular tachycardia at a rate of 250 beats per minute was induced with a high-energy ICD artifact terminating the tachycardia. Atrial pacing artifacts have been distorted by the ICD discharge. ICD systems incorporating ATP also include AV sequential pacing to protect against bradyarrhythmias.

PACEMAKER EVALUATION

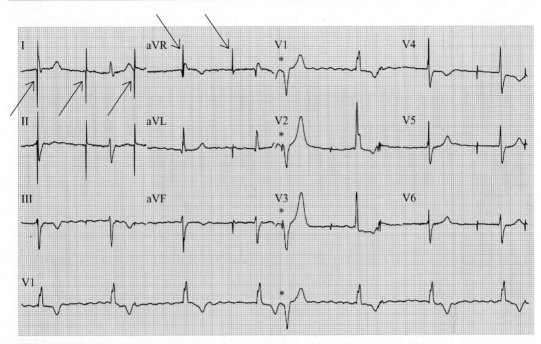

FIGURE 23.11. *Arrows,* pacing artifacts; *asterisks,* single instance of ventricular capture by the pacemaker.

The initial aspect of evaluation of any pacemaker system is the assessment of its pacing and sensing functions. Pacing failure is indicated by the absence of atrial or ventricular capture after a pacing artifact, and a pacemaker system may also exhibit either under- or *oversensing.*

Figure 23.11 shows the typical appearance of failure of both the pacing and sensing functions of a pacemaker. Pacing artifacts are seen continuing regularly (68 beats per minute), not sensing for the patient's intrinsic beats and usually not producing a QRS following paced beats. Only a single incidence of ventricular capture occurs. Failure of the sensing function is apparent from the absence of pacemaker inhibition by the patient's intrinsic ventricular beats.

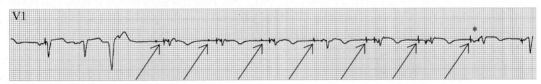

FIGURE 23.12. *First six arrows,* minimum-rate pacing without atrial capture; *asterisk and last arrow,* atrial capture by the pacemaker.

The evaluation of dual-chamber pacing systems must assess both atrial and ventricular capture and sensing.[7,8] Figure 23.12 demonstrates failure only of atrial capture; the ventricular pacing function is intact. Effective atrial sensing is indicated by the tracking of the first two sinus beats, with ventricular pacing at the sinus rate. During the pause after the VPB, minimum-rate pacing occurs, but with failure of atrial capture. Effective ventricular sensing is indicated by inhibition of ventricular pacing after the VPB.

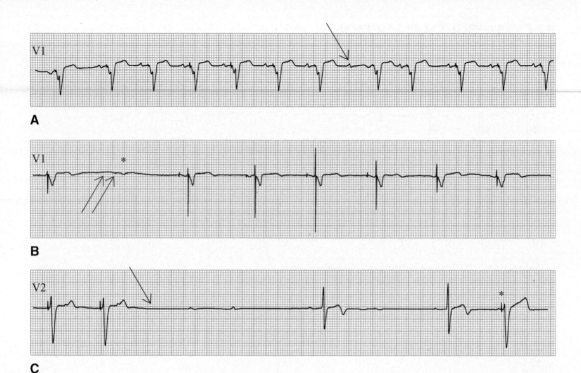

FIGURE 23.13. **A.** *Arrow*, single undersensed P wave. **B.** *Arrows*, expected locations of atrial and ventricular pacing artifacts; *asterisk*, P wave that fails to conduct owing to underlying AV block. **C.** *Arrow*, expected location of the next ventricular pacing artifact; *asterisk*, pacing artifact reappearance.

Figure 23.13 shows three examples of sensing dysfunction: atrial undersensing (see Fig. 23.13A) and ventricular oversensing (see Fig. 23.13B, C). A DDD device was present in Figure 23.13A and B and a VVI device in Figure 23.13C. In normal pacemaker function, ventricular sensing inhibits the pacemaker activity and atrial sensing triggers the pacemaker activity. The failure of atrial sensing in Figure 23.13A causes failure of the P wave (arrow) to trigger ventricular activity. A prolonged pause (continuing for >6 seconds in Fig. 23.13C) is typical of abnormal sensing occurring with broken pacemaker leads. The reappearance of the pacing artifact (asterisk) indicates that the lead break is only intermittent. Regardless, the abnormal sensing of either skeletal muscle (pectoralis) activity via the ventricular lead (see Fig. 23.13B) or noise from a broken lead (see Fig. 23.13C) pathologically inhibits the pacemaker activity.

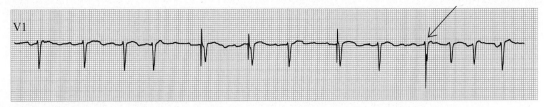

FIGURE 23.14. *Arrow*, pacemaker artifact 0.04 second into an intrinsic QRS complex.

"Failure to sense" may be incorrectly suspected when the pacing system has not had sufficient time to sense an intrinsic beat.[7,8] This occurs when the patient's intrinsic rate is similar to the instrument's minimum pacing rate, as in lead V1 rhythm recording of atrial fibrillation with intermittent slowing and ventricular pacing (Fig. 23.14). A period of >0.04 second is required for intrinsic activation to reach the pacemaker lead in the right-ventricular apex and to be sensed by the pacemaker. The apparent abnormality in fact represents normal pacemaker function.

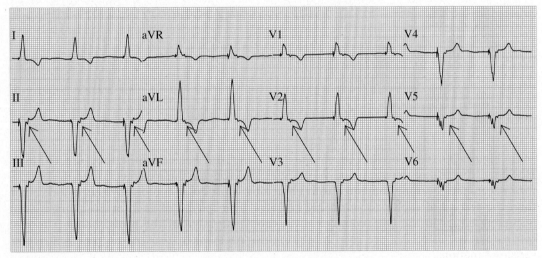

FIGURE 23.15. *Arrows*, retrograde P waves of 1:1 ventricular-to-atrial conduction.

At times, both the pacing and sensing functions of a pacemaker may occur normally in patients with symptoms that are typically associated with pacemaker dysfunction. Figure 23.15 documents normal pacing by a VVI pacemaker. Absence of competing intrinsic activity prevents evaluation of the instrument's sensing function. However, the occurrence of 1:1 ventricular-to-atrial conduction leads to the clinical probability that *"pacemaker syndrome"*[9]—vasovagal syncope caused by atrial dilation produced by the occurrence of atrial contraction with the closed tricuspid valve during ventricular contraction—is causing the patient's symptoms.

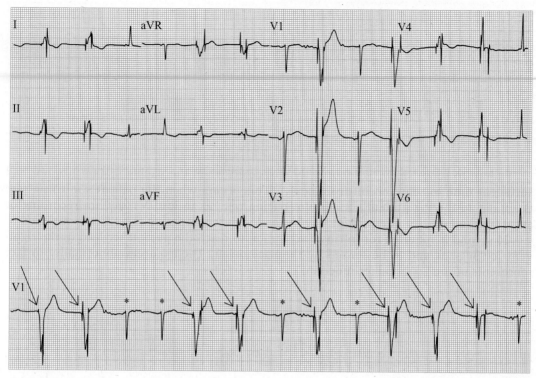

FIGURE 23.16. *Arrows*, effective ventricular capture by the first of two coupled pacing artifacts; *asterisks*, intrinsic beats.

In Figure 23.16, both the pacemaker's pacing and sensing functions are evident. However, reversal of the atrial and ventricular leads during their connection to the temporary pacemaker becomes obvious from observing ventricular capture by the initial rather than the second of each pair of pacing artifacts. The second of each of the pairs is seen occurring either in the QRS complex or in the ST segment of the paced beats. The five intrinsic beats (asterisks) are seen inhibiting the pacemaker, proving normal ventricular sensing function.

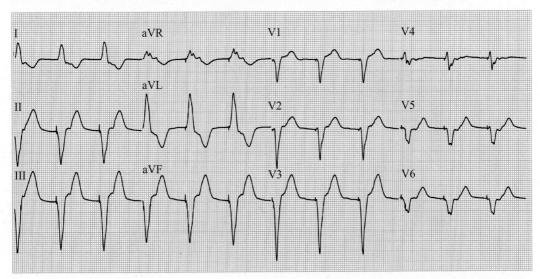

A

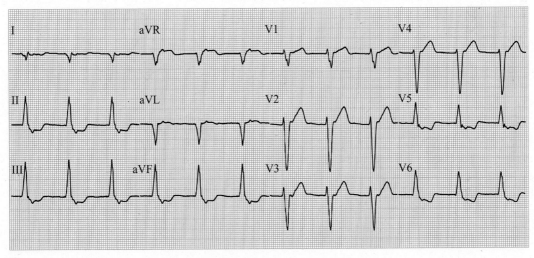

B

FIGURE 23.17. **A.** Right-ventricular apex pacing. **B.** Right-ventricular outflow tract pacing.

The spread within the heart of the wave fronts of depolarization from a pacemaker depends on the location of the stimulating electrode. Currently, most endocardial electrodes are positioned near the right-ventricular (RV) apex. This produces sequential right- and then left-ventricular activation and therefore a left-bundle-branch block (LBBB) pattern on the ECG. As activation proceeds from the RV apex toward the base, the frontal axis is superior, producing extreme left-axis deviation (Fig. 23.17A). Endocardial electrodes placed in the RV outflow tract produce activation beginning at the base and directed inferiorly. The frontal axis is then vertical (see Fig. 23.17B).

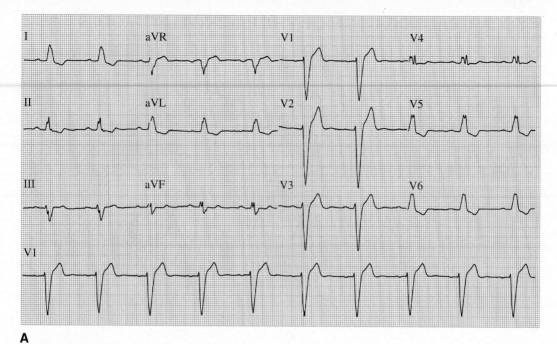

A

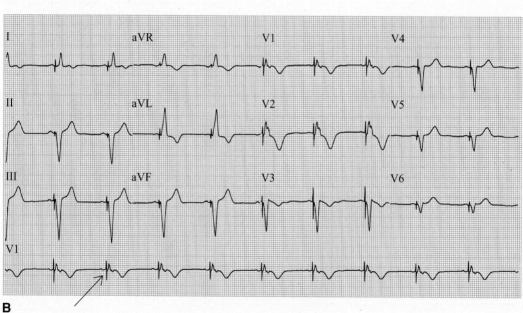

B

FIGURE 23.18. Three 12-lead ECGs with lead V1 rhythm strips from a 54-year-old man with heart failure caused by cardiomyopathy and LBBB, with a QRS duration of 190 milliseconds **(A)**. Recordings **(B and C)** were obtained at the time of implantation of a DDD pacemaker with *pacing electrodes* in both the right-ventricular apex and distal coronary sinus. Biventricular pacing **(B)** narrowed the QRS duration from 190 milliseconds to 155 milliseconds. An *arrow* indicates the ventricular pacing artifact tracking sinus rhythm. Intermittent right-ventricular pacing alone **(C)** extended the QRS duration to 210 milliseconds (*asterisks*) in contrast to the biventricular pacing effect.

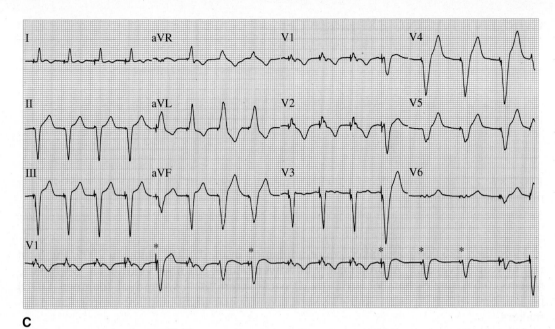

C

FIGURE 23.18. *(continued)*

LV epicardial electrodes or electrodes placed in the distal coronary sinus pace the left ventricle. This produces sequential left- then right-ventricular activation and therefore a right-bundle-branch block (RBBB) pattern on the ECG. Usually, pacing a single ventricle produces a wide QRS complex (210 milliseconds in Fig. 23.18C), but pacing of both ventricles simultaneously may narrow the QRS complex, as shown in the figure, from the baseline 190 milliseconds in Fig. 23.18A to 155 milliseconds in Fig. 23.18B.

Asterisks show wider complexes occuring with loss of left ventricular capture and only capture of the right ventricle.

CURRENT PACING EXPERIENCE

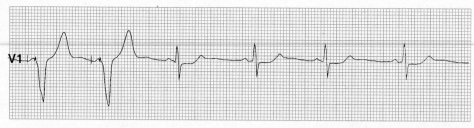

FIGURE 23.19. Dual-chamber (with right-atrial and right-ventricular leads) pacemaker minimizing ventricular pacing.

More than 225,000 pacemakers were implanted in the United States in 2009, the most recent year surveyed.[5,6] Approximately 14% were single-chamber ventricular (VVI) pacemakers, 0.5% single-chamber atrial (AAI) pacemakers, 82% were dual-chamber (DDD) pacemakers with RV pacing, and 4% were biventricular (right- and left-ventricular) pacemakers.

Although the majority (86%) of pacemakers are programmed DDD, the frequency of pacing and the number of paced ventricular beats on the ECG should vary greatly between subjects with RV leads and subjects with *biventricular pacemakers* and leads. The Dual Chamber and VVI Implantable Defibrillator (DAVID) study documented an earlier onset of heart failure secondary to LV dysfunction in patients that were aggressively paced with dual-chamber RV systems.[10] The MOST study comparing VVI and DDD pacing in patients with implantable defibrillators (but not pacemaker dependent) found that frequent RV (>40% to 50%) pacing was deleterious and increased mortality and heart failure admissions when compared with sinus rhythm.[11] Consequently, manufacturers have developed new algorithms to provide minimal use of ventricular pacing in dual-chamber pacemakers with only right-ventricular leads.

Figure 23.19 begins with AV sequential pacing with a short AV interval (110 milliseconds) followed by atrial pacing but with return of intrinsic AV conduction. The intrinsic conduction typically reduces the LV dyssynergy caused by pacing the RV apex. This is an example of "dual-chamber—right-ventricular pacing." The improved LV function in patients with normal intrinsic intraventricular conduction can be achieved by simply prolonging the AV interval of this dual-chamber pacemaker (see Fig. 23.19). However, in patients with underlying intraventricular conduction delays (LBBB, RBBB, etc.), the additional implantation of an LV lead is required, as in Figure 23.18.

Changes in the indications for pacing have influenced pacemaker function and consequently increased the variety of normal-paced rhythms. For biventricular pacing, studies[12-15] continue to show the benefit of *"cardiac resynchronization therapy"* (CRT), and manufacturers have developed algorithms to promote maximal ventricular pacing.[16]

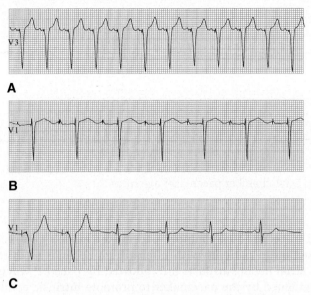

FIGURE 23.20. **A.** Biventricular pacing with a short AV interval. **B.** Dual-chamber pacing with a long AV interval. **C.** Dual-chamber pacemaker extending the AV interval.

Figure 23.20 includes three rhythm strips illustrating recent changes in pacing algorithms. Figure 23.20A is from a 55-year-old man with ischemic cardiomyopathy, left-bundle-branch block, and history of heart failure who was treated with biventricular pacemaker implantation for CRT. The short AV interval optimizes AV timing and promotes 100% ventricular pacing. Biventricular pacing coordinates right- and left-ventricular contraction and corrects delayed LV activation and septal dyskinesis previously caused by the native LBBB.

Figure 23.20B is a tracing from a 72-year-old man with a dual-chamber pacemaker implanted for symptomatic sinus bradycardia and near-syncope owing to sinus pauses of several seconds' duration. Testing during pacemaker implantation revealed a moderately impaired AV conduction with a first-degree AV block and 1:1 AV conduction during atrial pacing only to 100 beats per minute. Programming the pacemaker to a long AV interval is a simple way to promote intrinsic AV conduction and minimize ventricular pacing.

Figure 23.20C illustrates an algorithm included in newer dual-chamber pacemakers to promote intrinsic AV conduction. The first two complexes show both atrial and ventricular pacing with an AV interval of 110 milliseconds. The device periodically extends the AV interval, as occurs with the third complex allowing intrinsic ventricular conduction with a narrow QRS. This longer AV interval persists until ventricular pacing is needed. Ventricular pacing ensues if the intrinsic AV lengthens or AV block recurs.

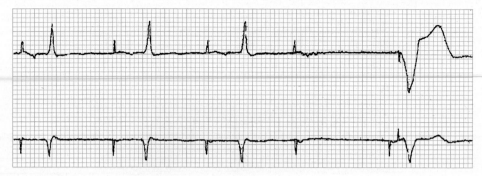

FIGURE 23.21. Dual-chamber pacemaker algorithm.

Algorithms used in recent dual-chamber pacemaker models can recognize and test for intrinsic AV conduction in patients with intermittent second- or third-degree AV block (Fig. 23.21). Three atrial pacing artifacts are followed by paced P waves, a long AV interval (previously lengthened by the pacemaker to promote intrinsic conduction), and a conducted QRS with a pacemaker spike superimposed on the QRS (see Fig. 23.14). Following the fourth atrial pace, ventricular pacing is suspended for a single cycle and no QRS is seen. The pacemaker algorithm allows a single "dropped" QRS before resuming both atrial and ventricular pacing with a short AV interval.

Expected Increase in Cardiac Resynchronization Therapy

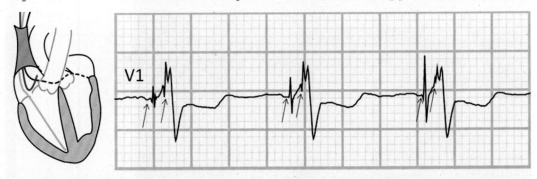

FIGURE 23.22. Biventricular pacing. **Left.** Schematic showing atrial, right-ventricular, and left-ventricular lead positions. **Right.** Rhythm strip showing two pacing impulses for each QRS, with an interval between pacing of the left and right ventricles. *Arrows* show the two pacing pulses for each QRS. This interval may be adjusted to optimize ventricular function for CRT.

Biventricular pacing is increasingly used for cardiac resynchronization therapy (CRT) in treatment of heart failure. In 2009, the last year surveyed, approximately 9,000 pacemaker devices and 48,000 pacing devices with an accompanying defibrillator were implanted yearly for treatment of heart failure.[6] The defibrillators were indicated for primary prevention of life-threatening arrhythmias in patients with a wide QRS, NYHA functional class II or III, and LV ejection fraction below 35%.[17] The number of CRT devices implanted yearly is likely to increase with an aging population, increasing indications from ongoing randomized studies, and many patients living longer with and without cardiac interventions and surgery.

The left of Figure 23.22 illustrates lead placement for biventricular pacing used for CRT. In patients without chronic atrial arrhythmias, a right-atrial lead is positioned in the appendage or lateral wall of the atrium. The RV lead is usually placed at the RV apex but may be positioned in the outflow tract. A transvenous LV lead is inserted through the coronary sinus and advanced to epicardial veins. Optimal position of the LV pacing lead is usually in the lateral wall, midway between the base and LV apex for most patients. The right of Figure 23.22 illustrates the separately programmable right- and left-ventricular pacing pulses of a CRT device.

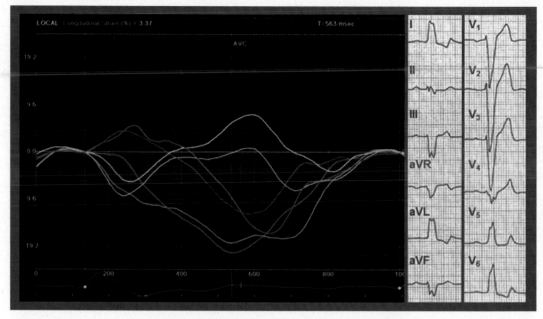

FIGURE 23.23. The early septal contraction (*blue line*) and early stretch of the LV free wall (*red line*) followed by the delayed contraction of the LV free wall associated with the classic mechanical impairment associated with a complete LBBB. (Modified from Risum N, Strauss D, Sogarrd P, et al. Left bundle branch block -The relationship between ECG electrical activation and echocardiographic mechanical contraction. Am Heart J. 2013;166(2):340–348.[18]

More than one in three patients with heart failure have an underlying LBBB which contributes to poor LV function by causing delayed contraction of the lateral LV wall, resulting in *dyssynchrony* between septal and free wall contraction (Fig. 23.23). The ECG is important in selecting patients most likely to benefit in follow-up of CRT and in improving site selection of the LV lead by recognizing areas of LV scar. Patients most likely to benefit from CRT are those with LBBB and a QRS width greater than 140 milliseconds for males and 130 milliseconds for females.[19] Forty percent of patients with LBBB with QRS duration of 120 milliseconds have underlying LV dyssynchrony. Seventy percent of those with LBBB and QRS width of 150 milliseconds have LV dyssynchrony.[3] Controlled studies show improved LV function, exercise performance, improved ejection fraction, and reduced LV diastolic size (reversal of remodeling) in the majority of patients. Randomized trials in patients with severe heart failure have shown reduction of symptoms, improved functional capacity, fewer hospitalizations for heart failure, and increased survival.[12-15] However, not all patients will benefit and up to 30% may fail to benefit from CRT.

The current consensus is that patients most likely to benefit from CRT must have mechanical as well as electrical dyssynchrony and that the LV pacing must reduce the delay and be capable of restoring the patient's LV synchrony.[20] The ECG and LBBB have been used as a surrogate for LV dyssynchrony, but this is not applicable for all patients. Echocardiographic methods may have improved recognition of LV dyssynchrony, but the optimal ultrasound technique has not been established. The classic mechanical pattern related to strain with LBBB includes three major elements. There is early contraction in the early activated septum, whereas the lateral or late-activated wall is stretched and shows late contraction. Recent application of regional strain analysis by speckle tracking stress improves recognition of this pattern, and responding patients show early reversal of the classic strain pattern.[21] Studies combining Doppler and electrocardiography may improve ECG criteria recognition of myocardial scars and prior myocardial infarction.

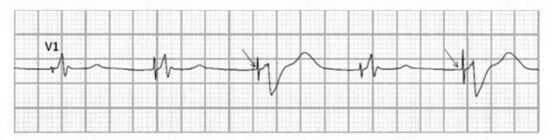

FIGURE 23.24. Biventricular pacing at follow-up. *Arrows* illustrate intermittent loss of left ventricular capture evidenced by loss of the RBBB pattern.

The ECG has a major role in follow-up of CRT patients in adjusting AV and RV-LV intervals to optimize pacing intervals, mode reprogramming in those subjects with only intermittent AV block, and to verify adequate capture of cardiac chambers.[22] Figure 23.24 shows intermittent capture of the LV as shown by the only intermitted RBBB pattern. The arrows show disappearance of the RBBB pattern with loss of LV capture. This should be corrected by increasing the pacing energy for the LV electrode.

Dual-Chamber Right Ventricular Pacing: Potential His-Bundle Pacing

Dual-chamber RV pacing will continue to have a role in patients with only intermittent bradyarrhythmias or intermittent AV block and normal LV function. Patients with persistent bradycardia and RV apical pacing continue to be at risk for earlier progression of heart failure. Patients with LBBB associated with frequent RV pacing may have even more dyssynchrony than patients with a native LBBB.[23] The RV lead may be placed in the RV outflow tract on the right side of the septum rather than at the apex in an effort to minimize the adverse effects of pacing at the RV apex. However, studies showing benefits have mixed results. A newer and promising approach is to anchor the RV lead near the His bundle and to pace the distal His bundle. The His-bundle deflection on the intracardiac ECG is localized by a catheter positioned across the tricuspid valve, and an RV lead with an anchoring helix is positioned at the site of the distal His bundle. Surprisingly, this often corrects the underlying LBBB in many patients with preexisting LBBB. Studies have confirmed stable anchoring of RV leads and satisfactory His-bundle pacing by this method. A recent study has found this approach functional in 9 of 13 patients.[24]

Newer Electrocardiograms

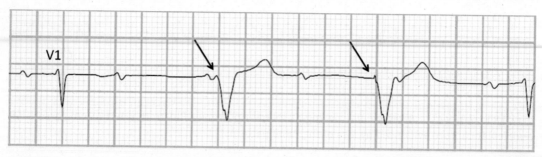

FIGURE 23.25. Sinus rhythm with second-degree AV block and ventricular pacing when the rate falls below 60 per minute. The wide QRS beats are paced. *Arrows* point to small pacing spikes. The pacing spikes are small and difficult to recognize for reasons discussed in the text.

Newer pacemakers and smaller lead electrodes allow pacing with greater efficiency and narrower pulses resulting in less energy use and longer pacemaker battery life. However, this makes the artifacts appearing on the ECG smaller and often difficult to recognize (Fig. 23.25). Digital ECG machines minimize the pacing artifact by routinely sampling the ECG electrical signal only once every 2 to 4 milliseconds (1/1000 of a second), whereas pulses of modern pacemakers are less than 0.4 millisecond. Recently, all major manufacturers of ECG machines have developed models that digitize the ECG signal at much higher frequency to recognize pacemaker artifacts and display the pacing spikes more clearly or on a separate lead.[25,26] We expect the newer ECG machines to be widely used in the near future.

GLOSSARY

Artificial cardiac pacemakers: devices capable of generating electrical impulses and delivering them to the myocardium.

Biventricular pacemaker: a pacemaker that paces both the right and left ventricles. Atrial pacing is also included unless the patient has chronic atrial arrhythmias that would prevent atrial pacing.

Cardiac resynchronization therapy (CRT): use of biventricular pacing to synchronize ventricular activation and contraction.

Defibrillation: termination of either atrial or ventricular fibrillation by an extrinsic electrical current.

Demand mode: a term describing an artificial pacemaking system with the ability to sense and be inhibited by intrinsic cardiac activity.

Dual-chamber pacemaker: a pacemaker that includes both atrial and ventricular pacing.

Dyssynchrony: loss of the normal synchronous mechanical contraction of the left-ventricular walls. The classic mechanical dyssynchrony with LBBB includes early activation and contraction of the septal wall with the late-activated free wall stretched and shows late contraction.

Fixed-rate pacing: artificial pacing with the capability only to generate an electrical impulse without sensing the heart's intrinsic rhythm.

Oversensing: abnormal function of an artificial pacemaker in which electrical signals other than those representing activation of the myocardium are sensed and inhibit impulse generation.

Pacemaker artifacts: high-frequency signals appearing on an ECG and representing impulses generated by an artificial pacemaker.

Pacemaker syndrome: a reduction in cardiac output caused by activation by an artificial pacemaker that does not produce an optimally efficient sequence of myocardial activation.

Pacing electrodes: electrodes that, in contrast with the electrodes used to record the ECG, are designed to transmit an electrical impulse to the myocardium. In pacing systems with sensing capability, these electrodes also transmit the intrinsic impulses of the heart to the pacemaking device.

Pulse generator: a device that produces electrical impulses as the key component of an artificial pacing system.

Single-chamber pacemaker: a pacemaker with one lead pacing and sensing one cardiac chamber.

REFERENCES

1. Ellenbogen KA, Wood MA, eds. *Cardiac Pacing and ICDs.* 5th ed. Hoboken, NJ: Wiley-Blackwell; 2008.
2. Hayes DL, Asirvatham SJ, Friedman PA, eds. *Cardiac Pacing, Defibrillation and Resynchronization: A Clinical Approach.* 3rd ed. Hoboken, NJ: Wiley-Blackwell; 2013.
3. Cynthia M, Tracy CM, Epstein AE, et al. 2012 ACCF/AHA/HRS focused update of the 2008 guidelines for device-based therapy for cardiac rhythm abnormalities: a report of the American College of Cardiology Foundation/American Heart Association Task Force on Practice Guidelines and the Heart Rhythm Society. *Circulation.* 2012;126:1784–1800.
4. Bernstein AD, Camm AJ, Fletcher RD, et al. NASPE/BPEG generic pacemaker code for antibradyarrhythmia and adaptive-rate pacing and antitachyarrhythmia devices. *Pace.* 1987;10:794–799.
5. Greenspon AJ, Patel JD, Lau E, et al. Trends in permanent pacemaker implantation in the United States from 1993 to 2009. *J Am Coll Cardiol.* 2012;60:1540–1545.
6. Mond HG, Proclemer A. The 11th world survey of cardiac pacing and implantable cardioverter-defibrillators: calendar year 2009—a World Society of Arrhythmia's Project. *Pace.* 2011;34:1013–1027.
7. Castellanos A Jr, Agha AS, Befeler B, et al. A study of arrival of excitation at selected ventricular sites during human bundle branch block using close bipolar catheter electrodes. *Chest.* 1973;63:208–213.
8. Vera Z, Mason DT, Awan NA, et al. Lack of sensing by demand pacemakers due

to intraventricular conduction defects. *Circulation*. 1975;51:815–822.

9. Ausubel K, Furman S. Pacemaker syndrome: definition and evaluation. *Cardiol Clin*. 1985; 3:587–594.

10. The DAVID Trial Investigators. Dual-chamber pacing or ventricular backup pacing in patients with an implantable defibrillator: the Dual Chamber and VVI Implantable Defibrillator (DAVID) Trial. *JAMA*. 2002;288:3115–3123.

11. Sweeney MO, Hellkamp AS, Ellenbogen KA, et al. Adverse effect of ventricular pacing on heart failure and atrial fibrillation among patients with normal baseline QRSD in a clinical trial of pacemaker therapy for sinus node dysfunction. *Circulation*. 2003;23:2932–2937.

12. Abraham WT, Fisher WG, Smith AL, et al. Cardiac resynchronization in chronic heart failure. *N Engl J Med*. 2002;346:1845–1853.

13. Bristow MR, Saxon LA, Boehmer J, et al. Cardiac resynchronization therapy with or without an implantable defibrillator in advanced chronic heart failure. *N Engl J Med*. 2004;350:2140–2150.

14. Moss AJ, Hall WJ, Cannom DS, et al. Cardiac resynchronization therapy for the prevention of heart-failure events. *N Engl J Med*. 2009;361:1329–1338.

15. Cleland JG, Daubert JC, Erdmann E, et al. The effect of cardiac resynchronization on morbidity and mortality in heart failure. *N Engl J Med*. 2005; 352:1539–1549.

16. Sweeney MO, Ellenbogen KA, Casavant D, et al. Multicenter, prospective, randomized safety and efficacy study of a new atrial-based managed ventricular pacing mode (MVP) in dual chamber ICDs. *J Cardiovasc Electrophysiol*. 2005;16:811–817.

17. Bardy GH, Lee KL, Mark DB et al. Amiodarone of an implantable cardioverter-defibrillator for congestive heart failure. *N Engl J Med*. 2005; 352:225–237.

18. Risum N, Strauss D, Sogarrd P, et al. Left bundle branch block: The relationship between ECG electrical activation and echocardiographic mechanical contraction. *Am Heart J*. 2013;166(2):340–348.

19. Straus DG, Selvester RH, Wagner GS: Defining left bundle branch block in the era of cardiac resynchronization therapy. *Am J Cardiol*. 2011;107:927–934.

20. Gorscan J III, Oyenuga O, Habib PJ, et al. Relationship of echocardiographic dyssynchrony to long-term survival after cardiac resynchronization therapy. *Circulation*. 2010;122:1910–1918.

21. Risum N, Jons C, Olsen JT, et al. Simple regional strain pattern analysis to predict response to cardiac resynchronization therapy: rationale, initial results, and advantages. *Am Heart J*. 2012;163:697–704.

22. Mullens W, Grimm RA, Verga T, et al. Insights from a cardiac resynchronization optimization clinic as part of a heart failure disease management program. *J Am Coll Cardiol*. 2009;53:765–773.

23. Park HE, Kim JH, Lee SP, et al. Ventricular dyssynchrony of idiopathic versus pacing-induced left bundle branch block and its prognostic effect in patients with preserved left ventricular systolic function. *Circ Heart Fail*. 2012;5:87–96.

24. Barba-Pichardo R, Sanchez AM, et al. Ventricular resynchronization therapy by direct His-bundle pacing using an internal cardioverter defibrillator. *Europace*. 2013;15:83–88.

25. Ricke AD, Swiryn S, Bauernfeind RA, et al. Improved pacemaker pulse detection: clinical evaluation of a new high-bandwidth ECG system. *J Electrocardiol*. 2011;44: 265–274.

26. Jennings M, Devine B, Lou S, et al. Enhanced software based detection of implanted cardiac pacemaker stimuli. *Computers in Cardiology IEEE*. 2009;833–836.

24

Dr. Marriott's Systematic Approach to the Diagnosis of Arrhythmias

HENRY J. L. MARRIOTT

DR. MARRIOTT'S SYSTEMATIC APPROACH TO THE DIAGNOSIS OF ARRHYTHMIAS

Doctor Marriott evolved the following approach to the analysis of arrhythmias during his first eight editions of *Practical Electrocardiography*. Regarding this approach, he observed: After analyzing the reasons for the mistakes I have made and those that I have repeatedly watched others make, this system is designed to avoid the common errors of omission and commission. Undoubtedly, we make most mistakes because of failure to apply reason and logic, not because of ignorance.

Many disturbances of rhythm and conduction are recognizable at first glance. Supraventricular arrhythmias are characterized by normal QRS complexes (unless complicated by aberrant ventricular conduction), and ventricular arrhythmias produce bizarre QRS complexes with prolonged QRS intervals. One can usually also immediately spot atrial flutter with 4:1 conduction or atrial fibrillation with a rapid ventricular response (see Chapter 17). However, if the diagnosis fails to fall into your lap, then the systematic approach is in order. The steps in the systematic approach are as follows.

Know the Causes of the Arrhythmia

The first step in any medical diagnosis is to know the causes of the presenting symptom. For example, if you want to be a superb headache specialist, the first step is to learn the 50 causes of a headache—which are the common ones, which are the uncommon ones, and how to differentiate between them. This is because "you see only what you look for, you recognize only what you know."[1] Knowing the causes of the various cardiac arrhythmias is part of the equipment that you carry with you and are prepared to use when faced with an unidentified arrhythmia.

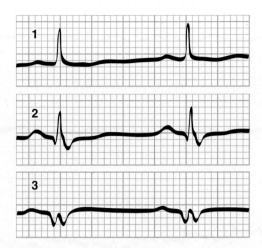

FIGURE 24.1. In lead I (1), the QRS complex appears to be of normal duration, but leads II (2) and III (3) reveal the true duration of the complex to be 0.12 second.

When a specific arrhythmia confronts you, you should first "milk" the QRS complex. There are two reasons for this. The first is an extension of the Willie Sutton law: "I robbed banks because that's where the money is." Second, milking the QRS complex keeps us in the healthy frame of mind of giving priority to ventricular behavior. It matters comparatively little what the atria are doing as long as the ventricles are behaving normally. If the QRS complex is of normal duration in at least two leads of the ECG (Fig. 24.1), then the rhythm is supraventricular. If the QRS complex is wide and bizarre, you are faced with the decision of whether this is of supraventricular origin with ventricular aberration or whether it is of ventricular origin. If you know your QRS waveform morphology, you know what to look for and you will recognize it if you see it.

During the past four decades, the diagnostic morphology of the ventricular complex has come into its own. This began with clinical observation and deduction in which acute coronary care nurses played an important role.[2-6]

Cherchez le P

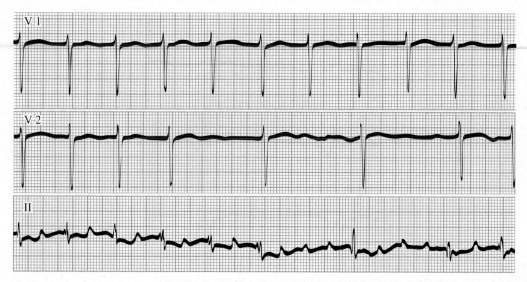

FIGURE 24.2. The top rhythm strip does not reveal any definite atrial activity. The middle strip shows the effect of carotid sinus stimulation with decreased AV conduction following the fourth QRS complex, revealing the slightly irregular baseline typical of fine atrial fibrillation. In contrast, there is obvious atrial activity following the sixth QRS complex in the bottom strip, identifying an atrial tachyarrhythmia with delayed AV conduction. However, the P waves are halfway between the QRS complexes and, indeed, carotid sinus massage reveals additional P waves concealed within each QRS complex.

If the answer to the source of an arrhythmia is not provided by the shape of the QRS complex, the next step is "cherchez (look for) le P." In the past, the P wave has certainly been overemphasized as the key to arrhythmias. A lifelong love affair with the P wave has afflicted many an electrocardiographer with the so-called P-preoccupation syndrome. However, there are times when the P wave holds an important diagnostic clue and must therefore be accorded the starring role.

In one's search for P waves, there are several clues and caveats to bear in mind. One technique that may be useful is to employ an alternate lead placement (see Chapter 2) with the positive electrode at the fifth right intercostal space close to the sternum and the negative electrode on the manubrium. This sometimes greatly magnifies the P wave, rendering it readily visible when it is virtually indiscernible in other leads. Figure 24.2 illustrates this amplifying effect and makes the diagnosis of atrial tachycardia with 2:1 block immediately apparent. If it succeeds, this technique is much kinder to the patient than introducing an atrial wire or an esophageal electrode to corral elusive P waves.

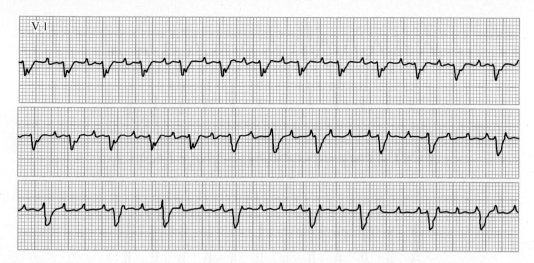

FIGURE 24.3. The rhythm strips are continuous. The top strip illustrates the Bix rule, and in the middle strip, the AV conduction spontaneously decreases, revealing that the atrial rate is twice the ventricular rate.

Another clue to the incidence of P waves is contained in the "Bix rule," named after the Baltimore cardiologist Harold Bix, who observed that "Whenever the P waves of a supraventricular tachycardia are halfway between the ventricular complexes, you should always suspect that additional P waves are hiding within the QRS complex."

In the top strip of Figure 24.3, the P wave is halfway between the QRS complexes and is therefore a good candidate for the Bix rule. It may be necessary to apply carotid sinus stimulation or another vagal maneuver to bring the alternate atrial waves out of the QRS complex. In the case in Figure 24.3, however, the patient obligingly altered his conduction pattern (middle strip) and spontaneously exposed the flutter waves. It is clearly important to know whether there are twice as many atrial impulses as are apparent because there is the ever-present danger that the ventricular rate may double or almost double, especially if the atrial rate were to slow somewhat. It is better to be forewarned and take steps to prevent such potentially disastrous acceleration.

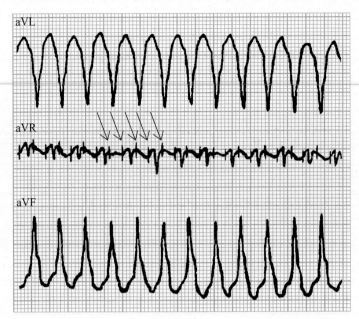

FIGURE 24.4. Only the prominent, wide QRS complexes are visible in leads aVL and aVF. However, in lead aVR, where the QRS complexes are much smaller, the extremely rapid rate (420 beats per minute) of a "runaway" artificial pacemaker (*arrows*) with 2:1 conduction to the ventricles is revealed.

The "haystack principle" can be of great diagnostic importance when you are searching for difficult-to-find P waves. When you have to find a needle in a haystack, you would obviously prefer a small haystack. Therefore, whenever you are faced with the problem of finding elusive items, always give the lead that shows the least disturbance of the ECG baseline (the smallest ventricular complex) a chance to help you. Some leads intuitively seem unhelpful when trying to identify the source of an arrhythmia (e.g., lead aVR). However, the patient whose ECG is shown in Figure 24.4 died because his attendants did not know or did not apply the haystack principle and make use of lead aVR. This patient had a runaway pacemaker at a discharge rate of 440 beats per minute, with a halved ventricular response at 220 beats per minute. Lead aVR was the lead with the smallest ventricular complex and was the only lead in which the pacemaker spikes were plainly visible (arrows). The patient went into shock and died because none of the attempted therapeutic measures affected the tachycardia when all that was necessary was to disconnect the wayward pulse generator.

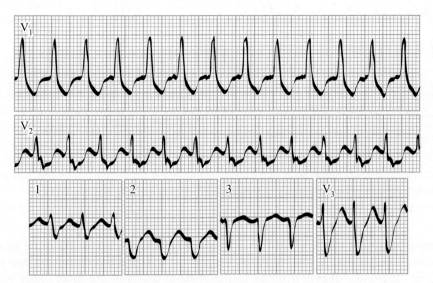

FIGURE 24.5. The small deflections before (lead V1) and after (lead V2) the large deflections, which are obviously from the ventricles, have the appearances of P waves. However, when the true width of the QRS complexes is revealed in leads I, II, and V3, it is apparent that the small deflections seen in leads V1 and V2 are really almost isoelectric parts of the QRS complexes.

The next caveat in identifying the source of an arrhythmia is to "mind your Ps." This means to be wary of things that look like P waves (Fig. 24.5) and P waves that look like other things (Fig. 24.6). This particularly applies to P-like waves that are adjacent to QRS complexes, which may turn out to be part of the QRS complexes. This is a trap for someone who suffers from the "P-preoccupation syndrome," to whom anything that looks like a P wave is a P wave. Many competent ECG interpreters, given the strip of lead V1 or V2 in Figure 24.5, would promptly and confidently diagnose a supraventricular tachycardia for the wrong reasons. In lead V1, the QRS complex does not seem very wide and appears to be preceded by a small P wave. In lead V2, an apparently narrow QRS complex is followed by an unmistakable retrograde P wave. However, the P-like waves in both of these leads are part of the QRS complex. If the duration of the QRS complex is measured in lead V3, it is found to be 0.14 second. To attain a QRS complex of that width in leads V1 and V2, the P-like waves need to be included in the measurement.

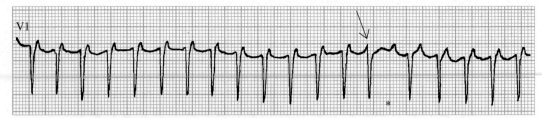

FIGURE 24.6. At the beginning of the rhythm strip, the small positive waveform following the large negative QRS waveform could be (a) a part of a wide QRS complex, (b) a retrograde P wave closely following a narrow QRS complex, or (c) an anterograde P wave with prolonged conduction to a narrow QRS complex. This sequence is broken during the 14th cycle (*arrow*), where the beginning of a small positive waveform is seen preceding the large negative QRS waveform, and in the 15th cycle, there is no QRS complex (*asterisk*). The pause (*asterisk*) produced by the blocked premature atrial beat is terminated by a normally conducted (PR interval = 0.20 second) beat.

Whenever a regular rhythm is difficult to identify, it is always worthwhile to seek and focus on any interruption in the regularity—a process that can be condensed into the three words: "dig the break." It is at a break in the rhythm that you are most likely to find the solution to the source of an arrhythmia. For example, in the beginning strip of Figure 24.6, where the rhythm is regular at a rate of 200 beats per minute, it is impossible to know whether the tachyarrhythmia is atrial or junctional. A third possibility is that the small positive waveform is part of the QRS complex and not a P wave at all. Further along the strip, there is a break in the rhythm in the form of a pause. The most common cause of a pause is a nonconducted atrial premature beat, and this culprit is indicated by the arrow. As a result of the pause, the mechanism of the arrhythmia is immediately obvious. When the rhythm resumes, the returning P wave is in front of the first QRS complex, indicating that the tachyarrhythmia is evidently an atrial tachycardia.

Who's Married to Whom?

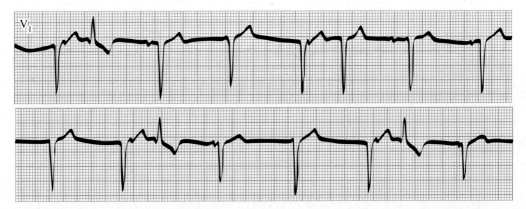

FIGURE 24.7. The rhythm strips are continuous. All of the early QRS complexes, but only some of the later QRS complexes, are preceded by P waves. The use of calipers reveals dissociation between the atria (which have a regular rate of about 50 beats per minute) and the ventricles (the later QRS complexes have a regular rate of about 60 beats per minute). The presence of P waves before each early QRS complex suggests intermittent capture of the ventricular rhythm by the atrial rhythm.

The next step is to establish relationships by asking yourself, "Who's married to whom?" This is often the crucial step in arriving at a firm diagnosis in a case of arrhythmia. Figure 24.7 illustrates this principle in its simplest form. A junctional rhythm is dissociated from sinus bradycardia. On three occasions, there are bizarre early beats with a qR configuration that is nondiagnostic. The early beats could be ventricular premature beats, but the fact that they are seen only when a P wave is emerging beyond the preceding QRS complex tells us that they are "married to" the preceding P waves. This therefore establishes the beats as conducted or capture beats with atypical right-bundle-branch block aberration.

Pinpoint the Primary Diagnosis

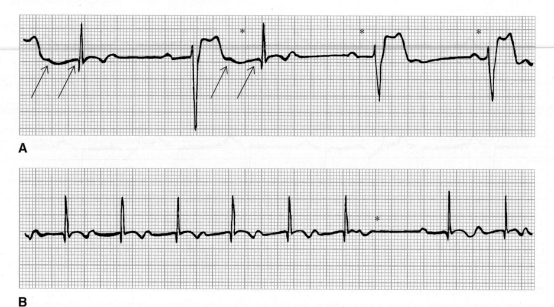

FIGURE 24.8.   Lead II rhythm strips from a patient with a recent inferior infarction. **A.** *Arrows* indicate the constant PR interval preceding each narrow QRS complex and indicate the varying PR intervals preceding the wide QRS complexes. **B.** An *asterisk* indicates the failure of conduction of P wave that identifies the single episode of second-degree AV block.

Figure 24.8 illustrates both the previous principle and the final one: "pinpoint the primary diagnosis." One must never be content to let the diagnosis rest on a secondary phenomenon such as atrioventricular (AV) dissociation, escape, or aberration. Each of these is always secondary to some primary disturbance in rhythm that must be sought out and identified. The ECG shown in Figure 24.8 was obtained from a patient shortly after admission to a coronary care unit. The basic rhythm (see Fig. 24.8A) is sinus rhythm with first- and second-degree AV block. The ECG showed wide QRS complexes that gave the coronary care unit staff concern. One faction contended that the QRS complexes represented ventricular escape beats, whereas another thought they were conducted from the atria with a paradoxical aberration in the critical rate (bradycardia-dependent bundle-branch block). If you ask yourself, "Who's married to whom?" it becomes obvious that the wide QRS complexes in question are not related to the P waves. The PR intervals preceding the last two wide QRS complexes are strikingly different, measuring 0.32 and 0.20 second, respectively, indicating that they are ventricular escape beats. When the patient's AV conduction improves to only occasional second-degree block (see Fig. 24.8B), there is never a sufficiently long pause for an escape beat to occur. These observations pinpoint the primary diagnosis as second-degree AV block. The normal ventricular escape beats are only secondary.

REFERENCES

1. Grodman PS. Arrhythmia surveillance by transtelephonic monitoring: comparison with Holter monitoring in symptomatic ambulatory patients. *Am Heart J*. 1979;98:459.
2. Judson P, Holmes DR, Baker WP. Evaluation of outpatient arrhythmias utilizing transtelephonic monitoring. *Am Heart J*. 1979;97:759–761.
3. Goldreyer BN. Intracardiac electrocardiography in the analysis and understanding of cardiac arrhythmias. *Ann Intern Med*. 1972;77:117–136.
4. Brodsky M, Wu D, Denes P, et al. Arrhythmias documented by 24-hour continuous electrocardiographic monitoring in 50 male medical students without apparent heart disease. *Am J Cardiol*. 1977;39:390–395.
5. Kantelip JP, Sage E, Duchene-Marullaz P. Findings on ambulatory monitoring in subjects older than 80 years. *Am J Cardiol*. 1986;57:398–401.
6. Harrison DC. Contribution of ambulatory electrocardiographic monitoring to antiarrhythmic management. *Am J Cardiol*. 1978;41:996–1004.

Index

Page numbers followed by "*f*" indicate figures; page numbers followed by "*t*" indicate tables